T0094207

**Complementary Medicine for
Veterinary Technicians and Nurses**

Complementary Medicine for Veterinary Technicians and Nurses

Second Edition

Nancy Scanlan
DVM (University of California, Davis), MSFP

WILEY Blackwell

Edition History: First edition © 2011 by Wiley Blackwell
Published by John Wiley & Sons, Inc., Hoboken, New Jersey.
Published simultaneously in Canada.

Limit of Liability/Disclaimer of Warranty
While the publisher and author have used their best efforts in preparing this book, they make no representations or warranties with respect to the accuracy or completeness of the contents of this book and specifically disclaim any implied warranties of merchantability or fitness for a particular purpose. No warranty may be created or extended by sales representatives or written sales materials. The advice and strategies contained herein may not be suitable for your situation. You should consult with a professional where appropriate. Neither the publisher nor author shall be liable for any loss of profit or any other commercial damages, including but not limited to special, incidental, consequential, or other damages. Further, readers should be aware that websites listed in this work may have changed or disappeared between when this work was written and when it is read. Neither the publisher nor authors shall be liable for any loss of profit or any other commercial damages, including but not limited to special, incidental, consequential, or other damages.

For general information on our other products and services or for technical support, please contact our Customer Care Department within the United States at (800) 762-2974, outside the United States at (317) 572-3993 or fax (317) 572-4002.

Wiley also publishes its books in a variety of electronic formats. Some content that appears in print may not be available in electronic formats. For more information about Wiley products, visit our web site at www.wiley.com.

Library of Congress Cataloging-in-Publication Data
Name: Scanlan, Nancy, author.
Title: Complementary medicine for veterinary technicians and nurses / Nancy
    Scanlan.
Description: 2nd edition. | Hoboken, New Jersey : Wiley-Blackwell, [2024] |
    Includes bibliographical references and index.
Identifiers: LCCN 2023053756 (print) | LCCN 2023053757 (ebook) | ISBN
    9781394172016 (paperback) | ISBN 9781394172023 (Adobe PDF) | ISBN
    9781394172030 (epub)
Subjects: MESH: Complementary Therapies–veterinary | Animal
    Diseases–therapy | Holistic Health | Animal Technicians
Classification: LCC SF745.5 (print) | LCC SF745.5 (ebook) | NLM SF 745.5 |
    DDC 636.089/55–dc23/eng/20240110
LC record available at https://lccn.loc.gov/2023053756
LC ebook record available at https://lccn.loc.gov/2023053757

Cover Design: Wiley
Cover Images: Courtesy of Nancy Scanlan; © Capelle.r/Getty Images

Set in 9.5/12.5pt STIXTwoText by Straive, Pondicherry, India
SKY10070506_032224

This book is dedicated to

R.B. Barsaleau, DVM, who taught me everything worth knowing about endurance riding and guided me into teaching veterinary technicians;

Carvel Tiekert, DVM, founder of the American Holistic Veterinary Medical Association, who warmly welcomed me into the association, introduced me to all aspects of complementary veterinary medicine, and inspired me to learn even more;

Sheldon Altman, DVM, who lured me into certification in veterinary acupuncture, promoting both scientific and clinical reasons for its use;

T.A. Holliday, DVM, PhD, who showed me how a specialist should behave;

And to my husband, Allan, who takes good care of my animal friends when I am gone and who puts up with all my projects.

And my sincere thanks to all the organizations who have helped expand the knowledge about complementary and alternative veterinary medicine.

Contents

Preface to the Second Edition

Complementary veterinary medicine has come a long way since this book was originally published. Some methods that were originally considered holistic modalities, not commonly used among conventional medicine, are now part of mainstream veterinary (and human) medicine. Veterinary technicians and nurses are allowed to perform more complementary medicine tasks and be a more active part of the complementary medicine team. The National Association of Veterinary Technicians in America (NAVTA) now recognizes veterinary technician assistants, and also has a Veterinary Technician Specialties program, promoting a higher level of recognition for advanced knowledge and skills in specific disciplines.

The purpose of this book remains the same. It is written as a reference book to help veterinary technicians and nurses answer common questions that owners may have about complementary medicine. This helps counteract the misinformation from "Dr. Google" that runs rampant among pet owners. It also frees up time for the veterinarian to get on with the basic job tasks of a veterinarian: diagnosing, prescribing, and surgery. To do that, it includes lists of complementary modalities, along with job tasks that technicians and nurses can do. In addition, commonly used herbs, supplements, and other treatments are discussed, to give enough of a background to help point a client toward some of the best options for their pets. It also includes a discussion of how to navigate through the pro- and anti-holistic opinions to make an informed decision about whether a treatment method is promising or useful.

It also has enough information that veterinarians who are curious about the field can get an overview of various modalities, where to go for more information, and where they and their staff can get further training. References, bibliographies, and webliographies are included throughout the book to further that purpose.

May this help you on your journey with integrative veterinary medicine.

Preface to the Original Edition

Although books on complementary veterinary medicine are becoming more plentiful, they are usually written for veterinarians and tend to be on the veterinary student textbook level. Other books on the subject are written for pet owners. They are good for an introduction to the subject but lack the depth needed to be useful for a technician in a practice. There are a growing number of owners who use natural methods for their pets. If a practice can't answer the questions these owners have, the owners often look for another resource who can. The other resource may be another veterinary practice, a well-meaning but misinformed neighbor, a poorly prepared lay practitioner, or even the Internet.

This book was written to help fill this information gap. It contains a description of the most common treatment modalities, with references supporting their use. It includes lists of commonly used herbs, supplements, and other methods. It also includes a discussion of how to navigate through the pro- and anti-holistic opinions to make an informed decision about whether a treatment method is promising or useful.

By opening informed discussions with pet owners about complementary medicine, it encourages owners to tell the technician or veterinarian about items their pets are being given, which they may never have mentioned to you previously. Being conversant with these methods will encourage your clients to ask before, not after, using herbs or supplements that may interfere with a pet's treatment. It will help technicians in responding to inquiries from clients of their practice as well as skeptics. It can also help those who want to whether if their clients are helping or hurting their pets.

This book can also answer questions for any veterinarian who is curious about the field but who does not yet need the depth of a textbook on the subject. The reference list in the appendices will help those who want to delve deeper into the subject and who want to find veterinarians well versed in this field. There is a discussion of how to judge research in JAVMA, Medline, and other sources to verify benefits of a treatment and how to spot fallacies in reasoning (by both regular practitioners and holistic ones). Finally, there is a list of training programs and certification courses that veterinarians, and sometimes technicians, can take to be trained in these subjects.

I hope you find this book useful.

About the Author

Dr. Scanlan taught veterinary technicians for 10 years in community colleges and at a 4-year college. She both absorbed the best of both cultures and learned how to help students become the best possible part of a veterinary health team.

Dr. Scanlan got her start in holistic medicine during her senior year in veterinary school when she read a book about the use of vitamin E for heart disease. One of the patients in her charge was a boxer dog with congestive heart failure. The dog had been given digoxin and furosemide for 1 year, and after the original successful treatment, the heart condition was just beginning to get worse. The supervising clinician did not want to increase the dose of digoxin for fear of side effects, and he was open to the idea of trying vitamin E. Dr. Scanlan guessed at a dose, and within 24 hours, she was introduced to all the main aspects of complementary medicine:

1) Vitamin E worked a little too well, and the dog showed signs of digitalis toxicity. (Just because it's natural does not mean it is harmless.)
2) A lower dose helped and the dog improved enough that more digoxin was not needed. (Natural methods, used properly at the correct dose, can be safer than conventional medications.)
3) The supervising clinician was impressed and wanted to publish the results, but he did not want it in a famous journal for fear of what his peers would think. (Some conventional veterinarians are interested and supportive but are worried about what could happen to their reputation if they become too involved.)
4) The cardiologist (who confirmed the digitalis toxicity) refused to believe that it was vitamin E even though he could not offer any better explanation. (Others do not believe in holistic medicine, do not believe it works, do not accept the connection between a symptom or improvement in disease, or may think it is dangerous.)

This was the beginning of Dr. Scanlan's studies in nutraceuticals. Years later, she heard a lecture by a medical doctor who also had learned acupuncture before it was recognized as a valid practice in this country. The doctor was a pain management specialist and used it only in his worst cases. He requested they not tell anyone (for the same reasons as the veterinary clinician had for not promoting vitamin E), but it worked so well that he found people lined up on his clinic's doorstep wanting treatment. Then she heard a presentation by a veterinarian who also promoted its use for pain control in dogs. Dr. Scanlan decided she needed to learn about this also.

She became certified in acupuncture, intending to use it only for pain. This worked for exactly 1 month, after which time a Doberman was brought in who "wanted to die," according to her owner. Blood tests were normal. An X-ray showed arthritis in one hip. A physical exam showed a lick granuloma on the hock of the opposite leg, which had been there despite treatment for 7 years. Acupuncture helped so much that the lick granuloma went away. However, the dog still was not acting normally: she did not want to leave the house, had to be pushed out the door to relieve herself (and came back in as soon as possible), clung to the owner, and did not want to go anywhere. Drugs did not work. There was no good Western diagnosis. In Traditional Chinese Veterinary Medicine (TCVM) theory, this dog was exhibiting very yin behavior. Because she had not really intended to use acupuncture for anything but pain, Dr. Scanlan's TCVM diagnosis did not go any further than the yin-yang part. She placed acupuncture needles in all the yang points she could remember.

The next week, the owner said, "I think maybe we overdid it." The dog was staying outside, refused to come in except to eat (then dashed back out), barked at everything, and had turned into an independent brat. This convinced Dr. Scanlan that TCVM theory was actually worthwhile, and it was useful as a different way of looking at things when Western medicine can't give an answer. (A second, more balanced acupuncture treatment got the dog back in balance.)

That opened the doors to other studies, adding holistic methods to the conventional methods she had already learned, authoring many articles on holistic veterinary care, speaking at holistic veterinary conferences, acquiring a membership in several holistic organizations, holding two executive director positions in holistic organizations, offering holistic help for women over the age of 50, and becoming part of both an integrative veterinary medicine college and the author of this book.

Introduction

> "It does not matter whether medicine is old or new, so long as it brings about a cure. It matters not whether theories be eastern or western, so long as they prove to be true."
>
> *Jen Hsou Lin, D.V.M., Ph.D.*

Holistic veterinary medicine, also known as alternative, complementary, or integrative veterinary medicine, is increasing in importance and use in veterinary practice. Conventional training of veterinary assistants and receptionists usually omits most methods of complementary medicine; thus, anyone working for a holistic veterinarian may have to learn by osmosis, so to speak. Pet owners are often more knowledgeable in this field than technicians or veterinarians, but they are also sources of misinformation. If you know at least a little bit about a subject, even if complementary medicine is not performed in your practice, clients are more likely to tell you about any complementary therapies they are using and to accept your advice about combining or dropping certain therapies. (This is especially important when the therapies they are using are interfering with useful conventional treatment.) Other pet owners have many beginners' questions that could be easily answered by a technician with a little knowledge, allowing the holistic veterinarian to spend time doing what he or she does best: applying additional methods of diagnosis and treatment to chronic conditions that do not respond well to conventional treatments.

Objectives

The objectives of this book are to help the technician to

- understand holistic veterinary medicine
- educate the public about holistic veterinary medicine
- understand his or her role in helping the holistic veterinarian
- understand what he or she can and cannot do in a veterinary practice
- learn about methods the technicians themselves can use either alone or in a veterinary practice
- gain some familiarity with what a holistic veterinarian can and cannot do
- learn about training and certification programs in various aspects of holistic medicine for technicians and veterinarians
- learn how to judge whether a nontraditional treatment shows promise even if it sounds crazy

The place of the technician can be especially important when performing the following tasks:

- answering general questions about holistic medicine
- discussing the practice's views on holistic medicine
- explaining what the veterinarian does and does not do
- explaining Chinese medical theory
- taking a holistic history
- designing, judging, and feeding holistic diets
- explaining the care and administration of homeopathic remedies and preparing those remedies
- explaining how to store and administer herbal medications
- preparing their veterinarian's prescription for herbal tinctures and ointments
- helping with hospice care and grief counseling
- designing and administering a physical therapy program

Overview of Holistic Medicine

Veterinarians are interested in holistic medicine for a number of reasons. Many holistic veterinarians became interested because they themselves were helped by holistic rather than conventional medicine. Others saw the results that a holistic veterinarian was achieving that they themselves were unable to achieve using conventional medicine.

Some methods used in holistic medicine can add income and clients to the practice with only a little study and a minimum of additional expense. At the other extreme, however, are methods that require more expensive education and lifelong study. A holistic veterinarian may use a single modality, a few, or a combination of many. In general, no matter how it is used, complementary medicine emphasizes wellness, natural methods, treating the whole animal (not just a single disease), and preventive medicine. The human–animal bond often plays a big part in holistic medicine.

To attract clients who are interested in holistic methods, both the technician and the veterinarian must understand the clients' viewpoints and speak their language. In addition, if the clinicians in a practice are recognized as being knowledgeable about complementary medicine, the practice's clients are more likely to turn to the veterinarian rather than the Internet as a source of information, which may prevent problems with malnutrition and misuse of herbs and other modalities. Instead of ignoring warnings about a dangerous practice, pet owners will act on the veterinarian's advice, perhaps preventing a catastrophe. For example, when grapes and raisins were first recognized as causing kidney damage in susceptible individuals, there was a message making the rounds of pet owner e-mail lists that this was just another example of veterinarians who thought all dogs should eat only commercial dog food and that grapes were a healthy treat for dogs. Holistic veterinarians answered those claims, spread the word about the very real dangers of possible kidney damage, gave supporting case studies, and their responses rapidly replaced those uninformed comments. Until a veterinarian who is respected in the alternative medicine community gives a valid response to this type of misinformation, there is a very real danger of problems such as this as well as the use of toxic herbs, improper detoxification procedures (which can lead to death), avoidance of veterinary care until it is too late, and other disasters.

Complementary Medicine for Small Animals

The goal of holistic medicine is to normalize the body, bring it back into balance, help it heal itself, and provide solutions that are more natural and have less side effects than those used in traditional medicine. Better food, the right kind of exercise, and treating the whole animal, not just the symptoms, are elements of practicing holistic medicine. Instead of giving medications that just counteract the symptoms without fixing the root cause, holistic medicine tries to heal the body and stop or reverse the cause itself.

Conventional veterinarians follow this practice to a certain extent and have begun using items that have been staples of holistic medicine for years. (See Chapter 4 for examples.)

For instance, to treat inflammatory bowel disease, special diets are often prescribed, some of which contain prebiotics. An increasing number of companies are now also marketing probiotics to conventional veterinarians to treat this disease as well as others. Veterinarians who are specialists in internal medicine are also incorporating all parts of this approach. Doing so is good for you, your pet, and the environment. Because complementary medicine aims to treat the whole animal, not just the disease, the idea of the holistic approach is to help the body heal itself (by correcting abnormal balance of bacterial species in the gut as well as by giving them prebiotics to help them thrive) rather than use methods to fight single problems (such as fighting bacterial overgrowth with antibiotics alone and inflammation of the gut with corticosteroids alone) and ignore others (including side effects brought on by those other methods).

To determine what is wrong in the whole animal, diagnostic methods and vocabulary may be used that are different from that to which conventional veterinarians are accustomed, including methods that have been used for thousands of years. These methods may bring insight by offering a new way of looking at a problem and may guide the veterinarian to a new treatment modality. This is especially true of chronic diseases. For example, irritable bowel syndrome (IBS) is a catch-all term for chronic inflammation of the gastrointestinal tract. Veterinarians will readily admit that what works for one animal will not work for all animals in the treatment of this disease. In fact, a diet that helps one animal (such as a high-fiber diet) may harm another animal (that requires a low-fiber diet). By using traditional Chinese theory, Ayurvedic medicine, or taking a homeopathic case study, this general diagnosis can be broken down into a number of different parts, each of which would require different herbs or remedies and diets. Instead of a hit-or-miss treatment method (if this doesn't work, try that thing next), a more precise treatment may begin right away.

Another tenet of holistic medicine is the idea that we and our pets are bombarded by unnatural substances: artificial flavors, colors, and preservatives, substances such as corn gluten meal, insecticides, air fresheners, cat litter perfumes, even nylon dog collars. These substances can build up in the body and cause reactions in sensitive individuals. Treatment consists of not only removing these from the environment but also removing them from the body by a procedure known as *detoxification*. Again, conventional medicine has now recognized problems caused by many of these substances.

Overvaccination is an issue of concern to many holistic veterinarians. Fibrosarcomas in cats have been linked to vaccination. Other less well-known problems may include autoimmune disease and chronic arteritis as well as other chronic inflammatory diseases (Hogenesch et al., 1999; Souayah et al., 2009). The American Association of Feline Practitioners (AAFP), the American Animal Hospital Association (AAHA), and the American Veterinary Medical Association (AVMA) all now recommend vaccinating less often than once a year for most diseases except for canine bordetella and canine influenza. Research that was in progress at the time of the first edition of this book has been completed and was published in 2020 (Dodds et al., 2020). It showed that immunity against rabies lasts longer than 3 years after vaccination with non-adjuvanted recombinant vaccine. The original Rabies Challenge Fund that was established to fund that research was disbanded, and the $6000 remaining was distributed to six other charitable organizations. (See https://www.rabie-schallengefund.org/ for details and a list of the organizations.)

Dogs and cats, originally considered servants (guard dogs and ratters) and then treated as employees (given a place in the house to sleep), are now increasingly looked upon as members of the family. Owners are more attuned to the human–animal bond, and more inclined to explore additional methods beyond conventional veterinary medicine, for any pet having chronic health problems.

With advances in veterinary medicine, dogs and cats (and other pets) are living longer lives, so the incidence of chronic conditions has increased. Owners are also increasingly concerned about a healthier lifestyle for themselves and for their pets. As a result of these concerns, owners are turning more and more to complementary medicine.

Integrative veterinarians usually practice both complementary and conventional veterinary medicine rather than only one or the other. Veterinarians may also use small parts of complementary medicine, or they may embrace most of it wholeheartedly. This can lead to confusion in the minds of the public. It is important for veterinary technicians and nurses to recognize the practice philosophy of the veterinarian with whom they work in order to be able to explain what the practice does and why, when taking questions by clients who are shopping for a new veterinarian.

Practitioners of complementary medicine emphasize that they don't practice in a vacuum. Proper nutrition and exercise are important parts of complementary medicine, and no single modality works for every situation. Holistic medicine for pets is like lifestyle medicine for humans. There are situations for which surgery is the best answer, and in an emergency, Western medicine, with its fast action, is best for saving lives. However, after the emergency is over and we need to get an animal back to homeostasis, complementary medicine is best to restore that balance.

Generally, when visiting a holistic practitioner, the first visit will last longer than does the average visit with a veterinarian who practices conventional veterinary medicine. For a holistic practitioner, the visit may last anywhere from 20 to 90 minutes. Clients are asked some questions that a conventional veterinarian might not ask, resulting in a more complete discussion of diet, supplements, exercise habits, and behavior. Because of the length of time and complexity of the visit as well as the additional training required for the veterinarian, fees are generally higher. The public needs to understand that this increased attention is the reason for higher fees.

Complementary medicine is most useful for chronic problems. Because of the chronic nature of the problem being treated, the total number of visits varies depending on whether the problem can be cured or if the goal is to control the condition. Initially, most conditions will require several visits spaced anywhere from twice a week to once a month. Later, they may be spaced farther apart.

As mentioned previously, veterinarians who practice complementary medicine usually have additional training and, often, special certification in their chosen modalities. Veterinary technicians may also receive additional training in some modalities. It is important that clients understand what the practice does so they are not disappointed by, for instance, a veterinarian's views on vaccinations, raw foods, or other controversial issues. It is also good for one practice to know about other practices whose knowledge may be complementary. For example, if a patient does not fully respond to one technique, such as acupuncture, they may do better when chiropractic, massage therapy, or time in an underwater treadmill is added. If a practice is able to freely refer to and accept referrals from other practices, as other specialty practices do, this helps the whole veterinary community as well as the patients.

Just as in Western medicine, complementary medicine can have side effects. Properly trained veterinarians and technicians are aware of potential side effects and which treatments can interfere with Western medicine. When conventional practitioners see that a holistic practice is aware of these matters, they will be more likely to support their clients' use of holistic medicine and often start referring them to a complementary or integrative medicine practice.

Complementary Medicine for Horses and Livestock

For large animals, holistic medicine has a different emphasis. For horses, a major emphasis of holistic medicine is that of sports medicine. Horse owners have been using physical therapy, including nutraceutical therapy, for many years. Stem cell therapy research started in horses (2003) before it was used in dogs (2006). Glycosaminoglycans have been available as products for horses longer than for dogs (1984 and 1997, respectively).

Reproductive problems are important for all large animals, and acupuncture plays a big part here. Some herbal medicine is also used. Large animals are most commonly treated by the veterinarian in stables or on farms, although owners may bring individual animals to a central clinic. Some horses are like family, but others are an investment for a specific goal (winning shows or races), and thus performance, rather than chronic care, is the emphasis for holistic medicine. For livestock, growth, and reproduction usually are the areas of emphasis, and any treatment must be economical enough that a farmer or rancher will still make a profit when an animal is sold or has offspring. Preventive care as well as reproductive care can be helpful here. A holistic approach to feeding and pasture management can make a big difference in the success of a practice.

What Technicians Can and Cannot Do

By law in the United States, only a veterinarian can diagnose, prescribe, or perform surgery. (In the UK, a Veterinary Nurse can perform minor surgery such as small growth removal, as long as it has been delegated to them by their veterinarian, but they cannot open a body cavity.) If a technician is involved in any of these procedures, it is only under the direct supervision of a veterinarian. For example, although a technician may be certified in physical therapy and may recognize that there is restriction in motion of a limb or a trigger point present in the neck, the initial diagnosis of the physical problem causing that restriction or trigger point must be done by a veterinarian. In many states, even licensed acupuncturists and chiropractors must work under the direct supervision of a veterinarian and will come to a veterinary practice to perform their services. Certification courses in rehabilitation are available for veterinary technicians, and, depending on the state, may allow certified technicians more leeway in what they can and cannot do.

Some other practices, such as Reiki, are in more of a gray area and may be allowed by a state without the practitioner having to practice through a veterinary office. Practitioners of complementary medicine should be familiar with their state's practice acts in order to avoid breaking the law. The fact that another practitioner is treating animals independently of a veterinarian does not mean that the practice is legal.

There are some areas of holistic medicine that are more controversial. These modalities may not be supported by research that conventional practitioners are aware of, either because research is difficult because of the way the modality is practiced or because most research may be in a foreign language such as Chinese, Japanese, or German, or because studies are few due to potential researchers having great difficulty obtaining research funds. Sometimes the methods just sound crazy, according to the way we understand the world. If a method has wide acceptance, there is a chance that there is something valid there, perhaps buried, perhaps different from what practitioners believe, but worth looking at. For example, there is no published double-blind research study showing an improvement in cancer using the Rife machine. However, it could have a place in cancer treatment: the machine has been reported to be extremely effective in relieving the pain of osteosarcoma. (This observation has been confirmed by holistic veterinarians questioned at conferences and meetings.) Conventional painkillers at very high doses do not do this. For humans, treatment for this pain is palliative radiation therapy, enough to temporarily kill cancer cells and some normal tissue. Instead of attacking the use of a Rife machine for what it does not do, it would be far better to explore the helpful things it might be able to do.

Finally, research on complementary or holistic medicine is much less common than research on conventional therapies. There are also many more associations devoted to facets of human holistic medicine than there are for veterinary holistic medicine. Therefore, in this book, references and websites for humans are often included, especially when they have more information (or sometimes, the only information) available.

References

Dodds W.J., et al. 2020. Duration of immunity after rabies vaccination in dogs: the Rabies Challenge Fund research study. *Can J Vet Res* 84(2):153–158.
Hogenesch H., et al. 1999. Vaccine-induced autoimmunity in the dog. *Adv Vet Med* 41:733–744.
Souayah N., et al. 2009. Small fiber neuropathy following vaccination for rabies, varicella, or Lyme disease. *Vaccine* 10:1016–1120.

Webliography

Luitpold, maker of Adequan, the first injectable glycosaminoglycan.
https://www.adequan.com/veterinarian_resource.aspx
A good source of information for Adequan. Includes package inserts, with research results.

I Love Veterinary blog
https://iloveveterinary.com/blog/vet-nurses-in-the-uk/
Source of information for and about veterinary medicine in the UK. They say "We are NOT an official veterinary medicine organization. We are a community that offers to share information between the veterinary enthusiasts. We are not here to give out veterinary advice, you should always consult your veterinarian."

UK government website Veterinary Nurse authorization page
https://www.gov.uk/find-licences/listed-veterinary-nurse-authorisation-all-uk
Includes information about what is required for a veterinary nurse to perform surgery

1

What Is Holistic Medicine?

Definition of Holistic Medicine

There are a number of terms used to describe holistic medicine. They have similar meanings but some subtle differences.

- Holistic medicine treats the body as a whole, using whole herbs, complete supplements rather than single chemical sources, etc.
- Natural medicine does not use artificial chemicals; rather, it uses natural methods such as acupuncture, massage, herbs, and nutritional supplements.
- Integrative medicine uses a combination of the best of conventional and holistic medicine.
- Alternative medicine uses nonconventional but valid methods, including such ancient methods as Ayurvedic medicine and traditional Chinese medicine.

Holistic medicine is also called *natural medicine, complementary medicine, integrative medicine,* and *alternative medicine.* There is currently no single accepted name for the concept. Each of these labels indicates a separate aspect of the idea of non-mainstream medicine. In addition, treatments that were originally considered alternative are now becoming part of mainstream medicine. This shift makes the term *alternative* less useful than some would think. *Complementary* or *integrative* medicine indicates the way that many holistic veterinarians practice this type of medicine: they rely on certain aspects of conventional medicine in their practice and use less conventional means for other aspects. In addition, mainstream veterinarians who adopt a treatment that was formerly alternative have integrated this into their practice. Many veterinarians prefer the "complementary" or "integrative" terminology.

The term *holistic* medicine reflects the idea that we need to look at a person or pet as a whole (body, mind, and spirit) and at healing methods as a whole (whole herbs, herbs plus acupuncture, methods that treat body/mind/spirit, etc.). Conventional medicine, especially as it is taught or presented in textbooks, tends to look at a single disease with a single treatment method. When multiple diseases occur simultaneously, treatment compromises are necessary, and the best treatment for one disease may not be the best for others. For example, treating elderly animals often results in a compromise: they may have kidney disease, which would indicate the ideal diet should be low protein, but also have cancer, for which a moderately low-carbohydrate diet is preferred. If an elderly animal is thin enough, with a poor appetite, often the general advice is to feed it whatever it will eat because weight loss for these animals is the most immediate threat.

Complementary Medicine for Veterinary Technicians and Nurses, Second Edition. Nancy Scanlan.
© 2024 John Wiley & Sons, Inc. Published 2024 by John Wiley & Sons, Inc.

The idea of reducing the problem to a single diagnosis of a single disease that has an ideal treatment, also known as the *atomic* or *reductionist* approach, seeks to reduce a problem to its smallest part and to fix that part. This is a powerful approach when only one thing is wrong or only one problem is life-threatening. Holism begins with all the individual problems and tries to see a pattern, believing that the whole picture is greater than the sum of its parts.

A tenet of holism is that the absence of a specific diagnosed disease does not necessarily mean that a body is healthy. (This is why people who just do not feel well, but have normal lab tests, are usually not helped by conventional medicine but are often helped by the holistic approach.) This approach looks at the animal, the health problems it may have, mental aspects such as anxiety or aggression, the owner, other pets in the household, the type of food being fed and any undesirable ingredients in that food, and the environment in which the animal is kept before recommending a treatment. Instead of a drug that has a single ingredient, herbs that contain a specific ingredient plus all its supporting factors may be preferred—or multiple antioxidants instead of one single vitamin, or a Chinese herbal formula with many herbs, etc. Even a single herb has many healing components that are synergistic rather than one single component that primarily treats one prob-lem, so the herb itself can have a greater range of beneficial effects. Humans and animals originally evolved along with the plants they ate or used and may respond better to them than to a drug.

History of Holistic Medicine

- Some types of holistic medicine date back thousands of years.
- Ayurvedic medicine is from India, dating from before 1600 BC.
- Chinese herbal medicine is more than 2000 years old.
- Kampo (Japanese herbal medicine) began in 562 AD.
- Homeopathy began in Germany in the late 1700s.
- Pulsed electromagnetic field therapy began in the 1930s.
- Chiropractic and osteopathy are more recent but were developed to address problems that con-ventional medicine does not address.

Much of what we think of as holistic medicine was at one time considered conventional medi-cine. Ayurvedic medicine has been described in the *Rig Veda*, compiled before 1600 BC. Written descriptions of Chinese herbal medicine and moxibustion date back over 2000 years (*Shen Nong Ben Cao Jing*). Kampo (Japanese herbal medicine and acupuncture) began in 562 AD when Chinese medical texts were brought to Japan. Homeopathy was developed in the late 1700s at a time when conventional medicine treated disease by bleeding, purging, and other unpleasant and even deadly methods. Homeopathic hospitals were common in the United States in the late 1800s and early 1900s, and some evolved into present-day hospitals.

W. K. Kellogg invented cornflakes as a nutritious way to start the day at his health spa in the early 1900s. He emphasized the need for exercise as well as proper nutrition to help people recover (Kellogg Co., 2010). This idea was revolutionary in its time and is an example of a holistic way of looking at things that resonated with the populace and improved their health, without being a part of general medical practice.

Other methods, such as chiropractic and osteopathic manipulation, have developed more recently as ways to help health problems that are not fully addressed by conventional medicine.

Holistic veterinary medicine has been increasingly incorporated into veterinary schools. A 2021 survey showed that 76.7% offered some level of instruction in integrative veterinary medicine (IVM)

Table 1.1 Comparing and contrasting holistic and conventional practitioners.

Holistic Practitioners	Conventional Practitioners
Holistic practitioners may consult sources that are hundreds or thousands of years old.	Conventional treatments are mostly those that have been recently discovered or that may be only a few decades old.
Holistic practitioners look at the human–animal bond and mind–body connection as part of their diagnosis and treatment.	Conventional practitioners tend to look at the human–animal bond as one of many behavioral diagnoses, with specific treatment depending on the problem.
Holistic practitioners are greatly concerned about side effects of conventional medicine.	Conventional practitioners are greatly concerned about the smaller amount of research done for holistic methods and their potential side effects.
Holistic practitioners worry about quality control and contamination of conventional pet foods.	Conventional practitioners are concerned about quality control and contamination of holistic remedies and holistic pet foods.

(combining holistic medicine with conventional medicine). About 74.4% provided clinical services in IVM, most commonly rehabilitation and acupuncture. About 30.2% offered a dedicated course in IVM, which was less than the previous survey, probably reflecting the fact the high number who offered clinical services. Additionally, the number of faculty who were trained in one or more aspects of IVM increased (Memon et al., 2021).

Holistic and Conventional Treatments

The holistic practitioner may use treatments that are not as well documented by scientific literature as conventional treatments but that have had hundreds or thousands of years of use behind them. Holistic practitioners may consult respected sources that may be 2000 years old. Conventional veterinarians look at modern published sources and place special confidence in double-blind studies. Holistic practitioners and holistic clients are more likely to look at the body–mind connection and to delve into areas such as hospice care for pets, pet–owner interactions and their effect on pet health, and the whole process of death, dying, and grieving, although this is now a growing field in conventional veterinary medicine as well (Table 1.1).

Another aspect that troubles holistic practitioners is the number of side effects or adverse effects of conventional medicine. A 2004 study showed that 1.2 million hospitalized patients experienced an adverse drug reaction. About 90% of these reactions were to drugs that were properly administered (AHRQ Agency, 2007). Conventional medicine may not be safe or very effective for chronic conditions. Although there can be side effects from holistic methods, when used correctly, these effects are generally much less serious than those from conventional medicine. For example, consider drugs commonly used for arthritis in veterinary medicine. NSAIDs commonly have deleterious effects on the gastrointestinal tract, liver, and/or kidneys (FDA, 2006). These side effects are not always reversible, especially any renal damage that may occur. Veterinarians are cautioned to perform laboratory tests regularly when treating animals with these drugs. Corticosteroids such as prednisone can cause long-term muscle wasting, weight gain, liver dysfunction, polydipsia, and polyuria (FDA, 1991). In contrast, side effects from acupuncture or homeopathy used for arthritis are extremely rare (Weidenhammer et al., 2007). Massage therapy also has few adverse effects but has almost immediate benefits. Side effects of herbs used for arthritis, when used as trained herbalists recommend, are few, milder than the effects of COX-2 inhibitors, and generally reversible (Setty and Sigal, 2005).

Conventional practitioners, in turn, are concerned about the lack of research available for a number of holistic methods. Quality control has been of concern in the past, but by using companies that control both quality and contamination, it is much less of a problem than it formerly was.

The term *evidence-based medicine* (EBM) is often used as the gold standard for judging treatment methods. It is usually interpreted strictly as referring to only research-supported methods and does not recognize the value of methods that have been used successfully for so long that research has never been done. For example, the use of fluids to help pets with renal dysfunction feel better is widely used but is not supported by research. Giving subcutaneous fluids is recommended for kidney failure, especially for stages 3 and 4 (Polzin, 2004). There are good theoretical reasons for doing so. Currently, there are no research studies published for either benefits or risks of giving subcutaneous fluids for renal failure, and the evidence supporting its use is grade 3. Yet for those who have seen fluids used, it is clear that it helps these pets feel better.

A better definition of EBM is rather "the integration of best research evidence with clinical expertise and patient values" (Sackett et al., 2000). Roudebush et al. (2004) believe that for veterinary clinical nutrition, the best clinical decisions are made when clinical expertise, research evidence, and owner/patient preferences overlap. This model is also valid for the practice of complementary and alternative veterinary medicine.

Holistic Veterinarians Versus Holistic Human Medicine Practitioners

- Pet owners will turn to holistic practitioners for humans if they cannot find a veterinarian who treats animals holistically.
- Just as medical doctors are not qualified to practice on pets, most holistic practitioners for humans are not qualified to practice on pets.

If no holistic veterinarian is available, owners will often turn to those practitioners who practice on humans. Conscientious practitioners will seek training or at least an understanding of animals before they treat them, or they will associate with a veterinary practice so they have the input of a veterinarian. Alternatively, practitioners will tell owners they have not studied animals and refer owners elsewhere. This is important because animals' anatomy and physiology are different from those of humans. This is especially true for cats: they lack the main liver enzyme used by humans and dogs to process various substances; thus, drugs and herbs that create no problems or that are only mildly toxic for a dog can be deadly for a cat. If a practitioner gains a client's trust, it may save an animal's life. (See the box Misinformation from a Chiropractor.)

MISINFORMATION FROM A CHIROPRACTOR

I once saw a cat that repeatedly suffered from levamisole poisoning. The owners, on the advice of their chiropractor, had been giving the equivalent of a sheep's dose of levamisole monthly. They were trying to get rid of the parasites that the chiropractor diagnosed and that he told them needed to be treated for a month. As a result, the cat kept ending up in the emergency hospital with liver disease, to the mystification of the treating veterinarian. The owners never told their veterinarian that they were giving their cat levamisole because their veterinarian was skeptical about all holistic treatments. They did tell me because I was willing to talk about anything and everything holistic. I educated them about levamisole poisoning, the difference between cats and sheep, the susceptibility of cats to poisoning by almost anything, the superior ability of veterinarians versus chiropractors to detect parasites, and the necessity to discuss with their veterinarian, or a holistic veterinarian, any treatment not recommended by a veterinarian. I also let their veterinarian know what was going on.

Practitioners should do what they are trained to do. Those trained for humans should not practice on animals without further training.

Use of Holistic Medicine in Human Patients

- One out of four human hospitals in the United States offered some type of complementary or alternative medicine services in 2006. This increased to 42% in 2010 (Ananth, 2011). By 2017, 82% of pediatric hospitals incorporated some type of CAM (Stubblefield 2017)
- Many pet owners use holistic medicine for themselves and their pets, but they often do not tell their veterinarian.
- Some interactions of holistic methods and conventional methods are possible, especially when clients use them without consulting a veterinarian. They can be beneficial, but they can also interfere with each other.
- Veterinarians need to know *everything* a pet is taking because of possible interactions.
- Holistic methods may look or sound strange unless the practitioner understands the background behind them.

In human medicine, musculoskeletal problems are the focus of much of complementary medicine. In 2007, 37% of hospitals surveyed stated that they offered complementary or alternative medicine services. Massage therapy, acupuncture, and relaxation therapy were the most popular outpatient therapies; the top three inpatient therapies were pet therapy, massage therapy, and music/art therapy. The top three reasons for offering these services were patient demand, clinical effectiveness, and organizational mission (Ananth, 2009). By 2010, the number had increased to 42%. The percentage has steadily increased since then.

These alternative methods were well received by patients despite the fact that few insurance carriers cover complementary medicine, which results in patients paying for these services out of pocket.

More than three-fourths of adolescents interviewed had already used some form of complementary or alternative medicine in their lives (Wilson et al., 2006). Veterinarians may be unaware that their clients use complementary medicine themselves and may already be using it for their pets. Interactions between some holistic treatments and conventional medicine are possible, however. If owners are not asked what alternative medicine therapies they are using for their pets, they will usually not volunteer the information to the practitioner, which may cause problems in the treatment of a patient.

MISSING INFORMATION FROM A CLIENT

A dog was referred to me that had problems with both oxalate stones and struvite stones. A diet for one type of stone increased the possibility that the dog would get the other type, and this patient had already had surgery twice: once for oxalate stones and once for struvite stones. I was the first veterinarian who had asked the owners about any supplements or herbs they might be giving. The dog was on three calcium supplements in addition to the calcium he was receiving in his food. When the supplements were stopped, the stone problem went away.

Methods used by holistic veterinarians may seem strange, especially when judged by conventional medicine. Acupuncture looked like some sort of voodoo until Westerners saw what it did for people in China. Chinese herbs do not look anything like what most Westerners think of as herbs. Homeopathy does not make sense to many people. Veterinarians who do not see evidence of arthritis on a radiograph often overlook the possibility of trigger points, muscle spasm, and decreased range of motion as contributors to lameness. Bad behavior in a pet may be attributed to anxiety, stubbornness, or willfulness when it actually is caused by pain that is not easily elicited or detected by conventional means.

Cases More Responsive to Holistic Medicine than to Conventional Medicine

- One reason humans and pet owners seek out holistic practitioners is that they or their pet has not responded to conventional therapy.
- Another reason is that they have a condition that does not match conventional medical diagnoses.

Measurements of health and response to medical treatment are usually considered to match a "normal" bell-shaped curve. When a curve is created with response to treatment ranging from poor to robust on the horizontal axis, and numbers of pets or humans responding to a treatment on the vertical axis, you will see that the majority will respond well to treatment. (In fact, those on the far right of the curve often respond well even if the treatment is not completed, or is stopped early.) However, the group on the far left is much less responsive and remains in poor health. (See Figure 1.1.)

Often the same individuals stay in the same unresponsive groups. When holistic veterinarians look beyond the conventional therapies for something else that might work for them, they find that many "unresponsive" patients will respond to holistic therapies, and many that do not have a conventional diagnosis will have a holistic diagnosis that has no correspondence to Western diagnoses.

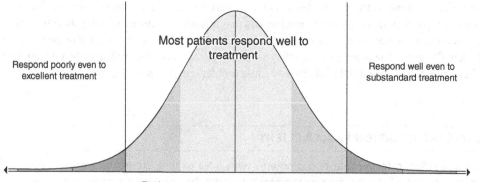

Figure 1.1 Normal curve featuring animal health and response to conventional treatments.

Lay (Unlicensed) Practitioners

- Some unlicensed practitioners are very talented and can be very helpful.
- Others do not have sound knowledge or are not familiar with the differences between animals and humans and thus can harm pets.

Lay practitioners can be both a help and a hindrance to the practice of veterinary medicine. This field covers a wide variety of talents and treatments for pets. Some, such as Linda Tellington-Jones (see TTouch in Chapter 6), have great talent, have studied their field carefully, and have evolved valid systems of treatment that can give amazing results. Others may use substances or amounts of substances that are toxic to animals. State boards of veterinary medicine are often overworked, underfunded, and understaffed, and usually focus on veterinarians rather than untrained lay practitioners who may do more harm.

POOR ADVICE FROM A LAY PRACTITIONER

Years ago in Southern California, there was a person who called herself an "herbalist" and advertised in the veterinary practice section of the Yellow Pages. She told her clients never to consult a veterinarian, not even holistic ones. One of her victims was brought to me for a second opinion. The practitioner had recommended an "herbal detox" for an ancient mixed-breed dog who developed severe diarrhea and dehydration. The owners had asked the "herbalist" for a change in treatment, and the practitioner refused, saying the dog was just detoxing and they needed to let it run its course. Fortunately, the owners could see that the dog was deteriorating rapidly and ignored her opinion. Some of the herbs were toxic, so I stopped her formula, rehydrated the dog, substituted herbs that were actually beneficial, and the dog rapidly recovered. When I reported the so-called herbalist to the state board, their response was to send the person a letter telling her to stop advertising in the veterinary section of the Yellow Pages.

On the flip side are those who may do unusual things that you may not believe in but that are harmless and may actually give you or your veterinarian some insight. Those who practice "animal communication" (and who do it well) may provide some amazing insights that can help point treatment in a new direction. Always be willing to listen to pet owners who have contacted a good communicator. Often, a communicator's reading agrees with what is being done (without having any contact with a practitioner beforehand), and sometimes it can give a veterinarian an idea that helps with the treatment. At the very least, it encourages the client to tell a practitioner everything possible that might have a bearing on the pet's problems.

Integration with Conventional Medicine

- There are times when holistic medicine works best and other times when conventional medicine works best.
- Conventional medicine has many useful diagnostic techniques unknown to ancient practitioners.
- Surgery can be life-saving.
- In emergency situations, conventional medicine works quickly and saves lives.

- Holistic methods work well for chronic disease.
- Holistic methods are ideal for whole-body support.
- Holistic practitioners can be useful as part of the veterinary holistic community.

Conventional and holistic medicine integrate well. Conventional medicine works best for most types of diagnosis. Also, there are many problems for which surgery is the only answer. For instance, currently there are no satisfactory substitutes for surgery in the sterilization of an animal. In an emergency or for immediate results, conventional medicine saves lives.

Although it is possible for holistic medicine to have rapid results, more often it takes longer for it to demonstrate its full effect. Holistic treatment also creates long-term results. Holistic medicine is ideal for chronic disease, musculoskeletal problems, and for general, whole-body support.

If a practice becomes known to other practitioners as one that does a good job holistically, achieving results that conventional medicine cannot and giving good advice without criticizing conventional practitioners, then those practitioners will begin to refer people to that practice for questions about herbs or other alternative treatments. Conventional medicine practitioners will no longer tell people to quit taking herbs, that large doses of vitamins are dangerous, and that complementary medicine is quackery. This is the best kind of integration.

Research

- Research in holistic veterinary medicine is difficult.
- Research funding is difficult to get. For some methods, there may be no good placebo to use as a comparison.
- Holistic methods work best where combinations of factors are used; research usually tries to isolate single factors, which ends in poor results for these modalities.
- Some holistic methods are highly individualized, and so there is no good way to quantify a single treatment for a single disease for research purposes.
- Meta-analyses may not be valid for some holistic methods. Much of conventional medicine is also not validated by the gold-standard double-blind research study.
- Well-written case studies may be the best way to show the validity of holistic medicine.

Research in holistic veterinary medicine is complicated by a number of factors. First, it is difficult to get funding for many facets of holistic medicine because such medicines use cheap, easily available ingredients. When vitamins or amino acids can be substituted for a currently patented drug, drug companies are less willing to fund this research.

Second, for some therapies it is difficult to properly devise a procedure using a placebo. For instance, using "sham" acupuncture as a placebo, where practitioners are directed to insert a needle into a randomly selected area of a body, may not be truly sham. There are hundreds of acupuncture points on the body. An experienced acupuncturist can find a point without using anatomical charts or point finders and can feel the point on the body without knowing or memorizing every single point. It is possible that an acupuncturist might subconsciously choose an acupuncture point if it is close to the sham point. In addition, some points come and go (especially Ah Shi points). A point that is a sham point for some may be a real point for others.

Reiki is another instance in which a placebo study would be nearly impossible. Reiki involves either touching a body with certain patterns of the hands or positioning the hands just above the body. Because the placement of the hands on or above the body is imperative for this modality, and the placement is so variable, no standard location could be used for the placebo. To do so would be likely to create a treatment.

Third, Western research tends to try to isolate one single item as *the* cause of a disease or a patient's improvement. Holistic medicine recognizes an interplay of factors as the cause of disease and looks for patterns. It also emphasizes the use of complex factors for treatment: whole herbs, not herb extracts, Chinese herbal formulas rather than single herbs, combinations of antioxidants rather than single antioxidants, etc. Some of this is validated in research (although it may be difficult to locate it) (Institute of Functional Medicine, 2008). For example, when vitamin E acts as an antioxidant, it is changed into a pro-oxidant form. Vitamin C is required to convert it back to an antioxidant. If large amounts of vitamin E are used alone in a cancer patient, the final result is an increase in pro-oxidants. This causes an acceleration of the disease and decreased survival time. If megadoses of both E and C are given at the same time, then often improved survival times are seen. Beta carotene, used as the sole high-dose antioxidant, will result in a higher incidence of three types of lung cancer and worsening of the disease. Carotenoids, used as a group or in whole foods, can improve cancer survival times. In addition, the action of an item in the body can be very different from that of the same item in an in vitro study. (All antioxidants will make cancer cells grow faster in tissue culture. However, in vivo, the beneficial effect on normal cells is greater than the effect on cancer cells.)

This last factor also confounds meta-analyses. If you combine all research articles on the effect of vitamin E on cancer, you may find the result says there is little to no effect, since the pure-E studies will cancel out the E-with-C studies and in vitro studies will cancel out in vivo studies. A careful selection of studies with specific criteria (such as in vivo only, in combinations only, always the same dose, used alone only) will generate the proper conclusion without selecting only the best cases.

Many holistic practices are used because large numbers of holistic veterinarians find them useful and valid, even without double-blind studies. These practitioners are criticized by mainstream veterinarians for doing so without proper research support. However, these conventional medicine veterinarians do the same thing. The earlier discussion about subcutaneous fluids is one example.

The best published articles for holistic medicine may well be in the form of rigorous case studies, conforming to specific criteria recognized as valid by the general scientific community. Unfortunately, the general public usually sees only the "testimonials," and even herb, pet food, and supplement companies often do not understand the difference. Without realizing it, licensed veterinarians may rely on one or two poorly designed studies for the off-label use of pharmaceuticals. It can take years before someone publishes a study demonstrating that these off-label uses are not effective.

The *Journal of the American Holistic Veterinary Medical Association* (JAHVMA) has published case studies in veterinary holistic medicine for years. The *Journal of the American Veterinary Medical Association* (JAVMA) published an article in November 2009, on EBM and the need for case studies (Holmes, 2009). Literature searches are only as good as the filters used to find the information you are looking for. Filters usually concentrate on gold-standard randomized controlled double-blind studies, and the Cochrane study filters are generally recognized as the best for this (Glanville et al., 2020). Artificial intelligence holds promise for biomedical research, especially if active learning and machine learning are included (Abdelkader et al., 2021).

Veterinary technicians and nurses can help veterinarians by keeping careful records and gathering information for the publication of such studies. Such published studies will go far to advance the cause of holistic medicine and help conventional veterinarians improve their practices. They can illustrate the need for further studies at the university level. Submission of case studies to the *AHVMA Journal* is a great way to share this information and to create a body of evidence for those who say there is no proof.

Telling the Difference Between Real and Fake

- You cannot judge whether a modality is real by its terminology.
- Modalities can be judged by other criteria:

Can you verify or falsify its claim (e.g., by laboratory tests)?
Can you relate its vocabulary or explanations to something else that is valid?
Is there actual proof (not testimonials) that the patient really got better?
Is there anything about the method that shows promise (whether or not the main method works as claimed)?

Because some explanations, such as traditional Chinese medicine theory, are so different from what we learn about the causes and treatments of disease in conventional medicine and because some names sound so different from the names we are used to, it is easy to get caught up in the terms and forget to look at the results of a treatment. There are several items we can look at to determine whether a holistic treatment is worthwhile.

First, are practitioners of a modality making a claim that we can verify (or disprove)? There is one theory about cancer that says that all cancer is caused by immature flukes. All we have to do is kill all the flukes in our body, and we will cure all cancer. There is one big problem with this theory: immature flukes are easy to see. They are multicellular organisms and thus are much bigger than single cancer cells. When a pathologist sections a small tumor, he or she can look at every section of the tumor. Looking at medical literature, lab reports, and veterinary textbooks published over the past 40 years, there has never been any report from a board-certified pathologist that noted the presence of any immature fluke in any tumor.

In contrast, there is the theory that low levels of iodine can cause or contribute to human breast cancer. You need three items to check this theory: a test to check for low levels of iodine, a survey to see if people with breast cancer have lower levels of iodine than those without cancer, and cases of breast cancer that improved after they were given iodine.

There is a test to check for low levels of iodine: Measure the amount of iodine in the urine for 24 hours. Swallow a big dose of iodine. Measure the iodine in the urine again. If you have enough iodine, you will urinate out the excess. If you do not have enough, you will absorb the iodine and very little will come out. After you have absorbed enough, iodine will start coming through into your urine. This test exists and has been validated (Abraham et al., 2006).

There are two ways to see if breast cancer victims have low levels of iodine: (1) do the test above, and (2) measure the amount of iodine in the cancerous breast tissue. Both tests have been done on breast cancer patients. Both have showed that many of these people have lower than average amounts of iodine in their body (Eskin, 1977).

The only way to know for sure if the rest of the theory is true is for doctors to perform the tests, give iodine to their patients, and publish the results in medical journals. This has been done, and the patients have improved (Derry, 2006). (This can be the hardest thing to convince a holistic veterinarian to do.) So it sounds crazy, but all the tests point to iodine as a good way to treat breast cancer in humans, and perhaps in dogs, if their blood iodine levels are low.

Second, if the explanation sounds crazy, can you relate it to anything else? A person in Southern California with a background in electrical engineering found out years ago he was able to help people improve their health. When he spoke of this, he talked in terms of grounding a part of their bodies and sending electrical energy through the body, which sounds crazy when you hear it. However, the places where he pressed to "ground" them are places that are also called acupuncture points, and the way he "sent energy" was by performing a maneuver that releases trigger points. He had developed this method himself without knowing anything about trigger points or conventional ways of detecting them. Others have to study books and attend classes and read research to accomplish the same thing.

Third, is there proof that the patient really got better? Did the cancer disappear (and are there biopsies to show it was cancer, and radiographs or pictures to prove it disappeared)? Did the infection go away (and are there cultures to prove it)? Did the paralyzed patient start walking? Did the patient stop trying to chew his foot off? Did the liver enzymes in his blood test improve after treatment with herbs that benefit the liver? One of the problems with "proofs" of cancer therapies working in humans is the lack of before and after data. Another problem is that there is not a long enough follow-up period for patients.

Henry Beecher, the first person to study the placebo effect, noted in his ground-breaking publication "The Powerful Placebo" that just feeling better is not enough. Up to 30% of improvement using some verified cancer treatments can be from the placebo effect (Beecher, 1955). (The mind is a powerful influence over cancer.) So if a treatment works for 30% or less of human cancer patients, you may be seeing the placebo effect. (Or you might be seeing a small sub-set of patients that respond to that treatment – but because it is so small, it would not be good to immediately recommend it for every cancer patient that comes in.) Study on placebos has continued at Harvard University to this day, and there has been some discussion about it being a part of the mind–body experience. Thus its effects can be useful when applied with treatments, even when the patient knows they are taking a placebo. The mind–body connection can also be useful for animals. The technician can help with this in the veterinary hospital, and help owners apply it at home (Jensen et al., 2015). (This is discussed further in Chapter 6.)

Because an animal's lifespan is much shorter than that of a human, it is easier to follow a case until the end of the pet's life. The biggest key here is good recordkeeping.

Finally, is there anything that shows promise, even if the claim itself is invalid? Rife's beam ray sounds crazy, looks crazy, and, in its current form, the equipment has not cured any cancer (or at least, no verifiable medical report has been published saying so). However, it has been known to instantly stop the pain of bone cancer. There is no other treatment that acts this rapidly, without side effects. Instead of believing the Rife treatment is worthless, we should be trying to understand how it stops cancer pain.

Conclusion

Holistic medicine is increasingly used by pet owners, both for themselves and their pets. In most cases, side effects are milder and less frequent than those for conventional medicine. Holistic medicine treats the whole body, not just one aspect of it. It is probably used by more clients than a practitioner is aware of, and if a practitioner in a conventional practice does not bring up the subject, the owner probably will not either. Knowledge of at least the basics of holistic medicine can help with client communication, with the effectiveness of conventional treatment, and to avoid interaction with any drugs that a pet may be given. A veterinary technician can seem less threatening to some pet owners than a veterinarian, and clients might open up to them better and disclose more about all the other things they are using. The owner might also be using something unfamiliar to the veterinarian or veterinary technician that turns out to be another valuable addition to the treatment toolbox. An open mind might lead a practitioner to new ways of helping patients.

Summary

What can a technician do?

1) Familiarize yourself with the types of holistic medicine your veterinarian practices.
2) Know what a technician can do and what can be done only by a veterinarian.
3) Know the reputable practitioners (both veterinarians and lay practitioners) in the area to whom your veterinarian refers clients and have their addresses and phone numbers on hand.
4) Be able to help clients determine whether an item or practice is legitimate.
5) Be able to explain why your veterinarian uses some conventional methods, such as X-rays, surgery, and lab tests, and why they prefer some conventional treatments over complementary ones.

References

Abdelkader W., et al. 2021. Machine learning approaches to retrieve high-quality, clinically relevant evidence from the biomedical literature: systematic review. *JMIR Med Inform* 9(9):e30401. doi: 10.2196/30401. PMID: 34499041; PMCID: PMC8461527.

Abraham G.E., et al. 2006. Simplified procedure for the measurement of urine iodide levels by the ion-selective electrode assay in a clinical setting. *Orig Internist* 13(3):125–135.

Agency for Healthcare Research and Quality (AHRQ). 2007. More than 1 Million Hospital Patients Experience Side Effects and Other Problems with Their Medications. *AHRQ News and Numbers*, April 12, 2007. Accessed online 9/6/2010 at https://www.ahrq.gov/news/nn/nn041207.htm.

Ananth S. 2009. CAM: An Increasing Presence in U.S. Hospitals. *HHN Magazine* Online. Accessed online 9/21/2010 at https://www.hhnmag.com/hhnmag_app/jsp/articledisplay.jsp?dcrpath= HHNMAG/Article/data/01JAN2009/090120HHN_Online_Ananth&domain=HHNMAG on 9/16/2010.

Ananth S. 2011. Complementary and Alternative Medicine Survey of Hospitals. Accessed online 7/16/2023 at https://allegralearning.com/wp-content/uploads/2015/06/CAM-Survey-FINAL-2011.pdf.

Beecher H.K. 1955. The powerful placebo. *Am Med Assoc* 159(17):1602–1606.

Eskin B.A. 1977. Iodine and mammary cancer. *Adv Exp Med Biol* 91:293–304.

Derry D. 2006. *Breast Cancer and Iodine*. Bloomington: Trafford Publishing. p. 88.

Food and Drug Administration (FDA). 1991. NADA 140–921 PrednisTab—original approval. Accessed online 5/22/2010 at https://www.fda.gov/AnimalVeterinary/Products/ ApprovedAnimalDrugProducts/FOIADrugSummaries/UCM054866.

Food and Drug Administration (FDA). 2006. Advice to dog owners whose pets take NSAIDs. *Vet Newsl* 21(1). Accessed online 5/22/2010 at https://www.fda.gov/AnimalVeterinary/NewsEvents/ FDAVeterinarianNewsletter/ucm093573.htm.

Glanville J, et al. 2020. Which are the most sensitive search filters to identify randomized controlled trials in MEDLINE? *J Med Libr Assoc* 108(4):556–563. doi: 10.5195/jmla.2020.912. PMID: 33013212; PMCID: PMC7524635.

Holmes M. 2009. Philosophical foundations of evidence-based medicine for veterinary clinicians. *J Am Vet Med Assoc* 235(9):1035–1039.

Institute of Functional Medicine. 2008. What Is Functional Medicine? What_is_FM_and_Working_with_a_FM_Practitioner_2pg.pdf. Accessed online at 9/16/2010 https://www.functionalmedicine.org/about/whatis.asp.

Jensen K.B., et al. 2015. A neural mechanism for nonconscious activation of conditioned placebo and nocebo responses. *Cereb Cortex* 25(10):3903–10. doi: 10.1093/cercor/bhu275. Epub 2014 Dec 1.

Kellogg Co. 2010. Kellogg Co. web site. "Our History." Accessed online 9/21/2010 at https://www.kelloggcompany.com/company.aspx?id=39.

Memon M.A., et al. 2021. Survey of integrative veterinary medicine training in AVMA-Accredited Veterinary Colleges. *J Vet Med Educ* 48(3):289–294.

Polzin D. 2004. *Optimizing Treatment of Chronic Kidney Failure.* Proceedings of the Western Veterinary Conference 2004. Las Vegas, Nevada: WVC Academy.

Roudebush P., et al. 2004. Application of evidence-based medicine to veterinary clinical nutrition. *J Am Vet Med Assoc* 224:1766–1771.

Sackett D.L., et al., ed. 2000. *Evidence-Based Medicine: How to Practice and Teach EBM*, 2nd edition. Philadelphia: Churchill-Livingstone.

Setty A.R. and Sigal L.H. 2005. Herbal medications commonly used in the practice of rheumatology: mechanisms of action, efficacy, and side effects. *Semin Arthritis Rheum* 34(6):773–784.

Stubblefield S. 2017. Survey of complementary and alternative medicine in pediatric inpatient settings. *Complement Ther Med* 35:20–24. doi: 10.1016/j.ctim.2017.08.009. Epub 2017 Aug 25. PMID: 29154062.

Weidenhammer W., et al. 2007. Acupuncture for chronic pain within the research program of 10 German health insurance funds—basic results from an observational study. *Complement Ther Med* 15(4):238–246. Epub 2006 Oct 30. Accessed online 5/11/2010 at https://www.ncbi.nlm.nih.gov/pubmed/18054725.

Wilson K.M., et al. 2006. Use of complementary medicine and dietary supplements among US adolescents. *J Adolesc Health* 38:385–394.

Bibliography

Wynnn S. and Fougere B. 2007. *Veterinary Herbal Medicine.* St. Louis: Mosby.

2

The Role of the Veterinary Technician or Veterinary Nurse in the Holistic Practice

Approaching all parts of the owner–patient–veterinary hospital interaction with a holistic approach, starting with the initial phone call and check-in process, sets the stage for a compassionate and low-stress clinic experience. Even asking owners to bring in pictures of the pet's environment at their first visit can provide valuable insights (especially for behavioral problems) and add to the whole-istic medicine approach. The technician can help by gathering information about all aspects of a pet's life, to aid in the process.

Many practices capitalize on the skills of the technician and offer "technician appointments," which include a technician fee. Technicians take an oral history (including CAM-oriented questions); record the temperature, pulse, and respiration; give routine care such as nail trims and expression of anal glands; and provide follow-up care, such as repeated blood or urine tests or bandage changes and other wound care and evaluation. For most states, as long as there is a valid veterinary–client–patient relationship (VCPR), the technician can perform these duties without the veterinarian being physically in the room. The veterinarian is involved in the part of the history taking involving more specific and probing questions, a complete physical exam, the diagnosis itself, and the actual final decisions, such as initial treatment or changes in follow-up care. If clients want a veterinarian to do the other procedures, an additional veterinary fee should be applied. In addition, technicians obtain blood and urine specimens and perform any tests that involve reading or operating equipment (e.g., EKGs, blood pressure, radiology, endoscopy, and cold LASER therapy). Often, technicians give injections and vaccinations, if called for by the veterinarian (and legal in the state in which they practice). After the examination and testing procedures are done, and the appropriate medications are prescribed, the technicians fill the prescriptions and explain to the client how they are to be given. The technicians are in charge of the pharmacy and order medications as needed. The veterinarian is involved when there is a new product, but the technicians keep items in stock without keeping too much inventory on hand.

Technicians may have similar responsibilities in a holistic veterinary practice, including using holistic equipment, asking different (additional) questions for the oral history, performing different types of testing, and ordering different items for the pharmacy. (See Appendix 5 for an example of a holistic oral history chart.) Technicians certified in physical therapy can also perform procedures such as massage therapy and can help with items such as gait analysis. In practices that dispense herbs or homeopathic solutions, the technician is often in charge of mixing them and then filling the appropriate bottles or vials. The owner and the pet get more total time at the practice and more personalized attention when the technician is involved in teaching about prescribed items and special procedures. The veterinarian is not involved in the technician's duties and, thus,

Complementary Medicine for Veterinary Technicians and Nurses, Second Edition. Nancy Scanlan.
© 2024 John Wiley & Sons, Inc. Published 2024 by John Wiley & Sons, Inc.

has more time for holistic diagnosis (which can initially involve more time interacting with the owner and additional aspects of hands-on examination compared to conventional medical diagnosis) and treatment. Technicians are used for their skills in assisting with diagnostic procedures, for general organization and administration of the pharmacy (including herbal and homeopathic items), for administering certain holistic treatments, for their ability to relate to clients, and to make the hospital client-centered.

Another way that technicians can help the veterinarian, as well as help the practice grow, is to check with the owner 3–5 days after the initial visit. This is especially important with new clients, who may be confused about the administration of remedies or who may be experiencing difficulties with changes in diet. Most of the time, the technician can reassure a client or clear up minor problems without having to interrupt the veterinarian. Sometimes a situation may need some early intervention by the veterinarian. Making these calls lets the clients know that you are truly a caring practice and allows for earlier additional treatment that the owner might not realize is needed.

What a Technician Can and Cannot Do

In general, the same constraints exist in a holistic practice as in a conventional veterinary practice. Only a veterinarian can diagnose, prescribe, or perform surgery in the US. In the UK, the situation is almost the same except that a veterinary nurse can also do minor surgery. For some critical procedures, holistic medicine embraces surgery, which can be lifesaving. Technicians still need to be able to help with anesthesia, surgical preparation, surgical assisting, and proper sterilization of equipment after its use, when surgery is part of the holistic practice.

Holistic medicine usually uses traditional methods of diagnosis, including radiography, urinalysis, fecal analysis, and analysis of blood, and a good technician with skills in performing radiographs, taking samples, and performing analyses is invaluable in a practice. Sometimes additional tests or laboratories are used that are specific for some types of tests, and the technician must be aware of what must be submitted, any special circumstances involved (such as fasting), any special collection items needed, how to submit specimens, and general information about the lab(s) themselves.

Some holistic methods have additional methods of diagnosis. The technician may be called upon, for example, to be a surrogate in an applied kinesiology examination or to help record tongue color and texture in a Chinese medicine examination. In some states, some techniques such as homeopathy or herbal medicine are omitted by law from veterinary practice, so an herbalist or homeopath may not need a veterinary license in order to use these methods. In most states, holistic systems such as chiropractic, acupuncture, or Traditional Chinese Veterinary Medicine (TCVM) may only be practiced by licensed individuals who have obtained post-graduate degrees in the subject. Sometimes they may be practiced either by a veterinarian or by an individual licensed in that practice. Other states may require that a licensed non-veterinarian practice only under the direct supervision of a veterinarian.

However, duties that specifically refer to nursing care (including some types of physical therapy) may be performed by technicians and nurses. Holistic nutrition is not as straightforward as standard pet food out of a bag or can, and a properly trained technician can help people interested in a "natural" diet (including finding out what the client means by that) and can help them formulate their own diet for their pet. They can also point out the benefits or dangers of adding or leaving out various supplements. A technician can be invaluable in helping set up an herbal dispensary, caring for and dispensing homeopathic remedies, and instructing clients on the use of herbs and homeopathic remedies. The technician is also invaluable in a holistic practice as the public's first introduction to holistic medicine. The public may ask general questions such as what holistic medicine is good for, how long a session will take, if acupuncture hurts, or even (usually in a conspiratorial whisper) if it really works. A veterinary technician who knows holistic terminology will be able to discern whether, when asked if the veterinarian is "homeopathic," a client really means "holistic."

If the veterinary technician or nurse has acquired certification in rehabilitation or has earned "specialist" status from the National Association of Veterinary Technicians in America (NAVTA), they may also be able to use most of their extra skills as part of the treatment procedure. This depends, in part, upon the veterinarian and the state, so be aware of what is legal at your practice.

Technicians or nurses can also gather information for the veterinarian when they check in a client. By asking the owner about diet or supplements or specific questions about how the patient has progressed, a technician can help an owner focus on items that are important in assessing the case in a holistic manner. Doing this will sometimes remind the owner about something he or she might otherwise forget to tell the veterinarian.

Holistic Examination Procedures

Veterinary technicians are usually part of the initial examination process, and they may also be called upon to perform a more complete holistic examination, before the veterinarian sees the patient. In a holistic physical examination, the technician and veterinarian are looking for clues about problems before they happen, and using some techniques not always taught in conventional courses. Rather than concentrating on examining primarily for signs of illness, the approach should also include examining for signs of lifestyle diseases and anything predisposing to chronic problems (such as gait and posture not usually termed abnormal in conventional veterinary medicine).

To conduct a complete integrative physical exam, here are the steps, along with tips on communicating with mainstream veterinarians and specialists:

1) Start with observation:
   - Before touching the patient, carefully observe how they move, breathe, and interact with their environment.
   - Look for signs of TCVM constitution, lameness, mental alertness, overall musculature, hair coat quality, and patient symmetry.
   - Simple observations like head carriage can provide insights into chiropractic malalignment of the atlas.
   - Asking insightful questions about the pet's behaviors before laying hands on them can impress clients and lead to important findings, such as the occipital malalignment caused by chasing balls.
2) Thorough evaluation:
   - Perform a comprehensive evaluation of the eyes, ears, nose, and mouth, including assessing the cranial nerves.
   - If the practice uses TCVM, pay attention to the patient's tongue, as it can provide valuable clues about underlying medical conditions and overall health.
     - A white-coated tongue may indicate phlegm or inflammation.
     - A purple or lavender tongue may suggest blood stagnation or deficiency.
     - A curled red tip of the tongue may indicate the need for careful auscultation of the heart.
   - The eyes can offer subtle cues about the patient's emotional well-being and can help identify conditions like allergic conjunctivitis or glaucoma.

3) Cervical region assessment:
   - Palpate the cervical region for pain, range of motion, and hypo- or hypermobility.
   - Continue palpation with attention to the hyoid apparatus, thyroid, and jugular fill.
   - Observations in this region, such as hyoid apparatus restriction, can provide early clues to underlying problems like cervical abscesses.
4) Lymph nodes, skin, musculature, and body condition:
   - Evaluate these areas thoroughly, looking for signs of blood deficiency, stagnation, or faulty peripheral circulation.
   - Utilize conventional muscle condition scoring to assess musculature and muscle wasting.
   - Body condition scoring is essential, since obesity in pets is increasing worldwide.
   - Auscultate the cardiopulmonary system and palpate the abdomen.
   - Assess pulses for TCVM characteristics, such as wiry, slippery, surging, or forceful pulses.
5) Orthopedics and neurology:
   - Perform a full orthopedic and neurologic examination on every patient.
   - Palpate shoulder tendons, digit joints, and other areas to identify specific conditions like tendinopathies or joint abnormalities.
   - Demonstrate myofascial trigger point work to the pet owner to provide pain relief and enhance the human–animal bond.
6) Conclusion:
   - Complete the physical examination by recording the temperature and conducting a rectal examination.
   - Be attentive to any fever or recto-anal masses, as they can significantly impact the chief complaint and guide further diagnostics or interventions.

Remember to approach each patient with a holistic mindset, considering their environment, social and emotional well-being, and implementing stress-reducing strategies. By asking specific questions about daily exercise, discussing consensual touch, and addressing a pet's mental health, veterinary staff can enhance the overall care provided to patients and foster a stronger human–animal bond.

The Holistic Pharmacy

When you were in school, learning about ordering, storing, and dispensing drugs, there was no discussion about special procedures for herbs or for homeopathic medicines. Most veterinarians dispense these in their tablet or capsule form, but some order homeopathic medicines, powdered herbs, or dried herbs in bulk and mix them to make their own capsules, tinctures, ointments, or mixes. A technician or nurse who works in such a practice needs to be aware of the differences, and how to order, store, and dispense them.

Herbs and homeopathic medicines should be stored in a different section of the pharmacy, apart from pharmaceutical drugs. They are usually ordered from companies that either sell only to licensed professionals, or which have a brand for licensed professionals that is different from their brand that is available directly for pet owners. Those companies and brands are more likely to have organically cultivated herbs, to only source endangered herbs from cultivated sources, and to take more care identifying the correct species for their products. You may hear about wildcrafted herbs being more potent than cultivated herbs. (Wildcrafted herbs are herbs that are growing naturally in the wild, and harvested to be made into herbal treatments.) Unfortunately, "ethical wildcrafting" has led to goldenseal, ginseng, and wild echinacea becoming endangered species. This is another reason to only use products that are organically cultivated.

Becoming familiar with the companies your practice deals with by reading their information, visiting their booths at holistic veterinary conferences, and talking to their sales reps will give you a better idea of why your practice uses (or should use) their products. It will also help you answer questions from clients about why your practice offers the expensive brand instead of the cheap one at the local health food store that appears to be the same thing. The best companies test for pesticides, heavy metals, and other contaminants; efficacy and safety; and are a member of NASC.

If you are in charge of ordering, do not be tempted by "specials" if your practice does not use a lot of the product. Even if you know, it will all be used before that 2-year expiration date, ordering a large amount ties up the money available to order holistic products, which means it will not be available for purchasing other items later. You can think of this as an herb money bank account. Save the account for specials offering the herbs or homeopathic medicines that are used the most in your office. The Japanese just-in-time system is ideal for a well-run pharmacy, and ordering a 3-month supply makes much more sense than a 2-year supply. The part of the office computer software devoted to dispensed items makes it easy to see how much of each item is sold, and how often. Check it once a month to guide you for future purchases.

When there are several forms of the same supplement, become familiar with the pros and cons of each form and why your practice recommends a specific one. For example, glucosamine is available as glucosamine HCl, or as glucosamine sulfate, with or without other substances. The other substances are most commonly chondroitin (and there are several versions of that). Next most common are other supplements or herbs that reduce inflammation, decrease pain, or both. Most practices do not dispense glucosamine itself, since veterinarians can't compete in price with an easily available supplement sold by large nationwide or international companies. But they might sell something else that is more effective for the same problem, that works in a similar way, that may or may not have glucosamine as one of the ingredients. When you have in-depth information about professional-level herbs compared to pet store herbs, you can help clients make the correct choice.

Another advantage of stocking practitioner-only products is that clients will return to you for refills. That gives you and your employer a chance to ask how the patient is doing and whether their guardian has seen any reactions they are concerned with. Your veterinarian can be notified, and, if necessary, an appointment can be set up for a problem that otherwise might be overlooked. Note your conversation in the patient's chart—both good comments and bad comments. It is an important part of monitoring the progress of the patient.

When your order arrives, make sure the herbs or supplements received are the ones you ordered. This is especially important if you are unfamiliar with the company you are ordering from. There are several ways that employees of an herb or supplement company can easily make mistakes. New employees of an herb or supplement company, who are unfamiliar with herbs or supplements, can get similar items confused. If they are in a hurry, they might also accidentally check the wrong box on a long form in their software. Or the person who is filling the order might accidentally choose the wrong herb to include in your order. This seems to happen most often with herbal products. If you received the wrong item, notify the company. They should give you instructions for how to return the item, and send the correct one in its place. They often will send an email with a return label to apply to the box you return the item in.

Herbal and homeopathic products should be kept in a clean, dry area away from heat and direct sunlight. Some herbs can get moldy more easily than most do (even if they are in capsules or tablets), especially if they are mucilaginous (such as slippery elm or marshmallow). It is even more important to keep just enough of these on hand to meet demand. Like drugs, rotate your stock on a first-in, first-out basis and store items in alphabetical order within their section. With proper storage, most herbs and supplements can last up to 2 years before expiring. No food or snacks should be kept in the dispensing area.

For practices that order herbs or herbal powders in bulk, do not store the new herbs on top of the old ones. Store them in a separate container or in the packaging they came in, and use up the ones in the old container first. When the container is empty, clean and dry it and place the new order in it. Check for foreign matter and remove it before storing the herbs or powders. If it is present throughout the product, discard the entire product or send it back to the company it was ordered from.

Tablets and capsules can be dispensed in plastic vials with child-proof tops. If you are mixing and dispensing items as a liquid (especially ones containing oils such as essential oils) or ointment, those containers should always be made of glass. On the dispensing label, single herbs should be listed with both Latin and common names, especially when more than one species shares the common name (such as skullcap or ginseng).

Some practices dispense tinctures of homeopathic or herbal combinations. There are specific procedures for mixing these, including how to shake them, how vigorously, how many times, and how much alcohol and water to add. The proportions and mixing methods vary, and so are not listed here. Become acquainted with the way your veterinarian wants it done, and do not vary from the method. Variations can make a difference, which can change the effectiveness.

When mixing a tincture, *always* use ethyl alcohol, *never* the alcohol used in hand sanitizers, or for sterilizing thermometers, etc. Vodka is most commonly used for the ethyl alcohol, although 100% ethyl alcohol may be used where it is legal. Use distilled water to dilute the tincture, not tap water. Always use a glass dropper bottle, never a plastic dropper bottle. Use brown or other dark colored bottles (such as dark blue), not clear glass, to minimize the chance of light causing oxidation.

If your practice makes creams or ointments, you will also need small jars (usually 2 oz or 50 ml size). These should also be made of dark colored glass. You might also need a small digital scale, depending on how herbs, etc. are measured for the final product.

If making oil infusions or creams or ointments, you will also need a good quality organic oil (such as olive oil or almond oil), vitamin E capsules (to add as an antioxidant and extend the life of the product), and beeswax (to thicken or harden the oil and create creams, ointments, or balms). Infusions are made by adding dried herbs to the organic oil, keeping it warm in sunlight or a crockpot or a 100° oven for 4–5 days, then strained or put through an herb press. Add the contents of one or two vitamin E capsules to each batch that you create. Add beeswax to the warm product, a little at a time, until you get the desired thickness, from creamy (just a little) to hard (like a lip balm). Store the unmixed liquid in a refrigerator. If adding essential oils, add after the liquid is strained. Your veterinarian can guide you through these procedures until you are familiar with them.

When you dispense ointments or balms, *be sure* to include "for external use only" on the label—people have been known to give these to their pets by mouth.

Often, all of these procedures are communicated by word of mouth to any new staff who might be helping dispense medication and herbs. Once you become familiar with the way your veterinary hospital runs a pharmacy, it is very helpful to write down everything in a Standard Operating Procedure (SOP)—especially for the parts that can vary from one practice to the next.

An SOP for staff in a veterinary practice gives detailed instructions for carrying out a specific activity. It should include names (or named positions) of people accountable for the activity, and who have final authorization (if not the veterinarian). It should be clear enough so it is easy to follow and not read like a legal document or make your eyes glaze over. This would include exact formulas and procedures for creating tinctures, etc., and a list of preferred companies to order from with phone numbers and (where applicable) specific salesperson to order from.

The SOP can be added to anything your practice already has that concerns dispensing medications. Or, if there is nothing, it can include everything, for drugs, supplies, and holistic items, and procedures from ordering and stocking, to filling prescriptions.

If you find yourself giving the same instructions to clients over and over, make a client handout. Go over them with the client, then include the handout when you give them the medication. Clients should be instructed to keep any dried herbs away from the stove, the refrigerator, the bathroom, and laundry. Client handouts can be stored on the computer and personalized for each patient before they are printed out.

(See also Appendix 15 Inventory Management.)

Summary

What can a technician do?

1) Be prepared to help with parts of the initial examination, if the veterinarian agrees.
2) Be prepared to include parts of a holistic exam, if the veterinarian agrees that you should do part of the initial examination (especially taking the temperature, pulse, and respiration).
3) Do call-backs to see how pets are progressing, note the answer in the charts, and have them ready for the veterinarian to review.
4) Know the requirements for setup and dispensing of holistic items. If the veterinarian agrees, keep track of inventory and order accordingly.
5) In an herbal and/or homeopathic pharmacy, know how to mix and dispense tinctures, solutions, and ointments.
6) Be able to answer general introductory questions from the public about holistic medicine in general and the practice in which you work in particular.
7) Maintain your skills at regular nursing care as well as other technician duties (such as anesthesia, drawing blood, etc.).

3

Legal Implications

Registered veterinary technicians should be aware of the legal implications regarding various holistic treatments. Technicians should know the law for their state and be aware of how their state board views various types of holistic treatments. They should also know the requirements of other professions' state boards regarding holistic treatments. For example, is direct supervision required for a chiropractor to practice on animals? Is the veterinarian the only person who may use or supervise chiropractic on animals, or may a chiropractor work on an animal without the involvement of a veterinarian? Are referrals to chiropractors allowed without direct involvement of a veterinarian? Herbalists, massage therapists, physical therapists, certified veterinary rehabilitation specialists, and acupuncturists are also treated differently from one state to another. The skill and knowledge of practitioners of these and other healing arts can vary greatly, which can cause concern in both conventional and holistic veterinarians. Knowing the law will enable the technician to explain to pet owners why referrals may not be possible if they want a specific kind of treatment that their veterinarian cannot supply. Keep in mind that laws change every so often, and sometimes local law affects what is allowed also.

Herbs

There are three important questions to ask when dealing with herbs:

1) Are they a drug?
2) Are they effective?
3) Are they dangerous or contaminated?

In the United States, if an herb is categorized as a drug, then it must go through all the testing that the FDA requires, which may cost millions of dollars. If an herb is tested through this type of research and is found to be effective for a specific disease, further restrictions may be placed upon its manufacture. After all this, these herbs can't be patented because they have been in use for so long. Thus, an herbal company will not be financially rewarded if they use this procedure.

If it goes in an animal's mouth and is not a drug, is it food? The Association of American Feed Control Officials (AAFCO) has published a list of items that are recognized as being safe to feed to an animal. AAFCO makes recommendations to state feed control officials, who apply recommendations in keeping with their individual state laws. If a substance is not on that list of safe items, then the state can ban its use, especially if it is incorporated into a treat or food.

Complementary Medicine for Veterinary Technicians and Nurses, Second Edition. Nancy Scanlan.
© 2024 John Wiley & Sons, Inc. Published 2024 by John Wiley & Sons, Inc.

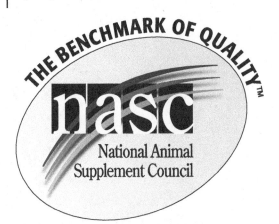

Figure 3.1 NASC (National Animal Supplement Council) seal.

For human use, herbs and supplements are considered a new category of food under federal regulations. To ban a human supplement, the FDA must prove it causes harm. For animals, herbs and supplements are considered either a drug or a food and as such are regulated by the FDA and an individual state's feed control officers. To be called a food, a supplement must be on a list of foods and supplements, which was developed by AAFCO. If it is not on this list, it is a drug and must undergo all the testing that other drugs do. Because of this, Bill Bookout, who has been active in the animal medical field for over 25 years, founded the National Animal Supplement Council (NASC), which helps manufacturers and the FDA work with each other to ensure the quality and safety of their products. Any company that is a member of NASC is allowed to use the NASC label on its products. (See Figure 3.1.) Members must keep track of all complaints reported and submit reports to the council regularly. In turn, the NASC acts as a go-between and helps notify its members and others of the FDA's actions and rulings.

If a company makes a specific claim for an herb or supplement, such as that it treats cancer, it has made a "drug claim." Such claims are not legal, even if research has shown that the specific herb does have some anti-cancer properties. Thus, companies use more general descriptions for their products. To learn about specific properties of herbs or supplements, technicians must consult textbooks (such as those listed in the appendix) and research literature (such as the articles available online on PubMed at https://www.ncbi.nlm.nih.gov/pubmed/).

Herb Safety

Besides the NASC label, the way that herbs are manufactured and tested will also determine herb safety. Imported herbs are especially a concern, particularly from countries such as China, which has been implicated a number of times in contamination of pet products and herbal products. The fact that a product is manufactured in the United States does not guarantee safety, however. There have been instances of contamination here as well. The situation has improved since the government has developed Good Manufacturing Procedures (GMP) required for the production of herbs.

To know if a product is truly organic, whether it comes from one or many sources, and what the quality control process is, read a company's literature, check its website, talk to its sales representatives, and go to meetings such as the annual meeting of the American Holistic Veterinary Medical Association, where you can meet the owners and representatives of the company.

Herb Quality

For all herbs, but for Chinese herbs especially, it is important that the correct parts of the plant be used and prepared correctly. If the person who prepares the formulas does not understand this, it can have disastrous results. For example, *ma huang* (ephedra), a Chinese herb, is used traditionally in small quantities in combination with other herbs to help with lung congestion, asthma, and respiratory disease. Instead of using it properly, in the United States, it was overdosed, resulting in illness, deaths, and banning of the herb. Again, by talking to the companies, you can determine whether or not they are following recognized principles and dosages. (See also Chapter 10 for a list of companies that follow safe practices.)

Companies that are dedicated to selling only to licensed individuals will make an extra effort to sell the correct herbs with the correct action. They usually have a veterinarian or certified herbalist on staff or as a consultant to make sure that formulations are created properly. Veterinarians who are trained as herbalists will recognize quickly if a product is not working as it should. There are products on the shelves of health food stores that have little or none of the ingredients listed on their labels. Until a laboratory such as consumerlab.com tests them, the consumer will not know this. That is why it is best for clients to use the products that the veterinarian keeps in stock, even though they may cost more.

Chiropractors, Acupuncturists, and Veterinarians

Many, but not all, states in the United States require that chiropractic and acupuncture be performed either by a veterinarian or under the supervision (direct or indirect) of a veterinarian. This means that for small animals, it must usually be performed in a veterinary practice, not at the office of the chiropractor or acupuncturist. All states require specialized education and a license to perform these methods. Veterinary technicians cannot perform acupuncture unless they are also licensed acupuncturists, and they cannot perform chiropractic unless they are also licensed chiropractors. However, with additional training, they may become certified in related practices such as Tui-na (a type of Chinese massage), and Chinese food therapy.

Homeopathy and Herbalists

Some states take the stance that any treatment of an animal for the purpose of helping a disease is the practice of veterinary medicine. Other states either ignore homeopaths and herbalists or they may specifically exclude them from the practice act. In those states, homeopaths and herbalists can practice their specialty on an animal without breaking the law.

Telephone Consultations

There are several types of consultations. For instance, in general, veterinarians employed by a university can legally be consulted by other veterinarians without a problem. Usually, a veterinarian who is a board-certified specialist is able to consult with veterinarians within a state. (The certification must be one that is recognized by the American Veterinary Medical Association. Therefore, holistic certifications do not count for this option.) There is some confusion over whether or not they can be consulted by veterinarians from other states.

If there is some question about the legality of one veterinarian speaking to another on the telephone about a case, imagine the confusion about telephone consultations between a veterinarian and a pet owner. In order to do phone consultations, it is usually required that some type of VCPR* exist within a specific time period or that there is a request for a consultation from the original treating veterinarian. A client–patient relationship happens when a veterinarian has seen the animal, in person. There is often a time limit for the visit—usually 1 year. After 1 year, the veterinarian must examine the animal again before they can prescribe for it, or refer it to a specialist. Again, this varies from state to state. This is one of the reasons that veterinarians don't just keep giving vaccinations over and over to a pet that the owner thinks is healthy, without having seen the pet within a year.

Teleconferences, where the owner and pet meet with a veterinarian over the internet, are not legal to create a client–patient relationship in the US, except in Alabama (as of 2023). Teleconference consultations have been used for years in human medicine, and other states might follow Alabama's lead. The veterinary profession is deeply divided over this issue. State boards, as of 2023, are against this. They fear that a video conference without the ability to actually touch a patient can miss critical information when examining a patient.

Release Forms (Consent Forms)

Whenever any treatment is performed that is outside the average or usual experience of a pet owner, it is best to obtain a signed release form, also known as a consent form. The purpose of a release form is to demonstrate that an owner has been told about a procedure, including possible side effects; notified that there is no guarantee of cure; and notified that the procedure might not be considered mainstream medicine. It may also specifically name or describe a procedure. Sometimes, the release form will specify the number of treatments recommended, especially for something such as physical therapy, where an owner might stop treatments before optimum benefit is established. Along with the release form, veterinarians may supply a cost estimate form, on which total charges are listed for procedures and any deposit is recorded. Another reason for a release form is when something is being done in a different way than is commonly recognized as "normal" veterinary procedure. For example, a practitioner may recommend vaccination at longer intervals than the manufacturer recommends or an owner may request they be given at longer intervals. Examples of release forms can be found in Appendices 6 and 7.

A technician can be of great help to a veterinarian here. An owner may consider a release form to mean that a procedure is more dangerous than it actually is, that the veterinarian takes no responsibility whatsoever, and that the owner will be financially liable for unlimited charges. The technician can ease the client's concerns by reviewing and explaining the form. This is a good time to review the actual procedure, discuss how the pet is expected to react, and explain what the owner can do if he or she is concerned.

---

*veterinary-client-patient relationship.

Summary

What can a technician do?

1) Be aware of what technicians can and cannot do in your state.
2) Be aware of what other lay practitioners can and cannot do in your state.
3) Be prepared to explain to clients the ramifications of items 1 and 2.
4) If your practice uses them, be sure that clients fill out all required release forms and disclosure documents, and help explain them to the client.

Webliography

American Holistic Veterinary Medical Association. https://www.ahvma.org
An organization for veterinarians interested in any aspect of complementary and alternative veterinary medicine. It also has good information for pet owners in general.
National Animal Supplement Council (NASC). https://www.nasc.cc/
A group of animal supplement manufacturers that works with the FDA to develop standards for the manufacturing of supplements for animals. (Includes a list of NASC members.)

4

Introduction to Modalities

Holistic medicine is a fluid field. What is new or unconventional today becomes mainstream medicine tomorrow. Examples of treatments that have crossed over into the mainstream include the following (see also Figures 4.1 and 4.2):

Antioxidants
Glucosamine and chondroitin
Longer intervals between vaccinations
Milk thistle
Omega-3 fatty acids
Physical therapy (including massage therapy)
Prebiotics (soluble fibers)
Probiotics
SAM-e
targeted pulsed electromagnetic field therapy

This fluidity is why there is no set definition of holistic medicine. Conventional veterinarians are practicing it, whether they know it or not!

All veterinarians are trained in conventional diagnostic methods. All use at least some of these methods, especially radiographs and blood tests and a good physical examination, as part of the initial evaluation. Holistic veterinarians may or may not include some extra diagnostic techniques such as static palpation (commonly used by those who perform chiropractic), identification of trigger points, examination of the tongue (by those who have studied traditional Chinese medicine theory), or a more thorough evaluation of the pulse to give some additional insight into the disease process. Again, as conventional veterinarians become more familiar with these methods, some will include them in their diagnostic regimens.

Some of the various modalities used by holistic veterinarians are relatively easy to master, whereas others may involve a lifetime of study in order to become a true master. This book explores the methods that veterinarians are most likely to use and to which clients are most likely to have been exposed. Being familiar with these terms will allow the veterinary technician to help clients choose the best ways to help their pets.

The following briefly lists and describes modalities and the chapter in this book in which they are found (in the order in which they are addressed; an alphabetical list can be found in Appendix 2).

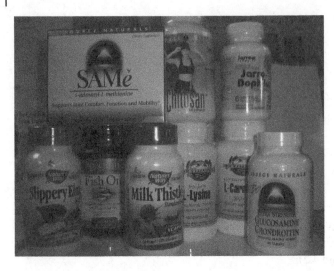

Figure 4.1 Items found in health food stores and holistic practices.

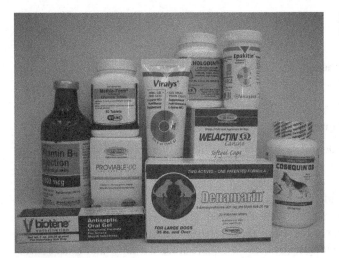

Figure 4.2 The same items found in conventional practices.

Modalities

Rehabilitation Therapy (Chapter 5)

Rehabilitation therapy is used to rehabilitate animals that have received injuries and to help strengthen animals that are disabled by age or disease. It consists of a number of different methods. Veterinary technicians and nurses can become certified in physical therapy and can perform some types of therapy themselves.

Cold Laser Therapy (Chapter 5)

A cold laser of a specific wavelength (usually at the red end of the spectrum) is used to reduce injury and speed healing. Lasers come in different classes, and the higher the class number, the more powerful the laser. Most lasers used by veterinarians are Class 3 or Class 4, with Class 4 becoming increasingly popular. Treatment with a Class 4 laser is faster, but it has a higher potential to cause damage. To prevent damage, both the therapist and the patient need to wear protective goggles, and the laser wand is kept in constant circulation over an area rather than keeping it on one spot continually.

Hydrotherapy (Chapter 5)

A general term including pool therapy and, especially, underwater treadmills. With pool therapy, dogs are fitted with life jackets and swim in a warm pool. Underwater treadmills can be horizontal, or they may be a type that allows the front part to be elevated in order to give more resistance and exercise for the dog. They especially help by decreasing the weight carried by injured or disabled limbs while allowing animals to rebuild muscle and improve balance after surgery or injury. Hydrotherapy pools and underwater treadmills are the main types of hydrotherapy used in small animals. Hydrotherapy pools are usually seen in physical therapy centers, whereas underwater treadmills may be in such centers or as part of a veterinary practice.

tPEMFT—Targeted Pulsed Electromagnetic Field Therapy (Chapter 5)

A magnetic field on an electric carrier wave is applied to an area to help relieve pain and swelling, and to speed up healing. tPEMFT is available as individual devices sold or rented by veterinarians for home treatment. The treatment is painless, and results can be seen after as little as a single treatment.

Hospice Care and Grief Therapy (Chapter 5)

All pet owners would like their pets to die peacefully in their sleep. There are owners who want to help their pets transition peacefully instead of bringing them to the veterinarian to be euthanized.

The pet hospice movement has come into being recently, and the most information available is usually from holistic veterinary meetings and in holistic veterinary journals.

Hospice care helps an animal stay comfortable and pain-free during this transition. The intent is to relieve pain and suffering without extensive treatment to prolong the life of a dying animal. Part of hospice care is to support the owners and help them through the grieving process. Pets may grieve also, and there is information that can help them, too.

Human–Animal Bond (Chapter 5)

Many pet owners have a strong bond with their pets that the human medical world may not recognize. Therapy dogs and service dogs have been ambassadors for this idea, and there are ways the technician can become involved with these animals and help support their use.

TTouch (Chapter 6)

Tellington TTouch is based on circular motions made by the fingers and hands in the form of gentle massage applied all over the body. It also includes specific exercises. Its purpose is not to physically massage muscles but rather to reconnect an animal with its body. It is used to speed up healing and to help with behavior problems.

Massage Therapy (Chapter 6)

Massage therapy comes in many forms and can be useful to help animals when done properly. Not all human massage therapists know how to properly massage an animal, so it is important to learn the technique from someone who is successful with animals. Massage therapy techniques include *shiatsu* (Japanese massage), *Tui-na* (Chinese massage), acupressure, and trigger point therapy. These methods may be used singly or as part of a general massage program. In addition, massage therapy is often a part of a program of physical therapy.

Traditional Chinese Medicine (TCM) Diagnosis (Chapters 6 and 10)

TCM diagnosis is a different way of looking at ways the body functions, and how that applies to health and disease. Many are superficially aware of some of the concepts—for example, the Yin/Yang sign is seen in many contexts. TCM is based on the idea of good health including the flow of energy through the body, removing obstruction to the flow of this energy, and also bringing the body back into balance, and looking at things we see as opposites (such as heat and cold) as being the extremes of one main factor.

Tui-Na (Chapter 6)

Tui-Na is the Chinese method of massage therapy, and among its goals is the restoration of balance and flow.

Acupressure (Chapter 6)

Acupressure is performed by massaging acupuncture points. Because it is based on acupuncture points, it can directly affect internal organs as well as muscles.

Shiatsu (Chapter 6)

Shiatsu is a Japanese form of massage. Its basis is a theory of medicine similar to TCM, but with a Japanese interpretation.

Trigger Point Therapy (Chapter 6)

Trigger point therapy locates trigger points (areas of tight and tender fibers) in muscles and releases them in a variety of ways. Some methods, such as chiropractic and acupuncture, must be performed by a veterinarian or licensed practitioner, but other methods, such as massage, can be performed by a veterinary nurse or technician.

Reiki (Chapter 6)

Reiki is a Japanese technique used to reduce stress and promote healing. It emphasizes the application of "life force energy" through the hands placed on or above the animal.

Detoxification and Fasting (Chapter 7)

Detoxification is done to eliminate various harmful substances (toxins) from the body. These toxins may be drugs that remain in the body or natural substances that the body has not yet dealt with.

Detoxification usually involves diet change (sometimes fasting) and various nutraceuticals and herbs to help the process.

Detoxification is recognized by a number of different holistic specialties, and the Institute of Functional Medicine has created a large body of research on this topic for humans.

Holistic Diet and Nutrition (Chapter 8)

Holistic nutrition is based upon the use of fresh, whole foods, with no artificial flavors, colors, or preservatives and no derivatives such as corn gluten meal. In addition, some types of diets attempt to recreate the ancestral diet of an animal. There are others that create balanced vegetarian diets for pets.

Special diets have been created to help animals with some specific disease problems. They have evolved so that some follow holistic principles of nutrition, along with the nutrients needed for those disease problems.

Nutraceuticals (Chapter 9)

Nutritional supplements are ingested products, not food, that add to the health of an animal. Vitamins, minerals, antioxidants, amino acids, and fatty acids are examples of nutritional supplements. Supplements are necessary in a "normal" diet, including holistic ones, to make up for potential imbalances. For example, because cats require large amounts of taurine, this substance should be added to all cat diets, including raw diets (even though raw meat has more taurine than cooked or processed meat). Nutraceuticals are nutritional supplements that are used for specific disease problems, often at higher doses than when used for supplementing a diet.

Traditional Chinese Medicine (Chapters 6 and 10)

Traditional Chinese medicine (TCM) is a system of medicine thousands of years old, based on the concept of yin and yang, and organ functions that go beyond the Western understanding of how they work. TCM uses acupuncture and Chinese herbs as the main methods of treatment. TCM aims to bring the body back into balance and restore the flow of the body's energy (qi). The terms used and the ideas behind TCM may sound like superstition, but they are actually just a different way of looking at the body and can lead to insights unavailable to veterinarians who use only conventional Western diagnostic methods. For example, the tongue is examined not only for paleness, but general color, shape, cracks, and coating. The pulse is taken on both sides of the body, not just the left (or right), and compared. One can sometimes make a diagnosis by using these methods alone (e.g., kidney failure). Sometimes, potential problems can be seen here before they are seen by other signs (e.g., pending heart problems from bloat surgery.)

Herbal Medicine (Chapter 10)

There are two main groups of herbal supplements used most commonly by holistic veterinarians: Chinese herbs and Western herbs.

Some other herbal systems, such as Ayurvedic and South American systems, are also beginning to be used. Ayurvedic herbs depend upon another ancient medical theory from India, whereas the South American herbs are used in a way similar to Western herbs.

Unless the veterinary technician or veterinarian is familiar with Chinese medicine, Chinese herbs should always be used in a balanced formula, not as individual items. They are best used if someone in the practice has a basic knowledge of Chinese medical theory. However, there are some formulas that are general enough to be used by a beginner. Western herbs are used more like conventional drugs: either alone or in combination for various disease problems. They are beginning to become a common part of conventional practice. If you use Denamarin, you are already using milk thistle, for example. Chinese and Western herbs have their own sections in Chapter 10.

There are some herbs that are well known by the general public. Because they are so common, they are found in herb or health food stores. Even if the veterinary practice does not dispense them, it is good for veterinary technicians to have some familiarity with these herbs and their uses so that they can properly advise clients rather than simply telling them to "stop because herbs can be dangerous." Owners will usually not stop when they hear this; they just stop telling the veterinary practice that they are using them.

Western Herbal Medicine (Chapter 10)

Based on a combination of European herbs and those found in North America, Western herbal medicine may use single herbs or combinations of them to treat various diseases. Common to other types of herbal medicine is the belief that the combination of dozens of factors in herbs has a more beneficial effect than a single drug used for a single purpose. In addition, herbs as a group have fewer side effects than do many drugs.

Aromatherapy (Chapter 10)

Aromatherapy is the use of essential oils from plants, usually diluted in carrier oils, to treat mental and physical problems. Oils are distilled from plant materials and hence are very strong. The dilute oils may be applied directly on the patient (carefully!) or to the environment.

Veterinary Orthopedic Manipulation (Chapter 10)

Veterinary orthopedic manipulation (VOM) uses instruments similar to those used by some chiropractors and adjusts all joints, not just those with fixations. Adjustments are not made by hand, however. Veterinary technicians can become certified in VOM techniques.

Homeopathy (Chapter 10)

Homeopathy is a system of medication based on several principles: (1) A substance that causes specific signs when used in high doses can be used to treat those same signs when used in low doses; (2) the more dilute the substance, the stronger its action; and (3) previous diseases may have been repressed rather than cured so that when one reverses the disease process, temporary recurrence of these previous conditions may be seen as the patient improves. (This is known as Hering's law, or regressive vicariation.) A very complete history of the patient is taken, and remedies are selected by how well they fit the disease pattern. Usually, single remedies are used.

Equine Osteopathy (Chapter 10)

Osteopathy looks for problems in both muscles and joints that impact the patient. These problems impinge upon both the nervous system and the circulatory system. By helping restore function to a local area, the rest of the body can be helped because of action on the nervous system and the circulatory system.

Acupuncture (Chapter 10)

An ancient Chinese practice, thousands of years old, acupuncture consists of inserting needles into specific spots on the body to create specific physiological results. Many of these points can be found with a pointfinder (actually just an ohmmeter that measures current flow in millivolts and microamperes), and others have common anatomical features (such as penetration of fascia by nerves and blood vessels). Most commonly used for pain, acupuncture can also help many other problems. It is the most commonly used part of TCM theory in the United States. Veterinary technicians and nurses can apply acupressure on points to accomplish specific effects, especially for pain relief.

Chinese Herbal Medicine (Chapter 10)

Chinese herbs are used in formulas that are designed using specific guidelines (for master herbs, helper herbs, etc.) and are usually used according to a TCM diagnosis.

Ayurvedic Herbal Medicine (Chapter 10)

Ayurvedic herbal medicine uses herbs from India and may also incorporate the Indian theory of disease. Indian theory is similar in some ways to Chinese medicine: *Purusha* and *Prakriti* correspond somewhat to yin and yang, respectively. *Prana* is life force, like the Chinese qi. Disease comes from an imbalance of three doshas: *Pitta*, *Kapha*, and *Vatta*, which correspond somewhat to the five-element theory of TCM. *Srotas* are similar to meridians, and some types of energy travel through them. Tongue and pulse diagnosis is also used in both.

Chiropractic (Chapter 10)

Chiropractic is a treatment system based on finding fixations in joints and treating them with fast acceleration, short-lever manipulations. Chiropractic emphasizes the effect of these fixations, the effect of their relief on the nervous system and, from there, on the entire body. Chiropractic is especially used for pain and lameness.

Applied Kinesiology (Chapter 10)

Applied kinesiology comes in various forms and uses the strength or weakness of a muscle (often by pressing down on an outstretched arm) to determine whether a substance is good or bad for a patient. It may also be used to determine whether a treatment has helped a patient.

Nambrudipad's Allergy Elimination Technique (NAET) (Chapter 11)

Nambrudipad's allergy elimination technique (NAET®) uses applied kinesiology and other methods to determine allergies and a form of acupressure to desensitize patients to those allergens. "Allergens" are any item that can cause hypersensitivity reactions and thus may include things we normally do not associate with allergens, such as emotional responses.

Bach Flower Remedies (Chapter 11)

Bach flower remedies are homeopathically prepared essences of specific flowers, each of which is used for a specific type of mental state (such as fear). Rescue Remedy is a commonly used combination of five of the remedies and is used for anxiety.

Glandular Therapy (Chapter 11)

Glandular therapy uses small amounts of tissue or tissue extracts (such as liver, thymus, and thyroid) orally administered to help heal that tissue or boost its function.

Magnetic Therapy (Chapter 12)

Magnets are used in therapy by placing them on the body or in a bed to help manage pain. Magnets may also be taped to specific acupuncture points to prolong the effects of treatment at those locations.

Ozone Therapy (Chapter 12)

Ozone is generated from oxygen by an ozone generator. It is usually administered rectally, although sometimes, a patient's blood is withdrawn, mixed with ozone, and the ozone-blood mixture injected back into the patient. It is used for pain and some degenerative diseases.

Hyperbaric Therapy (Chapter 12)

Hyperbaric therapy uses a 100% oxygen atmosphere with pressure of more than 1 atm to treat various diseases. Hyperbaric chambers were first used for deep sea divers suffering from decompression sickness (the bends).

Prolotherapy (Chapter 12)

Prolotherapy involves injection of substances (usually including a concentrated dextrose solution) to create scar tissue to help support joints. It is commonly used in the back, hips, and stifles.

Homotoxicology (Chapter 12)

Homotoxicology uses remedies that are similar to those used by homeopathy and shares some of the same theories of disease. However, homotoxicology uses combined low-potency dilutions instead of single remedies and places a major emphasis on detoxification. In addition, homotoxicology relies more upon a Western medical diagnosis.

Immuno-Augmentive Therapy (Chapter 12)

Immuno-augmentive therapy (IAT) helps boost certain components in the blood to fight cancer. This therapy is currently unavailable to veterinarians, although it is still practiced in the Bahamas for humans and there are references to it on the Internet.

Color Therapy (Chapter 12)

Colors are used to affect mood and the immune system of animals. Color therapy is used more often in people than in animals. It can be useful in setting the mood for clients.

Rife Machine (Chapter 12)

The Rife machine is based on Royal Rife's work. The machine emits various electromagnetic frequencies used to treat disease.

Electroacupuncture According to Voll, Biotron, and Other Electronic Diagnostic and Treatment Equipment (Chapter 12)

Various electronic equipment is often used by holistic veterinarians. This equipment often measures electric resistance of the skin in various parts of the body (especially, but not always, at various acupuncture points). Treatment may be performed by these machines, or it may be based on the readings from these machines.

Animal Communicators (Chapter 12)

There are people who have a deep bond with animals and believe they can communicate with them, usually using pictures rather than words. Animal communicators may give insight into a pet's behavior.

These modalities will be explored further in the rest of this book.

Summary

What can the technician do?

1) Familiarize yourself with short descriptions of all modalities, even if your practice does not use them.
2) Know which modalities may be practiced by a veterinarian only and which a technician can perform.
3) Be prepared to discuss any of these modalities with clients.
4) If appropriate, seek further training in any modality that a technician is allowed to perform. This makes you more valuable to your employer and can make work more fun for you.

5

Holistic Training for Veterinary Technicians: Rehabilitation and Hospice Care

Rehabilitation (Physical Therapy)

Definition

Rehabilitation (for animals) or physical therapy (for humans) is the application of various methods to rehabilitate an animal from sports injuries, or after surgery, or to help with lameness. These methods include (but are not limited to) swim therapy, underwater treadmill, chiropractic, acupuncture, massage therapy, special exercises, ball therapy, and elastic bands to increase muscle strength. Rehabilitation also includes diet and nutraceuticals to help these goals. Rehabilitation is now a recognized AVMA Board Certified specialty for veterinarians, officially known as Sports Medicine and Rehabilitation. Technicians can become certified in Veterinary Physical Rehabilitation (but not AVMA board-certified), and with the proper training and experience, can become a member of the NAVTA specialty group Academy of Physical Rehabilitation Veterinary Technicians (Figures 5.1–5.3).

Purpose

The ultimate purpose of rehabilitation or physical therapy in general is to restore strength and range of motion and to decrease or abolish lameness. Individual modalities chosen for each case are the ones that are most appropriate for each set of problems.

History

For humans, physical therapy in the United States evolved because of the polio epidemics that occurred from the 1800s through the 1950s, but especially in the 1920s and 1930s, and because of the needs of injured soldiers, beginning with soldiers in World War I. Originally, treatment for polio was immobilization, splinting, bed rest, and later, surgery. Elizabeth Kenny, an Australian nurse, developed a treatment for polio from her experiences in the bush, consisting of hot bandages for the paralyzed limbs and gentle massage. Sister Kenny ("Sister" is a title in the British Commonwealth for nurses) clashed with medical authorities of the day, who recommended splinting and casts instead. In 1940, Sister Kenny brought her treatment for polio victims to the United States. World War II brought improved methods of medical and surgical treatment of wounds for soldiers, resulting in more disabled soldiers surviving and needing further treatment. Physical

Complementary Medicine for Veterinary Technicians and Nurses, Second Edition. Nancy Scanlan.
© 2024 John Wiley & Sons, Inc. Published 2024 by John Wiley & Sons, Inc.

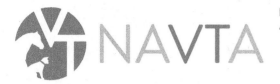

Figure 5.1 North American Veterinary Technicians Association.

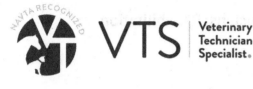

Figure 5.2 Veterinary Technician Specialist.

Figure 5.3 Veterinary Nurse Specialist.

therapists evolved from the role of a technician to a practitioner. In 1967, the Social Security Act was amended to recognize outpatient physical therapy as a valid treatment. Now, physical therapists for humans must undergo special training in a 2-year course, and over 40 states require that they be licensed.

Although for decades, much research has been devoted to repairing sports injuries in racehorses and sport horses, for most animals, rehabilitation as an individual modality has only relatively recently evolved. It wasn't until 2001 that the first International Symposium on Rehabilitation and Physical Therapy in Veterinary Medicine was held. There are currently several programs in the United States that train physical therapists, veterinary technicians, and veterinarians in the art of rehabilitation for canines or horses.

Description

Physical therapy addresses three main areas:

- Sports medicine
- Recovery from surgery
- Problems of geriatric dogs

Physical therapy consists of various procedures designed to speed healing and restore strength, flexibility, joint function, and general health. Physical therapists must know anatomy and physiology in order to help an animal properly, and their training courses include these subjects.

Diagnostic methods include examination and evaluation of areas and the patient's abilities beyond that which is employed by most veterinarians, such as the following:

- Range of motion (goniometry) and assessment of joint flexibility
- Measurement of muscle circumference
- Measurement of muscle strength

- Identification of trigger points
- Lameness evaluation (on a sliding scale), including gait analysis (force plates may be used as part of this evaluation)

Treatment may include a number of methods, depending on the needs of the patient and the willingness of the owner. Simple superficial heating and cooling of affected areas may be performed or its use explained. Many people who do not understand physical therapy often apply heat or cold at the wrong time, which can result in the worsening of the condition. For example, ice on a joint with chronic arthritis can make it stiffer, whereas heat may give relief and result in increased flexibility. The same joint, newly injured in an athletic event, may require ice to accomplish the same result.

A conditioning program will be recommended, beyond the general "take him for a walk for X minutes," which is often the advice of a regular veterinarian. These programs will vary depending on whether the problem is neurological or mechanical (joint and muscle), the age of the patient, and the type of injury (surgical, athletic, or age related). Certified therapists learn not only how to perform the procedures but also how to instruct clients, measure outcomes, document properly, educate the client, and understand legal and ethical issues.

The following modalities are all part of physical therapy. Depending on the facility, there may only be a few of these available.

- Therapeutic exercise
- Cold laser therapy
- Hydrotherapy
  - Whirlpool hydrotherapy
  - Swim therapy
  - Underwater treadmill
- Dry treadmill
- Massage therapy
- Therapeutic ultrasound
- Superficial heating and cooling of affected areas
- Electrical stimulation of muscles or acupuncture points
- Extra corporeal shock wave treatment
- Cold lasers
- Assistive devices, such as slings, carts, balance boards, Zuni and Hoyer lifts

Therapeutic exercises can include the following:

- Doggie dancing
- Wheelbarrowing
- Backpacks
- Weights
- Cavalettis
- Physiorolls/physioballs
- Stairs
- Sit-to-stand exercises

Veterinarian's Role

A veterinarian must make the initial diagnosis. If referring, the veterinarian must give the referral to a physical therapy center before a number of physical therapy treatments can begin (although some, such as Reiki, are in a legal gray area and usually can be performed without a referral). If the veterinarian is part of the physical therapy group, this is easy. If the veterinarian is certified in physical therapy, he or she may perform the initial examination and design the therapy program as well. A veterinarian may also be the person performing acupuncture and chiropractic.

Technician's Role

Regardless of the initial veterinary participation, technicians are the main workforce in a physical therapy setting. They are the ones who do the measurements and apply many of the physical procedures. Technicians are very important for the proper assessment of the patient and in modifying a program if it seems to be too difficult for the patient.

Where to Learn How

The following organizations provide training for veterinary rehabilitation for veterinary technicians in the US

Animal Rehab Institute
2457 C Road
Loxahatchee, FL 33470
https://animalrehabinstitute.com/
Certified Equine Rehabilitation Assistant (CERA) for Registered Veterinary Technicians

Canine Rehabilitation Institute
2137 S. Eastgate Avenue
Springfield, MO 65809
https://www.caninerehabinstitute.com
(For veterinary technician graduates of a 2-year veterinary technology program, they award a
  Canine Rehabilitation Veterinary Nurses certificate [CCRVN]; for non-credentialed veterinary
  technicians, it awards a Canine Rehabilitation Assistant certificate [CCRA]; for veterinarians
  and physical therapists, the institute awards a CCRT certificate)

Chi University
9650 W Hwy 318
Reddick, FL 32686
(800) 860-1543
https://chiu.edu/courses/vtec110_usa
register@chiu.edu
(Awards a Certification in Certified Canine Rehab Veterinary Technician—CCRVT)

Healing Oasis Wellness Center
2555 Wisconsin St.
Sturtevant, WI 53177-1825
US Toll Free: 866-203-7584
www.healingoasis.edu
(Awards a Certification in Veterinary Massage and Rehabilitation Therapy—VMRT)

The University of Tennessee
College of Veterinary Medicine
2407 River Drive
Knoxville, TN 37996
https://www.u-tenn.org/ccrp/
(Awards a CCRP certificate for canine rehabilitation, and a CERP certificate for equine rehabilitation. The labs are available worldwide, and classes are available online)

Summary

What can a technician do?

1) Certification is available for technicians
2) Additional certification is available from NAVA after certification and additional experience
3) Certified technicians can administer treatments authorized by veterinarians
4) Certified technicians can join with veterinarians to help design a rehabilitation program

Cold Laser Therapy (Also Called Photobiomodulation, Low-Level Laser Therapy, LLLT, and Therapeutic Laser)

Definition

A laser beam is a coherent light (light that stays in a tightly focused narrow beam with waves that are all in the same phase and usually all of the same color). In contrast, the average light beam from the sun or a flashlight spreads out and has many different colors of the spectrum. A cold laser is a low-level laser that does not cut and does not burn when it touches skin briefly. Cold lasers are used to help heal tissues.

Purpose

Cold lasers are used primarily for wound healing, pain (especially arthritic pain), and tendon and ligament injuries. Originally, they were used primarily by equine veterinarians, but their use for small animals has grown. Their acceptance was originally greater among holistic veterinarians, but now they are being increasingly used in small animal practices in general.

History

Laser (Light Amplification by Stimulated Emission of Radiation) light was conceived and named in 1957 by Gordon Gould, a graduate student at Columbia University. He is usually credited as the inventor, although there is some controversy over this.

In 1964, Andre Mester began experimenting with cold lasers at Semmelweis University in Budapest, Hungary. His initial thought was to prove that exposure to a cold laser could lead to skin cancer (as UV light from the sun does). He shaved mice to expose them to the laser. Instead, the mice treated with the laser grew hair thicker and faster than nontreated mice. He studied the cold laser's ability to treat other problems and, in 1968, found that indolent diabetic ulcers would heal when treated with cold lasers.

Cold laser therapy has been used for an increasing number of purposes in humans. They have been used to help heal cochlear hair cells and decrease deafness, help treat fungal infections by their actions on neutrophils, help periodontitis, help traumatic brain injury, increase muscle performance, and reduce muscle damage after exercise (Hamblin, 2016). They have been shown to accelerate deep foot ulcer healing in human patients with ulcers that had been unresponsive to standard-of-care therapy (Johnson et al., 2019). They help with oral mucositis in cancer patients undergoing radiation therapy.

Description

A cold laser light beam is:

- Coherent light
- Monochromatic (all one color, measured as a wavelength in nanometers, or nm)
- Red or near-infrared wavelength (usually between 635 and 970 nm)
- Low power (1–500 milliwatts—mW)
- Polarized

Lasers come in various wavelengths and different power levels. They may come with a single diode (like a lightbulb) or many diodes. Lasers are classed by their power, from Class 1 (weakest, like in a laser printer) to Class 4 (strongest).

A cold laser may be harmful if viewed directly, and protective eyewear must be worn by the operator and the patient. It must be equipped with a safety interlock. Therapeutic cold lasers are usually Class 4, although there are still a number of Class 3 lasers being sold and used.

Class 4 lasers can burn the skin if left in one site for a period of time. So when administering treatment, they are usually moved back and forth over an area. Class 3b lasers may be left over an area for longer periods of time.

Cold lasers used for healing use red or infrared laser light, generally between 630 and 970 nm wavelength, at a power from 10 to 500 mW. A 500-mW laser emits light 100 times faster than a 5-mW and 10 times faster than a 50-mW laser. The more power, the faster the total treatment dose gets delivered. However, higher power does not mean greater penetration of the skin—that is determined by the wavelength. The higher the wavelength, the deeper the penetration. The power depends partly on how many light-emitting units (diodes) are in the equipment. More diodes allow one to treat a wider area at one time, and deliver more laser light at a time.

A high-power laser with many diodes and low power is still a cold laser. A high-power laser with a single diode with 7,500 mW of power is generally not a cold laser.

Do not confuse Laser therapy with LED therapy. LED therapy is a type of phototherapy using red (and sometimes blue) LED lights, which are used to treat some skin conditions in humans. They have no effect on pain, arthritis, tendonitis, etc.

Doses of laser therapies are measured as Joules (J) per square centimeter of skin (or J/cm^2). The more power a therapeutic laser has, the higher the amount of Joules that are delivered per second. One reason Class 4 lasers are more popular than Class 3b is that it takes a lot less time to deliver the calculated dose in a therapy session.

The 904-nm sized wavelength, which is near-infrared, penetrates the skin the deepest and has the biggest general healing effect. The farther the penetration, the deeper the structures that are affected and the more profound the effect on healing. This wavelength can penetrate from 3 to 4 cm. With shorter wavelengths, most of the energy is absorbed close to the skin.

The best (and most expensive) therapeutic lasers have ways to modulate their power. The lifespan of the average high-quality laser unit is usually 10–12 years.

The effects of laser treatment include the following (Hochman, 2018; Lubart et al., 2005; Miller, 2017; Millis and Bergh, 2023; Prindeze et al., 2012):

- Improved collagen formation and decreased scar formation
- Increased ATP production
- Vasodilation, resulting in increased blood flow to an area
- Decreased swelling from doubled size of lymphatic ducts, from reestablishment of the lymphatic system, and from ridding the area of protein breakdown products
- Faster wound healing (including wounds that are indolent or not healing at all and proud flesh in horses)
- Pain relief by stimulation of endorphins and enkephalins

Laser light stimulates cytochrome c oxidase, the terminal enzyme of the mitochondrial respiratory chain. Cytochrome c oxidase is thus considered to be the photoacceptor. This generates a signal to the nucleus regarding the functional state of the mitochondria (Karu, 2008). The results include a release of growth factors and proliferation of multiple cells. The action is mainly through the activation of the mitochondrial respiratory chain and the initiation of cellular signaling (Shamloo et al., 2023).

The electron transport chain of mitochondria is sensitive to red and near-infrared light. When mitochondria are stimulated by light in these wavelengths, ATP production is increased, and there is a transient increase in reactive oxygen molecules (Ferraresi et al., 2015). The reactive molecules participate in redox (reduction/oxidation) signaling, which is involved in cellular homeostasis, including control of growth and proliferation. (Gene therapy research uses ultraviolet lasers to stimulate cells by redox mechanisms.) It is interesting that mitochondria have this ability, considering the theory that they may have been bacteria that became a part of cells eons ago. Perhaps they were originally photosynthetic and have retained part of the photosynthetic pathway.

It is recommended that laser therapy not be used on pregnant animals or on cancerous lesions, and not near the eyes or brain.

Treatment using a Class 4 laser usually takes 5–10 minutes, depending on the size of the area being treated and whether acupuncture points are being stimulated (at 1–2 minutes per point).

Cold laser therapy is considered to be safe, with very few contraindications. One should never look directly at the laser light and always wear protective eyewear specifically designed for laser light protection. Sunglasses do not work and can even increase eye damage. Pets should also wear eye protection (called "Doggles").

Veterinarian's Role

Class 3b and higher lasers are medical devices, so their use must be prescribed by veterinarians only, after a veterinary diagnosis.

Technician's Role

Technicians are usually the ones who administer the laser therapy itself. The job of the technician in the case of lasers also includes explaining their usefulness to the public. This can be critical because many people associate lasers with surgery and other Class 4 cutting laser uses.

Where to Learn How

There are no formal classes in laser therapy. Information and some training are usually supplied by the laser companies themselves and can be supplemented by talks at veterinary conferences and articles in technician journals.

Summary

What can a technician do?

1) Technicians can apply laser therapy after a treatment program has been designed for a veterinarian.
2) Technicians can ensure that as many safety goggles and doggles that are needed, are always available, clean, and always used.
3) Technicians can ensure that equipment is working, clean, and repaired when needed.
4) Technicians can ensure that goggles/doggles are immediately replaced when necessary.

Hydrotherapy

Definition

Canine hydrotherapy, also known as water therapy, consists of exercising in an aquatic environment, aimed at improving function in limbs during rehabilitation. Thus, it can be used for recovery from surgery, or from a wide range of injuries, and to help senior dogs improve mobility, regain some muscle, improve their balance, and improve their quality of life. It can also be used for weight loss. Hydrotherapy has been used for humans since before the Roman Empire, but hydrotherapy for animals was first used in the horse-racing industry, then in the dog-racing industry, and finally for pet dogs.

For dogs, it involves swimming (pool therapy) or walking in water to improve mobility, strengthen muscles, and aid in healing. The buoyancy of a body in water reduces stress on joints and helps decrease joint pain, especially when combined with warm water (for dogs) or cold water (for horses). It is one part of a complete physical therapy program, that can include herbs, drugs, massage therapy, and targeted exercise, among other methods.

Both pools and underwater treadmills are usually seen in a separate canine physical therapy facility. In a veterinary practice, you will usually encounter only the underwater treadmill.

Description

When dogs are in water, they become buoyant, reducing the weight they have to carry. This minimizes discomfort and helps them to move their legs through an increased range of motion. Water also provides resistance, requiring muscles to work harder and promoting strength-building at an accelerated pace. Additionally, hydrotherapy is typically conducted in warm water, helping dogs relax and preventing muscle spasms.

Pool-based hydrotherapy is an option that can be used when weight-bearing is painful for the dog or in cases of arthritis in more than one joint, or throughout the whole back. Swimming in a pool provides a cardiovascular workout as well as working muscles in general and can help increase stamina and endurance in athletic dogs. It offers a less concussive impact on joints compared to land-based exercises. It can be especially helpful for dogs with front leg problems, since the range of motion for the front legs is greater than seen when the dog is walking. The fee charged for pool-based hydrotherapy is usually less than the fee for an underwater treadmill. However, it is not possible to adjust buoyancy, and it is very difficult to regulate the amount of effort or exercise a dog is getting, so when it is important for the amount and type of exercise be more specific, an underwater treadmill is usually preferred.

During pool sessions, dogs must be closely supervised. Flotation or buoyancy jackets must be used to ensure their safety. A vigorous pool session using controlled fetch games and floating toys can be used to increase aerobic capacity and stamina for canine athletes, and increase calories burned when used for weight loss.

The other commonly used hydrotherapy for dogs is an underwater treadmill. An underwater treadmill resembles a treadmill in a very large fish tank. Dogs walk on the treadmill, and the tank is gradually filled with water. The depth can be adjusted to increase or decrease buoyancy, depending on how much pressure is desired on the legs. If the main objective is to increase muscle mass, it might only cover the legs to provide resistance without any buoyancy.

The speed of the treadmill can be varied, from very slow for dogs who are very painful, to faster as they improve from the therapy. In the more expensive versions, the treadmill can be inclined, to increase the effort the dog must make and so help build muscle.

Dogs often need a period of adjustment to become comfortable with the treadmill. Stigall et al. have published a protocol to help them do that, which worked well in seven out of eight dogs it was tested on (Stigall et al., 2022).

Underwater treadmills can be used to treat:

Neurological problems including those that results from nerve injuries and intervertebral disc disease
Anterior Cruciate Ligament (ACL) injuries (especially right after surgery)
Hip dysplasia
Elbow dysplasia
Osteoarthritis
Cushing's disease (to help the muscle atrophy associated with it)
Obesity (making exercise easier and less painful by decreasing pressure on the joints)

Underwater treadmills are not perfect for canine athletes. Muscle mass can increase to normal if it has been lost because the dog was recovering from an injury. But it cannot hypertrophy using the underwater treadmill, so other means must be used to increase muscle strength.

Understanding the limitations: While hydrotherapy has proven efficacy in many cases, it is important to recognize that it is just one component of a comprehensive rehabilitation program. Rehabilitation is not a one-size-fits-all approach, and hydrotherapy should be tailored to the specific needs of each dog. Over-reliance on underwater treadmills, for example, may not promote progressive loading or address underlying gait abnormalities. A holistic approach that includes manual therapy, therapeutic exercise, massage, and other modalities is crucial for successful rehabilitation.

It is crucial to consider the dog's comfort, fearfulness, and ability to move freely in the water. Flotation devices like life jackets can provide additional support and confidence to dogs during pool therapy sessions.

However, it's important to acknowledge that hydrotherapy is not a one-size-fits-all solution. While it can be a valuable tool in a dog's treatment plan, it should be approached with caution and as part of a comprehensive program that addresses the specific needs of each individual dog.

Not all dogs are comfortable with swimming or water sports, and it's important not to force them into hydrotherapy if they exhibit anxiety or fear. Seeking professional guidance can help teach dogs to feel more at ease in the water. Additionally, providing medical hydrotherapy at home is not advised, especially for dogs with underlying medical conditions. Professional hydrotherapy centers equipped with underwater treadmills and supervised by veterinary rehabilitation teams offer the best environment for safe and effective hydrotherapy.

Hydrotherapy is contraindicated for dogs with intervertebral disc disease, since movements associated with water-based exercises and swimming can place excess stress on the discs and possibly cause additional damage. Dogs with advanced cardiac disease can also have problems if the sessions are too aerobically taxing.

The underwater treadmill does not support progressive overloading beyond returning an under-used muscle to its original strength. So, although it is useful for canine athletes to increase aerobic capacity, other methods must be used to increase muscle strength. Constant repetition of the same gait in a restricted space can perpetuate and worsen any existing abnormal gait instead of improving it. So, any abnormal gaits or movement dysfunctions must be addressed before using an underwater treadmill to increase aerobic capacity and endurance.

Brachycephalic dogs can also have difficulties with underwater treadmills because their airway can be easily compromised.

Before a pool or treadmill session, the technician should:

Inspect the dog to make sure it is reasonably clean. If they have muddy paws, mud should be washed off before they enter a pool or treadmill.

Take the dog out to urinate or defecate. (The technician can also advise the owners that it would be good to take their dog for a walk before coming in for a hydrotherapy session. If a dog defecates in the pool or treadmill, there might be an extra fee charged.)

During the session:

Sometimes in the first session a dog might refuse to move forward or will bound forward all at once when the treadmill starts to move. The technician must be prepared to encourage a dog, calm it down, or retrieve it if it tries to go over the side. So it is imperative that the technician be there by the dog's side at the beginning of each session. (See also Stigall's paper describing a method of accommodating dogs to underwater treadmills–Stigall et al., 2022.)

If it is a short session, the technician should stay by the dog throughout the session. If it is a long session, the technician can do other things but should keep the treadmill within eyesight.

After the session:

Dry the dog well, first with a towel, and then put them in a cage with a cage dryer. Keep a close eye on them so they do not get overheated, and remove them as soon as their coat is dry.

Veterinarian's Role

The veterinarian will make the diagnosis of the problem that needs treatment. They will identify the primary part of the body that needs treatment, and the ideal outcome (e.g., repair an injury, increase muscle mass, treat lameness). If they are Board Certified in Sports Medicine and Rehabilitation, they will develop a complete treatment plan for the hydrotherapy part of rehabilitation, with specific treatment methods including the length of time for each session and specifications for underwater treadmill sessions. The veterinarian must refer a patient to a rehabilitation center before a technician associated with such a center can begin treatment.

Technician's Role

A technician who is certified in canine rehabilitation will actively contribute to the hydrotherapy treatment plan and to any subsequent changes. Regardless of certification, the technician is the main person who will be monitoring the dog and running the equipment. They will also be evaluating the dog's progress or lack of it and can recommend increasing or decreasing buoyancy or speed of the treadmill. In most states, a technician who is certified in rehab can also open a rehab center with hydrotherapy equipment available. State law usually requires that a veterinarian refer a patient to the center, so check with your state or province before making plans to open your own center.

Where to Learn How

The rehabilitation certification courses listed under the Rehabilitation section at the beginning of this chapter include information on hydrotherapy.

Summary

What can a technician do?

1) Technicians can apply hydrotherapy or underwater treadmill therapy after a treatment program has been designed by a veterinarian.
2) A technician can ensure equipment is in working order, dog life vests are available and do not need repairing or replacement.
3) If a technician is certified in rehabilitation, they can take a more active part in designing the specific hydrotherapy program.
4) If a technician is certified in rehabilitation, in most areas, they can open their own hydrotherapy center. (Check with local laws to make sure you can do this.)

targeted Pulsating Electromagnetic Field Therapy (tPEMFT)

Definition

Magnetic therapy may be static (where the magnetic field is stationary) or pulsating (a field in motion). PEMFT (pulsating electromagnetic field therapy, also known as pulsed signal therapy or PST) is used for pain and to speed healing (including nonhealing fractures).

Purpose

Most commonly, pulsating magnetic field therapy is used to decrease inflammation, restore circulation, speed healing, restore damaged nerves, and decrease pain. For humans, the FDA also recently approved a device for clinical depression. It is sometimes referred to as an NPAID (non-pharmaceutical anti-inflammatory device).

History

PEMFT is a type of electrotherapy, consisting of magnetic fields delivered by an electric carrier wave, through an antenna on the device. It has been around since the 1930's, when a diathermy machine which was designed for deep heat treatment was modified to deliver an electromagnetic field that did not generate heat. The result worked even better than the deep heat treatment for pain reduction and wound healing.

The FDA granted its first approval for the use of a PEMFT device for humans in 1979, to treat fractures that had failed to heal after 6 months of treatment. By varying the frequency and amplitude of the carrier wave, the general effects of PEMFT can be modified so it enhances specific biological effects, giving even better medical results. This type of PEMFT is called a targeted PEMF, or tPEMF. That is the type currently in common use in human and animal medicine.

Between 1994 and 1999, it approved tPEMFT devices specifically to treat fractures in the human lumbar spine. tPEMFT devices can be modified by changing the shape and strength of the electromagnetic waveforms and the size and shape of the antennas used. Treatments can be modified by changing treatment duration and frequency. As research found the ways in which the devices worked, and the parameters that would get various results, the FDA approved additional advices that had other effects. Currently, there are devices for humans that are approved for healing failed union fractures in the cervical spine, to stimulate slow-healing wounds such as pressure sores to heal faster, to relieve pain and edema, and to treat depression. A device called the Assisi Loop is now available for use in dogs and cats, as well as tPEMFT pads.

Meanwhile, about 30 years of research on magnetic therapy totaling over 200 referenced papers, a large number of which included PEMF, had been done in Eastern European countries. The countries included Germany, Russia, Ukraine, Bulgaria, Czech Republic, and Hungary, as well as others. Those results were published in English in 1998 (Jerabeck and Pawluk, 1998) and the publication is still available on the co-author's website as well as on Amazon.

The detailed technical research, shows scientific evidence for promising benefits from the use of PEMFT for a very wide range of applications including peripheral vascular disease, lung disease, gastrointestinal disease, neurological disease, rheumatic disease, pediatrics, dermatology, surgery, gynecology, oral medicine, otorhinolaryngology, ophthalmology, immunity, inflammation, reproduction, and tumors, based on those 200 referenced scientific papers involving both human and animal studies (Jerabeck and Pawluk, 1998).

In Australia, it has been used for arthritis (decreased pain and improved mobility), osteoporosis, chronic fatigue syndrome (increased energy, decreased pain, more restful sleep), migraines, sleep disorders, psoriasis, and acne (but only after prolonged treatment).

Currently, clinical experience and a few published studies support its use as an adjunct for bone healing, to decrease pain and inflammation, osteoarthritis, faster recovery from surgery, improve proprioception after spinal decompression surgery, faster wound healing (both surgical wounds and other problems like pressure sores), decreased pain, inflammation, and edema after surgery, mood and behavioral disorders, Alzheimer's canine cognitive disease, animal anxiety, chronic pain.

Description

A pulsating magnetic field is formed by a pulsing current flowing through a wire coil, creating a pulsating magnetic field around the wire. (A magnetic field is formed at right angles to the flow of electricity; this is how electromagnets work.) As the number of coils of wire increases, and as the current flow increases, the magnetic field gets stronger. The magnetic field penetrates the whole body unlike laser treatments, which only penetrate up to 2 in.

After tissue injury (surgical or traumatic), a complex inflammatory cascade occurs to avoid infection, enhance tissue remodeling, and start tissue healing. At the same time, an anti-inflammatory cascade is initiated, decreasing inflammation, increasing cGMP, and releasing growth factors to bolster vascularization, tissue regeneration, and remodeling.

Upon stimulation with tPEMFT, intracellular Ca^{++} is released. The calcium ion binds to calmodulin, causing a number of signaling pathways related to inflammation, vascular tone, and others (Cadossi et al., 2020). The most significant is the production of NO, which most know about for its function as a vasodilator in the heart. NO reduces programmed cell death, decreases inflammation, and enhances vasodilation (Bragin et al., 2014; Pena-Philippides et al., 2014; Rasouli et al., 2012; Rohde et al., 2010, 2015), which helps decrease edema and decrease the harmful effects of prolonged inflammation. In addition, NO can stimulate the immune system and directly influence the nervous system (and other places), and help with bone repair (Bodamyali et al., 1998; Petecchia et al., 2015; Tsai et al., 2009).

Benefits that are seen include the following:

- Increased blood supply
- Revascularization of a site
- Increased oxygenation of a site
- Improved immune function
- Decreased swelling
- Faster wound healing (including luxations)
- Healing of nonunion fractures
- Pain relief (in humans, this is almost instant, with onset of the field).

Initial effects last for 6–8 hours. For chronic conditions, treatment may have to continue for 6–8 weeks for maximum benefit. No serious side effects have been reported. In some human studies, there have been reports of dizziness or increased pain in a few people. PEMFT should not be used in pregnant animals, animals with pacemakers, or during acute flare-ups of autoimmune disease (Gaynor et al., 2018). There is some controversy regarding its use with cancer patients.

Results of using PEMFT therapy include decreased inflammation, increased blood flow, decreased pain, and increased circulation. Healing of nonunion fractures has been attributed in part to increased ion flow or increased availability of calcium to a fracture site.

Veterinarian's Role

This equipment is available to veterinarians only, and the veterinarian is the one who will diagnose the problem and recommend PEMFT.

Technician's Role

The technician is helpful in making sure the animal stays within the coil (although once a pet figures out it makes him feel good, most just stay there). Technicians are often the ones who administer the therapy, if given at the hospital. An informed technician can also discuss the treatment with owners and help answer their questions. The technicians can also help describe how to use any device that the veterinarian has prescribed for a patient.

Where to Learn How

No special knowledge is needed to apply tPEMFT devices. The device is placed on, around, or under the animal, according to its design and instructions.

Summary

What can a technician do?

1) After a diagnosis and recommendation for tPEMFT therapy, if it is to be applied in-house, the technician can apply the device and supervise the animal to make sure the device stays in place (if it is a loop, blanket, or neck wrap) during the time of administration.
2) If a tPEMFT device has been rented or sold to an owner to take home, the technician can explain its use and help answer general questions about the device itself.

Hospice Care

Definition

Hospice care is the decision to relieve pain and suffering but not to unnecessarily prolong the life of a dying being. Hospice care also supports the caregiver, making sure he or she is able to cope with the process of easing their loved one's transition. Although hospice care is equally available for conventional and holistic veterinarians, more information is generally available at holistic veterinary meetings and in holistic veterinary journals. The subject is not fully covered in textbooks for technicians and nurses. In the human medicine field, nurses are usually the primary medical personnel involved in administering hospice care to both patient and caregiver, as are technicians and nurses in veterinary hospice care. Hence its inclusion here.

Purpose

Hospice care is designed to ease the transition of a pet at the end of its life. This involves both the adequate use of painkillers as well as using palliative care instead of heroic measures. In addition, hospice involves grief therapy for owners, who may be surprised at the intensity of their grief after the pet has died.

History

The term *hospice* originally meant a place for weary or ill medieval travelers who were on a long journey to rest. The modern meaning was coined by Dame Cicely Saunders. Dame Saunders introduced the idea to the United States in 1963 at a lecture at Yale University. She included before and after pictures of patients, showing dramatic effects of palliative care (treatments designed to relieve them of symptoms, but not to try to cure their terminal disease).

Dame Cicely Saunders founded the first modern hospice in London (St. Christopher's Hospice) in 1967. She believed that doctors desert the dying, and that their role instead should be as the head of a support team. She recognized the physical, social, emotional, and spiritual dimensions of pain and distress for patients and believed that what they need most is care and compassion at the end of life. She gained this insight initially as a nurse and decided she could make a bigger impact as a physician, graduating from medical school in 1958 (Richmond, 2005).

In 1969 in the United States, the book *On Death and Dying,* by Dr. Elisabeth Kubler-Ross, was published. It described the five stages of grief that many terminally ill people go through, promoted the idea of death with dignity, and made a plea for home care instead of institutionalized care.

In 1984, hospice accreditation was begun. In 1986, hospice care was made a permanent Medicare benefit, and in 1991, it became a part of veterans' benefits.

For animals, once they were no longer viewed as property and instead seen as companions, owners began looking at the possibility of hospice care for their pets. The hospice movement for animals has been a much more recent phenomenon.

Description

Humans are eligible for hospice care when it is estimated that they have no longer than 6 months to live. The goal is comfort, not cure. The disease may still be treated but with the purpose of making the patient comfortable, pain-free, and with a minimum of side effects. This means that there will be no heroic measures taken. Hospice care may be at home or in a medical facility. Part of hospice care for humans is care for the caretakers, including counseling and group sessions.

Very few facilities offer hospice care for animals, so essentially all hospice care is given at home. When it is recognized that an animal has a terminal disease, everything is done to make the animal comfortable, but treatments are not forced on it. If the animal had originally been force-fed, this is stopped. Water is offered, but not forced. Subcutaneous fluids may or may not be continued, depending on the animal's acceptance and the fluid's role in its feelings of well-being. Painkillers are always appropriate. Acupuncture may be used for comfort and to ease pain. Vomiting and diarrhea may be controlled by drugs.

It is normal for many dying animals to stop eating, and then to stop drinking. From human hospice studies, we know that dehydration is not painful (Byock, 1995). Therefore, with hospice care, it is important to support the owners if they decide not to force food or water on a patient that declines to eat or drink.

Sometimes hospice care is inappropriate. Excessive, uncontrollable pain is not part of "hospice." Inability to breathe or inadequate oxygen supply is also not appropriate. For humans, we can more easily administer oxygen through respirators, and morphine controls the feeling of strangulation. It is difficult to quantify this for animals, and they may reject efforts to supply them with oxygen. If the animal is uncomfortable, and if there is no way to make the pet comfortable, then euthanasia should be considered.

Support of caregivers can be difficult. If they have made a choice of hospice care, then they should not be made to feel guilty. They should be helped in their decision to make their pet feel as comfortable as possible. There are websites that help caregivers process these feelings. There are also websites and hotlines to help them deal with their grief after a pet has died (See Webliography).

Veterinarian's Role

Most veterinarians feel uncomfortable with the idea of hospice care. We have been trained to consider euthanasia to be the kindest thing to do. However, if an animal is not suffering, but just fading away, the veterinarian can help by providing needed medications and stopping medication that adds to side effects.

Technician's Role

The technician can play a major role in hospice care. Technicians can go to a client's house to help them administer medications or fluids. They can help a client determine whether an animal is comfortable or uncomfortable.

They can help owners with information about websites and books appropriate to the subject. The attitude of the staff toward a pet owner can make a big difference in the quality of the experience for the pet and the owner.

Where to Learn How

Nikki Hospice Foundation for Pets
Rosemoor House
400 New Bedford Drive,
Vallejo, CA 94591
https://www.pethospice.org/
(Read their guidelines on veterinary hospice care at https://www.pethospice.org/HOSPICE%
   20FRAME.htm. This also includes a link to AVMA's guide for veterinary hospice care.)

Spirits in Transition
https://www.spiritsintransition.org/

Summary

What can technicians do?

1) Help with at-home or in-hospital end-of-life care, such as administering fluids or painkillers.
2) Familiarize yourself with local and online help for clients, especially regarding grief therapy.
3) Be sure all owners receive a sympathy card when their pet dies.
4) Make a charitable contribution to research and education in holistic veterinary medicine in memory of each pet that dies. The American Holistic Veterinary Medical Association has a program whereby your practice can make such a donation. Each donation is in the name of the pet and its owner and often is a source of comfort for the owners. If your practice does not do this, familiarize yourself with this program and talk to your veterinarian about implementing it, or something similar.

References

Bodamyali, T., et al. 1998. Pulsed electromagnetic fields simultaneously induce osteogenesis and upregulate transcription of bone morphogenetic proteins 2 and 4 in rat osteoblasts in vitro. *Biochem Biophys Res Commun* 250:458–461.

Bragin, D.E., et al. 2014. Increases in microvascular perfusion and tissue oxygenation via pulsed electromagnetic fields in the healthy rat brain. *J Neurosurg* 122:1–9.

Byock I.R. 1995. Patient refusal of nutrition and hydration: walking the ever-finer line. *Am J Hosp Palliat Care* 12:8–13. Accessed 2/20/2010 at https://www.dyingwell.com/prnh.htm.

Cadossi, R., et al. (2020). Pulsed electromagnetic field stimulation of bone healing and joint preservation: cellular mechanisms of skeletal response. *J Am Acad Orthop Surg Glob Res Rev* 4 (5): e19.00155.

Ferraresi, C., et al. 2015. Low-level laser (light) therapy increases mitochondrial membrane potential and ATP synthesis in C2C12 myotubes with a peak response at 3–6 h. *Photochem Photobiol* 91(2):411–416.

Gaynor, J.S., et al. 2018. Veterinary applications of pulsed electromagnetic field therapy. *Res Vet Sci* 119:1–8. doi: 10.1016/j.rvsc.2018.05.005. Epub 2018 May 7. PMID: 29775839.

Hamblin, M.R. 2016. Photobiomodulation or low-level laser therapy. *J Biophotonics* 9(11–12):1122–1124.

Hochman, L. 2018. Photobiomodulation therapy in veterinary medicine: a review. *Top Companion Anim Med* 33(3):83–88.

Jerabeck, J. and Pawluk, W. 1998. *Magnetic Therapy in Eastern Europe: A Review of 30 Years of Research*. Baltimore, MD: W. Pawluk.

Johnson, M., et al. 2019. Erbium: yttrium aluminum garnet laser accelerates healing in indolent diabetic foot ulcers. *J Foot Ankle Surg* 58:1077–1080.

Karu, T.I. 2008. Mitochondrial signaling in mammalian cells activated by red and near-IR radiation. *Photochem Photobiol* 84:1091–1099.

Lubart, R, et al. 2005. Low-energy laser irradiation promotes cellular redox activity. *Photomed Laser Surg* 23:3–9.

Miller, L.A. 2017. Musculoskeletal disorders and osteoarthritis. In: Reigel, R.J. and Godbold, J.C. Jr., eds. *Laser Therapy in Veterinary Medicine: Photobiomodulation*. Ames, IA: Wiley:132–149.

Millis, D.L. and Bergh, A. 2023. A systematic literature review of complementary and alternative veterinary medicine: laser therapy. *Animals (Basel)* 13(4):667. doi: 10.3390/ani13040667. PMID: 36830454; PMCID: PMC9951699.

Pena-Philippides, J.C., et al. 2014. Effect of pulsed electromagnetic field (PEMF) on infarct size and inflammation after cerebral ischemia in mice. *Transl Stroke Res* 5:491–500.

Petecchia, L., et al. 2015. Electro-magnetic field promotes osteogenic differentiation of BMhMSCs through a selective action on Ca^{2+}-related mechanisms. *Sci Rep* 5, 13856.

Prindeze, N.J., et al. 2012. Mechanisms of action for light therapy: a review of molecular interactions. *Exp Biol Med* 237:1241–1248.

Rasouli, J., et al. 2012. Attenuation of interleukin-1beta by pulsed electromagnetic fields after traumatic brain injury. *Neurosci Lett* 519:4–8.

Richmond, C. 2005. Dame Cicely Saunders, founder of the modern hospice movement. *Br Med J* 331:7509.

Rohde, C., et al. 2010. Effects of pulsed electromagnetic fields on interleukin-1 beta and postoperative pain: a double-blind, placebo-controlled, pilot study in breast reduction patients. *Plast Reconstr Surg* 125:1620–1629.

Rohde, C.H., et al. 2015. Pulsed electromagnetic fields reduce postoperative interleukin-1beta, pain, and inflammation: a double-blind, placebo-controlled study in TRAM flap breast reconstruction patients. *Plast Reconstr Surg* 135:808e–817e.

Shamloo, S, et al. 2023. The anti-inflammatory effects of photobiomodulation are mediated by cytokines: Evidence from a mouse model of inflammation. *Front Neurosci* 17:1150156.

Stigall, A.R., et al. 2022. A Formalized Method to Acclimate Dogs to Voluntary Treadmill Locomotion at Various Speeds and Inclines. *Animals (Basel)* 12(5):567.

Tsai, M.T., et al. 2009. Modulation of osteogenesis in human mesenchymal stem cells by specific pulsed electromagnetic field stimulation. *J Orthop Res* 27:1169–1174.

Bibliography

Cold Laser Therapy

Oshiro, T. 1988. *Low Level Laser Therapy*. Avon, UK: Wiley, Bush Press.

Tuner, J. and Hode, L. 2007. *The Laser Therapy Handbook*. Grangesberg, Sweden: Prima Books.

Al-Watban, F.A.H. and Andres, B.L. 2000. Laser photons and pharmacological treatments in wound healing. *Laser Ther.* 12, Special Millenium Edition.

Enwemmeka, C.S. and Reddy, G.K. 2000. The biological effects of laser therapy and other physical modalities on connective tissue repair processes. *Laser Ther* 12, Special Millenium Edition.

Gao, X. and Xing, D. 2009. Molecular mechanisms of cell proliferation induced by low power laser irradiation. *J Biomed Sci* 16(1):4.

Lopez, Q. 2009. Treatment of large skin necrosis following a modified avelar abdominoplasty with the Erchonia EML 635 nm laser and platelet-rich plasma. *Am J Cosmetic Surg* 26(1):29.

Reddy, G.K., et al. 1998. Laser photostimulation of collagen production in healing rabbit *Achilles tendons*. *Lasers Surg Med* 22(5):281–287.

Silveira, P.C., et al. 2009. Evaluation of mitochondrial respiratory chain activity in muscle healing by low-level laser therapy. *J Photochem Photobiol B* 95(2):89–92.

Tafur, J. and Mills, P.J. 2008. Low-intensity light therapy: Exploring the role of redox mechanisms. *Photomed Laser Surg* 26(4):323–328.

Wong, E., et al. 1995. Successful management of female office workers with "repetitive stress injury" or "carpal tunnel syndrome" by a new treatment modality—application of low level laser. *Int J Clin Pharmacol Ther* 33(4).

Hospice

Bittell, E. 2008. Veterinary hospice care. *J Am Vet Med Assoc* 27(2):25–28.

Bockstahler, B. 2004. *Essential Facts of Physiotherapy in Dogs & Cats—Rehabilitation and Pain Management: A Reference Guide with DVD*. Babenhausen, Germany: BE VetVerlag.

Flaim, D. 2008. A natural transition. *Dog Fancy Magazine* 39(7):21.

Millis, D., et al. 2004. *Canine Rehabilitation and Physical Therapy*. Philadelphia: Saunders.

Rivera, M. 2001. *Using Dogs to Help Humans in Hospice Care*. Herndon, VA: Lantern Books.

Stubbs, N.C. and Clayton, H.M. 2008. *Activate Your Horse's Core*. Mason, MI: Sport Horse Publications.

Pulsed Magnetic Field Therapy

Bassett, C.A., et al. 1982. Pulsing electromagnetic field treatment in ununited fractures and failed arthrodeses. *JAMA* 247(5):623–628.

Bessmel'tsev, S.S., et al. 2001. The *in vitro* effect of constant and pulsating magnetic field on immunocompetent blood cells of hematologic patients. *Vopr Onkol* 47(1):59–65.

Kroeling, P., et al. 2009. Electrotherapy for neck pain. *Cochrane Database Syst Rev* (4):CD004251.

May, K. 1992. Use of pulsating magnetic therapy in birds. *J Assoc Avian Vet* 6(3):146.

Mertl, T., et al. 2006. Regenerative effects of pulsed magnetic field on injured peripheral nerves. *Altern Ther Health Med* 12(5):42–49.

Morrow, T. 2009. Treating depression with a pulsating magnetic field. *Manag Care* 18(4):47–48.

Webliography

Cold Laser Therapy

Bioflex
https://bioflexlaser.com/
Cold laser company that sells lasers for both personal and professional use.
Cold Lasers.org
https://www.coldlasers.org/
A company that is a distributor of cold lasers. They stock many brands and will help a practice choose the one that is best for them. They also have a book list and cold laser articles.

Erchonia Laser Healthcare
https://www.erchonia.com/
Manufacturer of cold lasers. This page includes research articles on laser therapy.

Respond Systems Incorporated
https://respondsystems.com/laser/laser-how-it-works/
FAQs about medical lasers on the website of Respond Systems, which makes Class 3 and 4 medical lasers for large and small animals. They also make PEMFT systems for dogs and horses.

Two websites with inexpensive portable veterinary lasers developed and sold by Daniel Kamen, DC. Plain English FAQs about both: Vetrolaser (Class 3b laser) and Vetro4 (Class 4 laser)
https://www.vetrolaser.com/ and https://www.vetrolaser4.com/

Hospice

Angels Gate
https://www.angelsgate.org/animalhospiceguide.htm
An organization that rescues "special needs" animals (elderly, requiring special care, etc.). The Web page link above has a list of guidelines for hospice care. They do recognize that euthanasia might be necessary.

Association for Pet Loss and Bereavement
https://www.aplb.org/
Provides support, support groups and referrals for those with elderly animals and for those seeking help with memorials, memorial ceremonies, etc. Their site includes links to specific support for both veterinarians and owners, and training for those who wish to be pet grief counselors.

Human Animal Bond Association (HABA)
https://humananimalbond.net/
Promotes education and understanding of the human-animal bond

Spirits in Transition
https://www.spiritsintransition.org/
A site created by a veterinarian, devoted to the idea of hospice care rather than euthanasia for elderly pets.

Physical Therapy

(As of 2023, rehabilitation information is a little disconnected and may become more centralized in the near future, and websites for training and CE have changed in the past without automatically forwarding to a new site. Do an internet search to find them if these links do not work. The websites below for companies that sell equipment and supplies have remained stable for at least 10 years.)

Canine Rehabilitation Institute
https://www.caninerehabinstitute.com/Resources.html
This resource page includes products for canine seniors, recovering patients, and the handicapped, as
   well as lists of organizations.

Handicapped Pets.com
https://www.handicappedpets.com
A site for products, services, and support for handicapped pets. Their About section has links to videos,
   articles, and forums.

Online Pet Health
https://onlinepethealth.com/resources-for-the-veterinary-rehabilitation-therapist/
This page has a long list of links to various resources for veterinary rehab. They are the current source
   of all continuing education for the University of Tennessee. Their aim is to be THE CE source for all
   rehabbers. It has three membership plans: free (which offers a large amount of information), single
   focus for a deeper dive into an area (either Hydrotherapy, Small Animal, or Equine), or multi (for
   access to two or all three areas). Though it is based in South Africa, they are worldwide-friendly.

Senior pet products.com
https://seniorpetproducts.com
Web site for items for senior dogs and cats: braces, stairs, raised bowls, etc.

Pulsed Magnetic Field Therapy

Assisi Animal Health
https://assisianimalhealth.com/
Manufacturers of the Assisi loop with some information about how PEMFT works, as well as a source
   for their Assisi Loops and pads.

Dr. Pawluk
https://www.drpawluk.com/
Web site of an MD who has amassed a large amount of information about PEMF.

Respond Systems
https://respondsystems.com/pemf/how-it-works/
A few faqs about PEMF. The company makes PEMFT beds for dogs and blankets and wraps for horses.

6

The Touch Therapies

Introduction

TTouch, massage, trigger point therapy, and Reiki are all helpful types of body work. TTouch helps animals get in touch with their bodies and can help with both physical and mental problems. Virtually everyone knows the benefits of massage, and one technician who is a Reiki master can be considered invaluable in helping pets both before and after surgery. A technician or nurse can legally perform any of these methods on a patient once they have obtained proper training.

TTouch

Definition

TTouch is a therapy developed by Linda Tellington-Jones in the 1970s (thus is sometimes referred to as "Tellington Touch," or "Tellington Ttouch"). The method grew out of her work training horses and working with their riders. What riders perceived as behavior problems, Linda saw was often related to a horse's movement problems and its surroundings. Linda was influenced by the Feldenkreis method. Often characterized as the practice of making little circles on the skin, TTouch goes far beyond this and includes ground work, mazes, and other movement exercises.

Purpose

TTouch aims to improve behavior and movement by reprogramming the way the brain directs the body to move. The reprogramming is accomplished by making circular motions on the skin using the fingers or hands, by moving the limbs in various ways, and by ground exercises.

History

- 1949–1972: Moshe Feldenkrais published the influential *Awareness Through Movement* as a follow-up to his 1949 publication *The Body and Mature Behavior*. This latter publication discusses reestablishing movement in his damaged legs by activating unused brain and peripheral neural pathways.
- 1970s: While attending training in the Feldenkrais method with the intention of using it to help riders at her equestrian school, Linda Tellington-Jones quickly saw its potential for horses also.

She developed ideas based on the Feldenkrais method and created a technique that came to be known as TTEAM, or The Tellington-Jones Equine Awareness Method. (Awareness in this case refers to Feldenkrais's work increasing awareness of the body and its movements.) Her methods developed for use with other animals evolved from her work with horses.

- 1983: Linda was inspired while giving a TTEAM workshop to add the circular motions that are a hallmark of the TTouch system – and so TTouch was born
- 1985: *The Potent Self: A Study of Spontaneity and Compulsion* by Moshe Feldenkrais was published. The book explains the theory behind Feldenkrais's techniques for improving the human motor system. The work is somewhat based on F.M. Alexander's work.
- 1988: *An Introduction to the Tellington-Jones Equine Awareness Method: The T.E.A.M. Approach to Problem-Free Training* by Linda Tellington-Jones was published.
- 1988–2023: Over 56 books about TTouch (including translations) published.

Description

Moshe Feldenkrais developed the Feldenkrais method after he successfully learned to walk again after an accident crushed his legs. His work involved establishing new neural pathways to help program new movements. He discovered that this also often involved new emotions or new ways of thinking when these new pathways were established. As a result, the Feldenkrais method emphasizes health as functioning well, both physically and mentally. It encourages self-exploration and awareness.

The Feldenkreis Guild of North America emphasizes that they do no diagnosis or prescribing for illnesses or disease. Instead, their method emphasizes self-discovery and mind–body development, rather than manipulation.

When a baby or young animal learns to walk and react to stimuli, the motor patterns gradually become an established circuit, including behaviors as well as movements. This allows the movement and behavior to become automatic. However, if the pattern is learned in response to fear or pain, then it is often not beneficial, may not be appropriate, and can even become ineffective (in the case of injury). However, it can be difficult to break this pattern.

When the nervous system is stimulated in new ways, especially with non-threatening movements and gentle manipulation of the body, behavior and motor patterns can be reprogrammed, and new motor patterns can be learned (Ullmann et al., 2010).

Tellington-Jones wanted to help animals in this way. With the help of what she learned with training in the Feldenkrais system, she created a method to stimulate the nervous system of horses in a way that it had not previously experienced. This new stimulation would help the brain establish new connections and new patterns of movement and behavior. In TTouch, this occurs by making circular patterns on the skin all over the body with the fingers or the whole hand, using varying pressures. This method also includes calming techniques for the animal, and it helps owners become more aware of their own posture, breathing, and other actions. Animals pick up very subtle cues from humans, and the animal's owner may be subconsciously adding to the problem.

In addition to this technique, animals may be asked to walk in various patterns, their limbs may be moved in specific unusual ways, or they may perform other exercises. This is all done in a low-key, minimal-stress way. They are not forced; instead, they are asked to discover the way to do this themselves. It is interesting to watch a horse or pet go through these exercises and see them figure things out for themselves instead of panicking. The exercises improve balance and coordination. With better balance, animals gain self-confidence and become more sure of themselves. This confidence lets them concentrate better on the task at hand. The changes are permanent, lasting far beyond the time of the gentle massage.

This method is based on cooperation and respect. It shows owners a new way to cooperate with their pets. It has been shown that the nervous system, including the brain, is much more plastic than formerly believed. TTouch evolved before research proved this, but the results demonstrate this fact.

In addition, certain postures are associated with certain emotions. Humans who tense up or adopt a tense attitude will be more anxious than if they intentionally use a relaxed posture.

Because the pattern is applied over the entire body, it is not necessary to know anatomy in order to be able to change performance and behavior or to improve motor patterns. It also allows handling of an animal in a way that decreases tension and avoids creating fear or anxiety. Because they are less anxious, animals can more easily learn new responses and behaviors. It decreases fear and anxiety in situations that were previously frightening. Thus, TTouch is an ideal tool to help pets with separation anxiety or other behavior connected to fear, such as excessive barking (in dogs) or shying (in horses). It also helps the owner to bond with his or her pet and to quickly connect with the pet on a deeper level, even after many months of misbehavior.

TTouch has been helpful for other problems such as the following:

- Pulling on a leash
- Digging
- Jumping up on owners and others
- Showing aggression toward people or other dogs
- Biting or showing resistance when being groomed
- Car sickness

Because it "reprograms" the pet's motor responses, TTouch is also useful after an injury or surgery, especially one involving nerves or muscles. In addition, the emphasis of this method is on the pet and owner working together as a team. This philosophy is in alignment with the general holistic view of animals as friends and companions rather than owned objects. The approach encourages a more intuitive view of pets and helps owners interpret their pets' reactions more correctly.

Tellington-Jones is a keen observer of horses, and one of her books (*Getting in Touch: Understand and Influence Your Horse's Personality*) shows horse owners how a number of personality traits of the horse are related to their conformation, including head swirls. In the book, she suggests how to interact with each type to get the most out of the horse.

Veterinarian's Role

Some veterinarians are trained in TTouch, but not many use it in their practice. Equine practitioners may use the method to help calm a horse. If veterinarians are interested in getting clients to use TTouch, they may recommend training or even demonstrate it to their clients. Likewise, small animal veterinarians will sometimes use it to calm animals. However, veterinarians usually do not teach the method, and even holistic veterinarians are not very cognizant of its methods.

Technician's Role

The TTouch method is an ideal method for technicians to learn and to apply to anxious pets in the initial part of the exam. It fits in with the holistic concept of the mind–body connection, and the concepts are easy to learn and teach. Short courses and certification are available online and at in-person workshops. TTouch practitioners can also have a career independent of a veterinary practice, as TTouch practitioners and teachers.

Where to Learn How

Tellington TTouch Training
1713 State Rd 502
Santa Fe, NM 87506
866-4-TTouch
https://ttouch.com/
https://learn.ttouch.ca/

Summary

What can technicians do?

1) Technicians can become trained in TTouch
2) Technicians can become certified as a TTouch practitioner
3) Technicians can use TTouch within a veterinary practice as a way to calm animals and also as part of a rehab program
4) Technicians can become a TTouch practitioner and use it outside of a veterinary practice (as long as you do not specifically diagnose a disease).
5) Technicians can become a TTouch teacher and teach the method to owners of horses, dogs, or other animals

Massage Therapy

Definition

Veterinary therapeutic massage is the manipulation of the animal's soft tissues by a practitioner trained in anatomy, physiology, and veterinary disease processes as a component of a holistic therapeutic intervention. This section includes both Western and Oriental massage therapies. Acupressure is considered by some to be a form of massage, and thus it is included here.

Purpose

Massage is an often-neglected part of physical therapy. It can help release trigger points, decrease muscle pain, and increase flexibility, as well as decreasing anxiety.

Animal massage is the use of pressure in various forms administered by hand to the musculoskeletal system with the intention of facilitating good health. Interest in this field has been on the rise over the past few years. Many countries and some US states recognize massage as a health-care service for animals, and each state has its own guidelines regarding training and recognition of practitioners. Although massage is an old tradition, it is still considered a fairly new "science." Consequently, many states are still defining its use and standards of practice.

Massage therapists are only one group of people who provide massage for animals. Veterinary technicians, horse guardians, grooms and trainers, physical therapists, and others offer massage for relaxation, well-being, and rehabilitation when appropriate (Shumway, 2007).

Massage is believed to facilitate health and balance in many ways. Massage eases tension in the soft tissues, promotes good circulation, provides relaxation, and stimulates the function of the immune system. Massage may be used for competition horses and dogs in the same way that it is used by professional athletes. Due to advances in veterinary care, many companion animals live longer lives, and massage can be a helpful tool in maintaining an animal's youthful exuberance.

History

3000 BC: The Chinese Cong-Fu of the Toa-Tse is the oldest known book written about massage. It was translated into French in the 1700s.

2760 BC: Nei Ching describes therapeutic touch.

2500 BC: Egyptians create reflexology.

1800 BC: The Ayurvedic *Art of Life* book includes massage techniques. In India, the focus is on sensual aspects of massage.

1000 BC: Homer writes about an oily medium used for massage.

776 BC: In the Olympic Games, athletes are massaged prior to their events.

200 BC: Greek physician Galen uses natural magnets to relieve pain in treating many illnesses.

600: The Japanese develop Shiatsu (finger pressure or acupressure); *anma* is massage in Japanese.

368–1644: In the Ming Dynasty, pediatric massage (which, for the first time, was referred to as *tuina*) evolves into a highly systematic treatment modality that is still popular today.

World War I: Swedish massage is used for rehabilitation of injured soldiers.

1939: The Florida State Massage Therapy Association Inc. (FSMTA) is first organized on June 15, 1939. It is one of the oldest massage organizations, with 85 charter members.

1943: Chicago American Association of Masseurs and Masseuses forms, later to become American Massage Therapy Association. Dues were $.50. The first Massage Act is passed by the Florida Legislature.

1991: The Touch Research Institute is created.

1992: National certification is required for human massage therapists. (Adapted from www.thebodyworker.com/history.htm.)

Description

Depending on the technique employed, massage may be used to affect the circulatory system (including lymphatics), muscles, skin, pain sensation, flexibility, healing, and scar tissue. It has effects locally in the skin, underlying tissues and muscles, and in the autonomic nervous system that regulates the body's response to such things as pain, disease, and injury.

While there are general types of massage, such as Swedish massage, that are recognized for humans, the term "massage" for animals usually refers to a combination of them if used for non-oriental types. Tui-Na, a type of Chinese massage, acupressure, a method for massaging specific acupuncture points, and Shiatsu, a type of Japanese massage, are oriental methods that are referred to separately and have distinct methods of applying them. Classes in the types are generally taught the same way.

Some massage techniques are taught in rehab courses, but a technician can get training in the general type and each of the oriental types without going through a rehab course. Although massage therapy can be very helpful in rehab, sports medicine, and geriatric medicine, there is no formal AVMA or NAVTA recognition of the individual trainings. "Massage" is a gray area in veterinary medicine, usually not included in practice acts. A technician who is trained in one or more types of massage therapy might be able to use their skills outside of a veterinary practice. You might need a referral from a veterinarian to do so, although not all states require the referral. Check with your veterinary state board to find out what is permissible in your state.

Role of the Veterinarian

Some veterinarians use massage therapy in their practice. Others refer pets to animal massage therapists. Some massage techniques can be taught to owners, and it is highly beneficial for musculoskeletal problems. Veterinarians may prefer to teach clients themselves, or they may prefer to have a technician demonstrate these techniques. Licensed human massage therapists usually need a referral from a veterinarian in order to legally massage animals.

Role of the Technician

A technician or nurse can include questions about massage therapy when providing a history of the pet to their veterinarian. If a pet is getting massage therapy from a licensed massage therapist, be sure that the therapist and the veterinarian are in communication. A technician trained in massage techniques can evaluate the animal's overall soft tissue and postural condition, just as a physical therapist would, before discussing appropriate physical therapy or massage technique with a veterinarian. The technician can answer questions about massage therapy, its benefits, and its application to that particular pet. The technician, if properly trained, can perform massage and may also offer instruction in follow-up techniques to be used at home.

For those interested in performing massage on animals, it is important to understand anatomy, physiology, biomechanics, and massage techniques relevant to the type of animal one wishes to work with. Most animal massage training programs offer these topics as well as animal behavior, first aid and handling, proper stretching techniques, and related subjects.

Where to Learn How

General Massage Techniques
Equissage
P.O. Box 447
Round Hill, VA 20142
https://www.equissage.com/
(Equissage is the oldest trainer of animal massage therapists in the world.)

International Association of Animal Massage & Bodywork
https://iaamb.org/directory/iaambacwt-preferred-educational-provider/#!directory/map
Provides a list of member schools

Northwest School of Animal Massage
https://www.nwsam.com/programs/
(Provides distance learning classes and training. Has a certification course for Animal Massage)

Summary

What can technicians do?

1) Courses are available for veterinary technicians in general animal massage and specific oriental massage techniques.
2) Massage therapy is a valuable addition to veterinary practices, which include sports medicine or rehab, and training in animal massage can add to the value of a technician for that practice.

3) "Animal massage" is in somewhat of a gray area legally. In some areas, a technician can practice animal massage independently of a veterinary practice. In others, they must use their skills in a veterinary practice.

Oriental Massage Therapy

Theory Underlying Oriental Massage Therapies

The aim of Oriental massage techniques is to restore balance and flow in the body. Chinese theory assumes a flow of blood along blood vessels and other fluids and energy (*qi* in China, *ki* in Japan) along certain pathways or meridians. The meridians are associated with organs in the body and with functions ascribed to the organs. (The functions match the Western ideas of organ functions, but they also include others such as resolving dampness.) A blockage of energy, fluid, or blood flow will result in disease.

In addition, there can be other problems, such as an "invasion of cold," or a "deficiency of blood," which cause imbalance and pain. (Painful areas or trigger points in muscles are often ischemic locally, with resultant cooler temperatures than surrounding muscle tissue.) By stimulating acupuncture points along the meridians, or in the case of Shiatsu and Tui-Na, in general areas along the meridians, the flow of qi (ki) resumes, bringing heat and reducing pain. (Colder areas often heat up during massage therapy.) Other types of imbalances are also treated: deficiencies are treated by acupressure and kneading and rubbing lightly, whereas excesses require more vigorous methods of rubbing, scrubbing, squeezing, or pressing. Cold problems are resolved with heat-generating methods (heat or rubbing with friction) and excessive heat is helped with cooler methods. TCM theory also states that anmo eliminates pathogens. Research has shown that lactic acid buildup is reversed during Shiatsu and anmo.

Shiatsu uses specific acupuncture points to help this process, and points that are painful during therapy are treated also. A big part of Shiatsu methodology is diagnosis by palpation and treatment, and painful points (which are not always acupuncture points) are located, treated, and if pain is resolved, the point was considered a diagnostic one. During Shiatsu, diagnosis and treatment are constantly changing, depending on how the body responds.

Of the three types of Oriental massage therapy, acupressure is the best known among Westerners. There are 300 books on acupressure listed at Amazon.com. Many of the books seem to imply that all one needs to do is identify a specific problem, look up the corresponding points in a table, and then practice acupressure. This is a very crude way to practice acupressure, but it can have some beneficial effects.

Diagnosis in Oriental medicine includes observations that are lacking in Western medical methods, such as the flow of qi and problems including blood, cold, damp, etc. However, there are some methods that are more easily mastered. One valuable aid to pain detection is motion palpation, used to a much greater extent than in the traditional veterinary curriculum. Often, the conventional veterinary practitioner is looking for wincing, crying, biting, or other indicators of pain, but it is equally (or more) useful to note a stiffness in specific areas. If veterinarians limit themselves to watching for overt signs of pain, they will miss evidence in more stoic individuals. For instance, to check the back, gently bounce it at each intervertebral joint, beginning at T1-T2 and continuing down to the lumbosacral joint. In general, lumbar vertebral joints should be more mobile than thoracic joints, and lumbosacral and T13-L1 areas should be the most flexible of all. The neck should be easily flexed dorsally, ventrally, and laterally to an equal extent. One should be able to extend and flex joints equally easily on both sides. Animals should stand squarely, and dogs and cats should sit squarely. Horses should turn equally well in both directions. If a joint is stiff compared to the corresponding joint on the other leg, there is some discomfort there.

Dogs who are reluctant to sit squarely and horses who are reluctant to bend to one side are often illustrating pain, not stubbornness. Another sign can be excessive grooming parallel to the spine, on the flanks, and on joints below the painful one. This last problem is also known as a lick granuloma.

Neck, shoulder, back, and leg muscles should be palpated. Stoic animals may not show signs of pain, but they often flick an ear or tense up when a painful region is palpated. Regions where muscles are hard, stiff, lumpy, stringy, hot, or cold all indicate problem areas. When a problem area is identified in the front, the rear is also often affected because the animal shifts weight to the less painful areas and puts additional stress there. Pain on one side can also result in problems on the opposite side. For example, right-front pain will often result in problems in the left rear and in the lower back. In addition, problems that manifest in lower limbs may actually demonstrate pain further up the body. For animals noted for lick granulomas (such as Doberman pinschers), resolving pain in the hip or lumbosacral area often results in a resolution or decreased severity of the lick granuloma.

Note that veterinary technicians cannot diagnose problems, but knowing some TCM signs can help give the technician some insight and more to look for when doing an initial or follow-up exam for a veterinarian. It is also useful to know in rehab practice, as a way to fine-tune rehab procedures and judgment of progression of the patient's response.

Development of Oriental Massage Therapy

Acupressure, Shiatsu, and Tui-Na all have their roots in traditional Chinese medicine (TCM), including ancient Chinese massage therapy *anmo* (known as *anma* in Japan). Originally, only the term *anmo* was used for therapeutic massage. The term *Tui-Na* is not seen in Chinese literature until it was used in a book on pediatric Tui-Na during the Ming dynasty (1368–1644).

The first references to anmo therapeutic massage in China, inscriptions on bones and tortoise shells, date back to the Shang Dynasty (16th to 11th centuries BC). References to anmo are included in many of the texts. The text, *Fifty-two Medical Formulas*, contains references to specific anmo techniques such as compression (*an*), gliding (*mo*), scratching (*sao*), scraping (*gua*), rubbing (*fu*), and percussing (*ji*). Although Confucius (551–479 BC), with his ideas of balance and yin and yang, was accepted at that time, the theory of Chinese medicine was still shamanistic. Despite this, acupuncture, anmo techniques, and herbal remedies from the Ma Wang Dui tomb texts are similar or the same as those used in current practice.

The *Yellow Emperor's Classic of Internal Medicine,* compiled between 200 and 100 BC, is the earliest surviving text of TCM, and contains the ideas of balance, yin and yang, etc. In it, anmo is referred to in 30 different chapters.

In general, modern-day Oriental massage therapy incorporates the main ideas of TCM, including the use of meridians and acupuncture points. Methods such as Nuad Bo'Rarn (Thai traditional massage) may incorporate other methods, such as Ayurvedic medicine, yoga, and Buddhist meditation techniques. The three methods that are closest to the Western concept of acupuncture and massage are acupressure, Shiatsu, and Tui-Na.

Acupressure is a form of therapy using pressure on acupuncture points. Shiatsu is a gentle therapy that includes pressure on these and other points and areas, as well as some stretching, stroking, and gentle rubbing techniques and, occasionally, Qi Gong methods. Tui-Na is a more vigorous treatment, combining elements of acupressure, chiropractic, Western massage techniques, herbal poultices, compresses, liniments, and salves to enhance the other methods, and it sometimes includes aspects of Qi Gong as well. It emphasizes points, meridians, and surfaces (such as fingers) connected with various organs.

Contraindications for any type of massage include conditions involving fractures, phlebitis, infectious conditions, inflammation, open wounds, or lesions.

Massage therapy can relieve pain, stiffness, loss of functional mobility, muscle spasm, swelling, and circulatory problems and can help with remodeling of scar tissue. It facilitates physical therapy and rehabilitation.

For Oriental massage, Shiatsu, Tui-Na, and acupressure are used to treat many problems by various practitioners, but the treatment of most medical problems by these massage techniques requires a good working knowledge of Chinese medical theory. In contrast, pain relief can be obtained by using these methods in local areas where pain occurs.

Tui-Na

Tui-Na – Development

Tui-Na flourished from the Three Kingdoms period (220–280) up until the Tang Dynasty (618–907). The Imperial Medical College included anmo as a separate department. Practitioners who specialized in anmo during the Tang Dynasty were divided into three levels: anmo doctorates, masters, and technicians. At that time, the scope of the anmo specialty included therapeutic gymnastics and bone-setting. In Tang literature, a number of anmo ointments are described for use with massage. In Tang medical textbooks, anmo was often prescribed for disease prevention, using self-massage techniques (Halliday, 1997). It was in the 6th century during the Tang Dynasty that Chinese medicine was first brought to Japan by Buddhist monks, where it developed into Japanese amma and Shiatsu, as well as Japanese acupuncture techniques.

In the Song Dynasty (960–1279), the use of anmo in the treatment of bone fractures and dislocations was further developed, including a description of manipulations (including traction) used for setting various types of fractures. Anmo was also used in obstetrics to help difficult deliveries and to correct breech presentations. In addition, more wellness techniques were described.

The term *Tui-Na* first appeared in the Ming Dynasty (1368–1644) as a description for pediatric massage, a separate branch of anmo or Tui-Na. It has been suggested the term *Tui-Na* (pushing and pulling) was originally a description of the movements required to pin down the squirming babies.

During the Qing Dynasty (1644–1911), a number of different versions of anmo arose, and the diversification continues today. One type is associated with the martial arts, emphasizing the treatment of trauma, including fractures and dislocations. Another version, the "rolling method" school, uses variations of a single technique, a form of oscillating compression using mainly the thumb. A third method, the "spine-pinching" school, uses the technique of rolling the skin between the thumb and fingers over the vertebral column. In 1830, allopathic medicine was introduced to Japan, and traditional Japanese medicine went into decline until the early 1900s. In 1919, Tamai Tempaku published *Shiatsu Ho,* influencing teachers of the 1920s who then developed various styles of Shiatsu. The Japan Shiatsu Institute was opened in 1940. In 1955, Shiatsu was legally approved as part of anma therapy, and in 1964 was finally recognized as a treatment independent of anma.

However, in China, after the establishment of the National Republic of China (1912–1949), TCM of all types went into decline, and schools teaching TCM were closed. In 1929, at the first meeting of the Central Health Committee, a resolution was passed to totally abolish TCM. In 1936, the government claimed there was no scientific basis for TCM, and its practice was banned. Tui-Na went underground, although anma was still practiced. Mao Tse-Tung's armies used TCM herbs, acupuncture, and Tui-Na, and after 1949, with the establishment of the People's Republic, clinics, research organizations, and colleges were established to standardize, teach, and promote traditional Chinese medicine. The term *Tui-Na* was then used to describe the current version of the method, with aspects of acupressure, massage, and chiropractic, to distinguish it from traditional techniques using massage only (now called anma) without TCM diagnosis. In 1958, a Tui-Na clinic and school were established in Shanghai. Despite setbacks during the Cultural Revolution in the 1960s and 1970s, Tui-Na is currently well-established in China as a basic therapeutic technique.

In 1979, the Shanghai College of Traditional Chinese Medicine established an acupuncture/Tui-Na major. In 1982, Beijing and many of the other colleges of TCM across China followed suit. Most of the Chinese-language journals of traditional Chinese medicine regularly feature articles and research on anmo, and at least one national journal (*Anmo Yu Daoyin*) is devoted exclusively to news and research in the field. A good deal of research has been done in China on the biomechanical and physiological principles of anmo treatment, and numerous trial studies have been done on its clinical applications.

Currently, Tui-Na is taught as a separate but equal field of study in the major traditional Chinese medical colleges. Tui-Na doctors receive the same demanding training as acupuncturists and herbalists and enjoy the same level of professional respect.

Tui-Na – Description

Chinese Tui-Na is a more vigorous therapy and less well-known. The definition of Tui-Na incorporates parts of acupressure, chiropractic, and massage therapy. In addition, the various schools of Tui-Na methods have resulted in subsets of treatment that are more specialized toward massage, acupressure, or chiropractic techniques.

Tui-Na is commonly used in humans for the treatment of specific musculoskeletal disorders and chronic stress-related disorders of the digestive, respiratory, and reproductive systems. Tui-Na methods include the use of hand techniques to massage the soft tissue (muscles and tendons) of the body, acupressure techniques, and manipulation techniques to restore muscle function. Massage techniques include the rolling method, which emphasizes soft tissue techniques and specializes in joint injuries and muscle sprains; the one-finger pushing method, which emphasizes techniques for acupressure and the treatment of internal diseases; and Nei Gung method, which emphasizes the use of Nei Gong Qi energy generation exercises and specific massage methods for revitalizing depleted energy systems.

Tui-Na rolling school techniques include effleurage (gliding), petrissage (kneading), vibration, shaking, rocking, tapotement (percussion), friction, and foulage. They also include a number of unique techniques, especially the oscillating compressions such as *yi zhi chan* and *gun fa* (rolling). In performing Tui-Na, practitioners use their fingers, thumbs, palms, knuckles, forearms, elbows, knees, and feet. Joint manipulations, include traction, circumduction, stretching, and *ban fa*. "Ban" literally means a trigger, wrench, or lever. It refers to sudden mobilization (wrenching) of the vertebrae or other joints following relaxation of the surrounding soft tissue with gliding, kneading, etc. It is traditionally performed with the patient in a side-lying position, seated position, or even borne on the back of the practitioner (back-to-back, with elbows interlocked). When done with the hands, the practitioner often uses palpation skills to direct the impulse to a specific vertebra.

In a typical human session, the client, wearing loose clothing and no shoes, lies on a table or floor mat. The practitioner examines the specific problems of the client and begins to apply a specific treatment protocol. The major focus of application is upon specific pain sites, acupressure points, energy meridians, and muscles and joints. Advanced Tui-Na practitioners may also use Chinese herbs to facilitate quicker healing. Sessions last from 30 minutes to 1 hour. Depending on the client's specific problems, he or she may return for additional treatments.

Tui-Na massage therapy is a very effective way to relieve muscular tension and spasm; it not only relaxes the muscles but also rids the body of the trigger points causing the muscular tension. The function and mechanism of Tui-Na massage therapy consists of three parts: first, it can locally promote blood circulation and raise body temperature. Second, it can increase the pain threshold of tissue with appropriate stimulation. Third, it can extend the tense and spasmodic muscles so that the illness can be eliminated.

Tui-Na can also help reduce luxations and relax muscle spasm and pain accompanying the dislocation. It is also used to break down adhesions, especially involving muscles, ligaments, and tendons, and remobilize stiff joints. It is used to help problems such as carpal tunnel syndrome, freeing up tendons within a constrictive sheath.

Tonification is accomplished by soft manipulation of structures, in the direction of channel flow, with slow frequency of movements. More vigorous manipulation, opposite the direction of channel flow, using a higher frequency of movements, will purge the area of pathogens and calm the body. Manipulations between these two extremes help regulate yin and yang and organ function.

The basic techniques of Tui-Na massage include the following:

Tui: To push
Na: To pull or drag
An: Rapid and rhythmical pressing
Tao: Strong pinching pressure
Nie: Kneading
Nien: Nipping
Moa: Rubbing
Pai: Tapping

Acupressure

Acupressure – Definition

Acupressure is pressure on acupuncture points. Everything that can be accomplished with acupuncture can, in theory, be accomplished with acupressure. There are several differences, however. Acupuncture is a stronger stimulus than acupressure. With acupuncture, many points can be stimulated at once, whereas with acupressure, the practitioner is limited by the number of fingers on his or her hands and by the location of the points. In a human or large animal, it is difficult to stimulate points on the head, anterior and posterior thorax, and lower legs at the same time. On the other hand, in humans, one can determine a finer gradation of pain in specific acupuncture points, as well as a specific timing of pain relief. This is much harder to do with animals. Touch itself is much more reassuring than the puncture of a needle and can help relax an animal enough so that diagnosis and treatment are done more easily.

Acupressure – Purpose

Acupressure can be useful for those animals that might not tolerate needles. Acupressure can also be used for animals that cannot be transported to the hospital, such as those in hospice. Ear acupressure can be used to decrease pain in post-surgical patients.

Acupressure – History

It is unclear when acupressure itself started to be used. Points and meridians were established first, with special stone tools and later needles used on specific points. (For a discussion of the history of acupuncture, see Chapter 10. For a discussion of Oriental massage in general, see the section on the development of Oriental massage therapy, above.)

Acupressure – Description

Once a problem has been diagnosed by the veterinarian and a spot or area has been identified that needs treatment, the veterinarian can show the client the appropriate acupuncture points as the first step in treatment.

There are three methods related to acupuncture points that are appropriate: treating ah-shi points, treating local points, and "surrounding the dragon." In addition, gentle massage of the affected area can also help. An ah-shi point is a painful point. The pet will let you know where it is. Local points are acupuncture points in the area of the problem. The "dragon" is the painful area, and by treating points around it, you are treating the area itself. There are a number of sources for dog and cat charts. One of the best, with good descriptions of appropriate points is *Four Paws, Five Directions* by Cheryl Schwartz, DVM (see the bibliography).

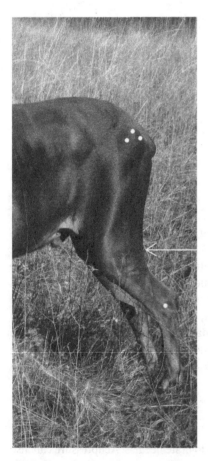

Acupressure is usually done with the tip of the thumb or forefinger. Pressure can be applied without motion, with a circular motion, or with a brushing motion. A gradually increasing pressure just on the borderline of discomfort is very effective for pain. One should start by just resting the fingertip or thumb tip on the acupressure point and gradually increase pressure until the animal becomes restless or otherwise indicates discomfort. Slightly decrease the pressure and hold for 5 seconds. Some animals will regulate the pressure themselves, pressing into the pressure or retreating from it until the pressure is comfortable for them. No more than 12 pounds of pressure is needed for a large dog.

The amount of pressure to use varies with each individual. As a general rule, large, heavily muscled bodies need deeper pressure than thinner-muscled animals, and phlegmatic animals need a heavier touch than highly excitable animals. This does not always hold true, however, and it is best to start with a light touch, then apply increasing pressure. One of the biggest benefits of acupressure in veterinary practice is that a veterinarian can identify specific points for an owner, and the owner can treat those points by acupressure between regular visits. It is hard for an owner to harm an animal with acupressure.

Acupressure Points

Four basic acupressure points that can help hip pain are Gall Bladder 29, Gall Bladder 30, Urinary Bladder 54, and Urinary Bladder 60 (also known as the "aspirin point") (see Figure 6.1). The first three points are depressions

Figure 6.1 Some acupressure points that may help hip pain.

found in a triangle immediately anterior, dorsal, and posterior to the greater trochanter of the femur. They are most easily found in large dogs suffering pain from hip dysplasia. These dogs have atrophy of the muscles surrounding the hip joint. After these points are located on this type of patient, it is easier to see where they are in smaller animals. One should hold the points for 15 seconds or use small circular motions. Urinary Bladder 60 is found on the outer surface of the hind leg, between the base of the Achilles tendon and the lateral malleolus of the tibia, just above the tibial tarsal bone (Figure 6.1).

Pressure should be applied directly on the area on the lateral and medial side or may be gently pinched. (This will also apply pressure on Kidney 3, which can help the kidneys.)

For an in-depth discussion of acupressure points and how to apply the proper pressure, see the book *Four Paws, Five Directions*, by Cheryl Schwartz, DVM.

Shiatsu

Shiatsu – Definition

Many people mistakenly believe that Shiatsu is just a Japanese form of acupressure. Although it does incorporate techniques of acupressure, it also includes some stretching and gentle massage techniques and, depending on the school, some Qi Gong. Unlike acupressure, diagnosis occurs at time of treatment. The look and feel of the body, as well as the patient's comments (for humans), are part of the diagnosis–treatment technique, which can change during the course of a treatment.

Shiatsu means "finger pressure," but the thumb, fingers, palms, elbows, and feet may all be used in humans to perform shiatsu. Shiatsu points, or *tsubo*, mostly correspond with acupuncture points, but there are also additional points. There is an emphasis in Shiatsu on communicating with the patient by touch and on modifying the treatment according to the response from the previous treatment. For a Shiatsu master, diagnosis and treatment can change with each point treated. Physical contact is believed to create total communication between practitioner and patient. The compassion and support from the practitioner, felt by the patient during physical contact, will help uncover other problems and emotions that cause the patient to feel vulnerable. In Shiatsu, *setsu-shin*, or touch and massage, is the most important part of diagnosis. *Bun-shin* (listening and smelling), *mon-shin* (asking—about the problem and general habits and preferences), and *bo-shin* (looking—especially at the shape and color of the body) are also used, along with pulse and tongue diagnosis.

Different schools of Shiatsu emphasize different methods of treatment. Some may consider Shiatsu to be only acupressure-like finger pressure, and others may be more familiar with another school that uses steady pressure, bouncing, gentle rubbing, and vibrations as well. Gentle stretching and manipulation of joints are also included. Treatment of humans is done with clothes remaining on the patient. Two hands are used, either simultaneously when treating bilateral points or with one hand as an anchor for the other point. Centering and strengthening exercises are encouraged, both for the practitioner before treating patients and for the patient, between treatments. There is an emphasis on imbalances. *Kyo* (deficiency) at one point in a meridian can create a *jitsu* (excess) at another site in the same or a different meridian. Although the jitsu area may manifest the main symptoms, the practitioner usually tries to identify and treat the kyo that is responsible.

For pain relief, *kori* (areas of stiffness and constriction with discomfort) are first identified by palpation. These areas block lymphatic, arterial, and venous circulation and nerve transmission. The most tender spot in this area is the spot treated by finger pressure as well as *moxa* (an herb that is burned on the site). The emphasis is on finding and treating the tender spot, not the specific acupuncture point, even if the spot is not precisely on an acupuncture point. (These tender spots usually are at an area of high electrical conductivity and can also be found by acupuncture point detectors.) These areas may also give rise to referred pain, which will not fully respond until the original point is identified and treated. For example, on the back of the neck, lateral to the spine, between the base of the skull and the beginning of the shoulders, there are four pairs of tsubo points but only one pair of acupuncture points.

The Shiatsu practitioner is encouraged to start with meditation and deep breathing exercises before beginning treatment. Practitioners should remain mindful of the patient at all times, concentrating on the treatment, not intruding thoughts. A short exercise for deep breathing is to raise the arms upward and outward while breathing in slowly, then exhaling while lowering the arms.

Shiatsu – Example

For back pain, the back is first gently stretched, then pressure is applied to points beside each vertebra and to gluteal muscles in a line between the lumbosacral space and the hip. The patient should be lying down, in a prone position. Stretching is accomplished by placing a palm at the cervical–thoracic junction and the other palm at the lumbosacral junction and gently stretching. (This can be modified for very small animals.) This is repeated on each side of the spine and then diagonally.

Next, using the tip of the left thumb on top of the tip of the right thumb, gentle pressure is applied to the areas on each side of the vertebrae for 5 seconds in each spot, from the area beside T1 to the area beside the last lumbar vertebra. Using the same technique, pressure is applied down the middle of the sacrum. Divide the back mentally into four sections. The spine is gently bounced from anterior to posterior along the spine with the flat of two fingers, the palm, or two palms (depending on the side of the animal), two times in each quarter. Finally, one palm is placed on top of the other, fingers pointing toward the head, and placed on the anterior thoracic spine. The palm gently sweeps down to the sacrum rapidly, three times.

Veterinarian's Role

Generally, veterinarians will perform acupuncture, not acupressure. In such a case, the role of a veterinarian in the case of acupressure is one of direct supervision of the person applying acupressure. In such a case, they might prefer to demonstrate acupressure to the owner also, as an at-home treatment, the owner can do to follow up or reinforce their treatment. They may perform Tui-Na or Shiatsu, but are more likely to leave them up to a trained technician.

Technician's Role

Acupressure is a gray area in veterinary medicine. In some states, any treatment of an animal's problem is considered the practice of veterinary medicine. In other states, where acupressure is considered an extension of acupuncture, only a licensed individual (veterinarian or licensed acupuncturist) is allowed to perform acupressure, but Tui-Na and Shiatsu might not be included in this ruling.

In still other states, acupressure, Tui-Na, and Shiatsu may be grouped with massage therapy. If this is the case, the technician may be able to perform all types of Oriental massage in a practice or in a client's home. Check with your veterinary licensing board to determine which case applies to you.

Where to Learn More or Learn How

Oriental Medicine Theory
Introduction to Veterinary Chinese Medicine
Online course for anyone interested in basic ideas of Veterinary Chinese Medicine

The College of Integrative Veterinary Therapies Pty Ltd (CIVT)
PO BOX 352
Yeppoon 4703
QLD, Australia
collegeoffice@civtedu.org
https://civtedu.org/courses/introduction-to-veterinary-chinese-medicine

TCVM for Veterinary Technicians
Lectures available online, but wet labs and demos are only available on-site
Chi University
9650 W Hwy 318, Reddick, FL 32686
(800) 860-1543
https://chiu.edu/courses/vtec100_usa_en

Acupressure
Northwest School of Animal Massage
PO Box 670
Fall City, WA 98024
(877) 836-3703
https://www.nwsam.com/courses/introduction-to-animal-acupressure/

Tui-Na
Chi University
9700 West Hwy 318
Reddick, FL 32686
https://www.tcvm.com/
(Provides classes in Tui-Na.)

Summary

What can the technician do?

1) Rehab courses are open to technicians if they are working in a practice with a veterinarian who is certified in it. There are classes in animal massage, Tui-Na, and acupressure that are also available for technicians. With this additional training, a technician can acquire the skills necessary for some types of massage therapy.
2) Learn the laws of your state. They may allow you to perform animal massage therapy under the supervision of a veterinarian. If so, you can use your skills in your practice, or you might be able to become part of a physical therapy practice.
3) Your local laws might allow you to practice animal massage therapy without the supervision of a veterinarian. If so, you might be able to open an animal massage practice independent of a veterinary practice.

Trigger Point Therapy (Myofascial Release)

Definition

Trigger points are often ignored in veterinary medicine because veterinarians, like medical doctors, may be unaware of their existence. Chiropractors and massage therapists, however, locate and treat trigger points regularly.

A trigger point is an area of tight, tender muscle fibers within a muscle. The muscle feels tense and fibrotic. A trigger point will spasm with slight provocation, and when it remains in spasm long enough, it will bring its own muscle into spasm. Eventually, it can cause other muscles to spasm and can create secondary trigger points. Trigger points are especially seen in the neck, shoulders, and back. (See Figures 6.2 and 6.3.) They will amplify and be affected by any form of stress—physical, chemical, or emotional.

Trigger points have been described primarily in dogs and horses. They are rare in cats, but they do exist. Trigger points are more prevalent in older animals and in those used in sports or competitive events such as agility trials, fly ball, Frisbee competitions, and in all sport horses. Trigger points are found in the same place in different dogs and in different horses. Thus, they can be described and identified anatomically. Many, but not all of them, are close to acupuncture points.

When located at the surface of the body, trigger points can easily be palpated as hard, painful nodular structures within muscle or fascia. They may be from 1/4 inch to 1 1/2 inches in diameter, but most are between 1/2 and 1 inch in diameter. When located in a deeper muscle, they are harder to feel, especially if the covering musculature is tense. If the muscle is relaxed a little with light massage, a trigger point can be palpated as a round, rubbery nodule.

Trigger points can also be found with magnetic resonance imaging (MRI) and with thermography. Contrary to what one might think, trigger points have a lower temperature than surrounding

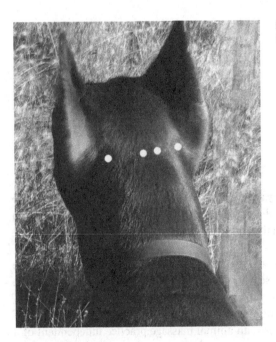

Figure 6.2 Four areas where a trigger point may be found in the upper neck.

Figure 6.3 Common trigger points in the body.

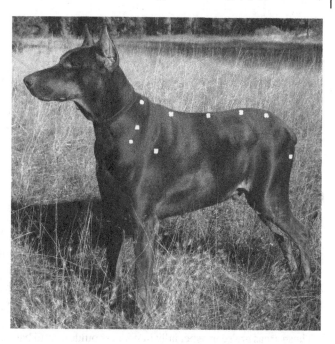

muscle. In humans, instruments are used to measure the amount of pressure on skin required for the sensation of pain. Trigger points are hyperirritable and very painful with normal digital pressure (dogs may bite, horses may kick, and cats may attack when a trigger point is pushed on, even gently). Some animals may present with shuddering and crying out at various intervals.

Histologically, a trigger point has excessive collagen fibers and abnormal muscle fibers with clusters of nuclei, knots of myofibrils, loss of cross striations, swollen mitochondria, and ragged red fibers. There is local vasoconstriction and hypertonia of the area.

Trigger points weaken the muscle without causing atrophy and prevent full lengthening of the muscle in which they are located. Weakness is reversed after trigger point therapy, and the full range of motion is restored. Trigger points cause referred pain, so the apparent pain may lead away from the site of the causative point. When the site of referred pain is treated, no cure is obtained. If the trigger point is squeezed, the referred pain becomes more severe. In animals, front leg lameness with pain radiating to the foot may be caused by a trigger point in the middle of the supraspinatus. Lick granulomas are sometimes created because of referred pain from trigger points. This is especially true with lick granulomas of the carpus and hocks. If the lameness goes away when the referring trigger point is treated, then the point is the cause of lameness. Primary trigger points can induce secondary points. Secondary points can't induce other points, but they can cause more pain than did the primary point originally.

Purpose

Trigger point therapy plays a big part in helping animals with lameness and can help solve problems that are refractory or unresponsive to corticosteroids or NSAIDs (nonsteroidal anti-inflammatory drugs). Even narcotics may have little effect. A knowledge of trigger point therapy can result in helping lameness that other methods have been unable to help.

History

1952: Janet Travell researches trigger points.

1960s: John Barnes develops myofascial release therapy.

1976: Bonnie Prudden develops the myotherapy method and publishes a book on the subject.

1985: Jack Meagher publishes *Beating Muscle Injuries,* a book on trigger point therapy for horses.

1990: Protocol for fibromyalgia syndrome (FMS) is defined by the American College of Rheumatology. (People with FMS may have many trigger points involving large areas of the body.)

Description

High-intensity stimuli from active trigger areas can produce, by reflex, prolonged vasoconstriction with partial ischemia in areas of the brain, spinal cord, and peripheral nerve fibers, as well as in the muscles themselves. The spinal cord is facilitated because of abnormal sensory or afferent inputs. This keeps a trigger point area in a state of constant increased excitation. Stimuli that are normally ineffectual or subliminal have a major effect on the area, which in turn affects the trigger point, keeping it in a state of overactivity. Trigger points are very sensitive to pressure and will spasm with minimal pressure, cold air, or a sudden muscle stretch.

These areas are seen especially in neck, shoulders, and back muscles. Affected muscles feel tense and fibrotic and often, but not always, have active trigger points. Trigger points will amplify and be affected by any form of stress—physical, chemical, or emotional.

Signs of a trigger point are extreme pain or lameness, which is unaffected by steroids or non-steroidal anti-inflammatory drugs. Usually, the only relief is from narcotics. When a trigger point involves the neck, a dog will hold the neck rigid and may scream when touched. When it involves the shoulder, lameness is often profound and may cause severe muscle wasting. When it involves the back or hindquarters, a dog may suddenly be unable to rise. Radiographs usually show nothing.

Trigger points are most often seen in stressed muscles. Stress on muscles can be caused by the following:

- Postural imbalance (especially in amputees)
- Congenital factors (such as short legs or a front end lower than the hind end)
- Overuse (especially in agility dogs)
- Emotional states (especially in fearful dogs, dogs suffering from separation anxiety, or dogs who are chronically aggressive)
- Trauma

Other causes for trigger points include the following:

- Acute and chronic infections that stimulate sympathetic nerve activity
- Excessive heat or cold
- Changes in atmospheric pressure (especially before a storm)
- Drafts
- Mechanical injuries (both major injuries and minor microtraumas)
- Allergies
- Endocrine factors (especially hypothyroidism)

- Hypooxygenation of tissues (for example, from injuries)
- Inherited factors
- Arthritic changes
- Visceral diseases

Trigger points are enhanced by nutritional deficiencies, especially B complex, iron, and in humans, vitamin C. They are aggravated by tension, stress, and inactivity. The owner of a dog with trigger points is often apprehensive about the pet's condition. The dog may echo the owner's fears and develop worse problems.

In humans, there are two syndromes involving trigger points. The first, myofascial pain syndrome, has a few trigger points that refer primarily to one area, and its symptoms are primarily pain and decreased mobility. People with this syndrome respond well to trigger point therapy. Most dogs and cats fall into this category. In these cases, trigger points are usually unilateral.

The second syndrome, fibromyalgia (FMS), involves many more trigger points affecting large areas of the body. People with FMS also have sleep disturbances and depression. Although trigger point therapy helps this group somewhat, these people also need treatment with tricyclic antidepressants, some types of benzodiazepines, or herbal equivalents. Animal patients of this type do best when therapy is combined with other natural relaxants, such as Rescue Remedy or herbal therapies. In extreme cases, a drug such as clomipramine may be necessary. These patients often have bilateral trigger points.

In dogs, trigger points have been reported in the triceps, infraspinatus (at acupuncture points SI 10), quadriceps, pectineus (at LIV 10, 11), iliocostalis lumborum, peroneus longus (at GB 34), semitendinosus, semimembranosus, tensor fasciae latae, gluteus medius (at GB 30), paravertebral muscles, and the extensor carpi radialis (at LI 10). They can also be seen in the supraspinatus. They may initially be bilateral, but often, one side has a more pronounced trigger point than the other side. They may alternate after treatment, especially during the first two or three sessions.

To locate a trigger point, feel for tight muscles and feel gently for painful lumps within muscles. Tight muscles may feel almost like pieces of wood, especially when palpating paravertebral muscles. At first, one might feel only tight muscles without individual trigger points. In such a case, move the skin on top of the muscle without applying any pressure on the muscle. One of three things will happen:

- the muscle will begin to relax and a hard lump (the trigger point) will appear;
- one area of the muscle will become warmer than the rest (this is also a trigger point); or
- the patient will start to push against you, indicating that more pressure is needed. (In this case, feel up and down in the area; when the trigger point is reached, the patient will push against you. When the point is left, the patient relaxes. Some dogs brace themselves against the wall in order to increase the pressure as much as possible.)

Let the patient determine the pressure; don't automatically increase it until there is some indication to do so. If the patient moves away, tries to bite, or otherwise indicates displeasure, there is too much pressure. Continuing to press can cause the point to become worse instead of more relaxed.

When the point is located, there are a number of different ways to relieve the spasms. After treatment, a trigger point often flares up again. With repeated treatments and some local heat and massage at home, flare-ups become less severe and occur further apart in time. In addition, the trigger points become less sensitive to minor stimuli.

Methods of Relief

There are several methods of trigger point relief. One method is to place an acupuncture needle in the trigger point. This is usually done in three treatments, 1 week apart, for 5 minutes each. It is somewhat painful.

Another method is to inject 0.2–0.25% lidocaine, water, procaine, B vitamins, DMSO, or long-acting corticosteroids into the point. This is very painful.

Heavy pressure may be applied (20–30 pounds) with thumbs, elbows, or special equipment for 7 seconds. This will drop human patients to their knees, but it is a quick release. In this case, patients should immediately stretch the affected muscle (slowly).

Digital ischemic pressure may be applied. This is painful if done with heavy pressure, but is pleasurable if done with gradually increasing pressure (Conarton 2019).

Digital ischemic pressure is the only method a technician can use. If a specific trigger point cannot be located, but an entire area feels stiff and hard, treat the entire muscle. Start by moving the skin only, in gentle circles, over the entire area, using a featherlight touch. Along the back and neck, this is primarily in the paravertebral area. The neck usually has points around C2-3 and/or C6-7. For the shoulder, it is often dorsal and anterior to the scapular spine. Some dogs have problems in the middle of the triceps. If there is a hind leg problem, it is often in the gluteals or in the area of the semimembranosus and semitendinosus.

Gradually increase the pressure, up to 5 pounds of pressure, at most. If pressure increases too quickly at the beginning of treatment, a reflex spasm may occur and make things worse. The patient will let the practitioner know if there is too much pressure by ducking away, rolling over, or biting. If there is a sudden inrush of heat into the area, a spasm has just been relieved.

When the muscles loosen up, specific trigger points are felt. They will vary in size from the size of the end of a finger to the size of an egg. The same trigger point may be different sizes at different times. To treat the point, start the same way as when treating a whole area, but concentrate on the trigger point itself. In the areas of the neck and shoulder, pressure can be increased up to about 10 pounds, or more if the patient starts leaning into the finger. Pressure should be held on each point for a minimum of 30 seconds. Stop when the point melts away or decreases (though a human patient usually will ask for more).

Show the owner how to do this. It is often more effective when combined with local heat (before the treatment) from a heating pad or a heating device warmed in the microwave.

When a patient has severe pain, treatment should be done at least twice a day until the pain stays away. A single treatment may only require 5 minutes to provide full relief of the spasm. Acupuncture can also help, especially with a "surround the dragon" pattern. Best results are achieved when acupuncture is combined with this technique, with the acupuncture following the trigger point therapy.

Chronic trigger points will return, especially in the beginning of treatment, but they will not be as extreme. Trigger points will also go away more easily and stay away longer, until relief lasts for many weeks or months. Warn an owner that trigger points may come back, but if the owner immediately starts therapy at home, he or she may be able to avoid another veterinary visit.

Veterinarian's Role

In most states, only veterinarians can use injections to treat a trigger point. Only a veterinarian or licensed acupuncturist can use acupuncture needles to treat a trigger point. Only a veterinarian may make the diagnosis, but once a problem has been identified, a technician can treat trigger points with massage or manual release techniques.

Technician's Role

In a physical therapy facility, this is one aspect of muscle therapy that can be performed by a technician.

Where to Learn How

Trigger point therapy may be included in a physical therapy certification course or a massage therapy course. (See those sections for specific courses.)

Summary

What can a technician do?

1) See if you can find a place where you can get hands-on training. If not, and you have a problem with painful trigger points, pay attention to the massage therapist who is treating you to get an idea of how to locate the points and how to massage them.
2) Books are very helpful for learning this procedure, especially if you or a friend have trigger points.
3) If it fits within the practice, trigger point therapy is an ideal addition to other methods of pain relief, such as acupuncture. The technician cannot use injections or acupuncture needles to relieve a trigger point but can use massage therapy.

Reiki A Mind-Body Connection

Definition

Reiki is also called a form of energy work. It can be applied both by laying hands on the patient and also by holding the hands over the patient and moving them in specific patterns. It is used to reduce stress and to induce relaxation and thus help healing.

Reiki is not a religion or belief system. There are a number of forms of Reiki, and the original is known as Usui Reiki, after its original founder, Dr. Usui. Other forms were developed by subsequent practitioners, including some in the United States.

Purpose

In veterinary medicine, one of the primary ways it can be used is for stress reduction for anxious patients.

History

- 1914: Reiki is first developed by Dr. Mikao Usui, a Japanese philosopher and Christian seminary educator.
- 1915: *Kenzen no Genri* (Health Principles), written by Dr. Bizan Suzuki and published in March 1915, contains the Reiki ideals.
- 1925: Dr. Hayashi develops a system of more complex hand positions, with specific positions for specific conditions. He also simplifies the attunement process.

- 1937: Takata-style Reiki is developed by Hawayo Takata, adding a foundation treatment (four positions on the abdomen and three or four positions on the head, with a few others for the back).
- 1989: Karuna Reiki system is developed by William Rand.

It is widely stated that the Reiki principles were adapted from the five principles of the Meiji emperor Mutsuhito. Dr. Usui did admire the emperor and included 125 of the emperor's *waka* (poems) in his Reiki handbook. However, there are no "five principles" that closely match Dr. Usui's Reiki ideals. The *Imperial Rescript on Education* (1890) contains the emperor's most important edict on moral education, but it does not enumerate five principles. The following quote appeared in *Kenzen no Genri* by Dr. Bizan Suzuki: "Just for today, do not anger (others), do not fear, work hard, be honest, and be kind to others." (This is almost an exact quote of the Reiki Ideals presented below.)

Later versions of Reiki were much more organized and structured. Dr. Hayashi, a physician who was attuned by Dr. Usui in 1925, developed a system of more complex hand positions, with specific positions for specific conditions. He also simplified the attunement process.

Hawayo Takata, born in Hawaii, traveled to Japan after the death of her sister. She did so to tell her parents of her sister's death and to seek treatment for her own illnesses. She received treatment at Dr. Hayashi's clinic and then received Reiki attunement from him. In 1937, she was finally initiated as a Reiki master by him after both Dr. Hayashi and Mrs. Takata moved to Hawaii.

Mrs. Takata added a foundation treatment (four positions on the abdomen and three or four positions on the head, with a few others for the back; Streich, 2007). These additions are the Takata-style Reiki.

Dr. Hayashi also gave Reiki training to Mrs. Yamaguchi. William Rand received his Reiki I and II training from Mrs. Yamaguchi and his Reiki master training from five Reiki masters. Rand developed the Karuna Reiki system of training and has authored several books. He is editor-in-chief of the Reiki News Magazine.

Reiki is believed by some to date back to early Tibetan healing practices. Some web sites connect it to Buddhism. However, Dr. Usui, in his *Reiki Ryoho Handbook*, says, "our Reiki Ryoho is something absolutely original and cannot be compared with any other (spiritual) path in the world" (Usui, 1925).

Description

The "ki" in Reiki refers to the body's *ki* (Japanese), known as *qi* in Chinese medicine, and is roughly translated as life force or life energy. "Rei" has a number of different meanings in Japanese, among them, a higher power, but also one's own soul. So the word *Reiki* can be interpreted as helping the flow of one's own ki, and it can also incorporate the idea of a higher power as the giver of the ki, or of this method. In Oriental medicine, when we are mentally and physically healthy, ki flows freely in the body. One cause of illness is a decrease or blockage of this flow. There are several types of ki. They can be depleted by environmental factors such as poor nutrition, as well as by disease. Some can be renewed. All can be blocked. Reiki aims to restore the flow and the amount of ki in the body. It does so in a way that does not deplete the ki of the Reiki practitioner.

Because Reiki treats both mental and physical well-being, it is ideal for treating agitated animals. Anxiety can interfere with the examination of a patient, but it can also delay healing. Humans who have had a Reiki treatment often feel warmth where the hands of the practitioner have been placed. Humans report feelings of peace and security, as well.

The ability to use Reiki is transferred from one person to another by a method known as "attunement," given by a Reiki master during a Reiki class. This attunement allows the student to tap into a universal source of ki, and this is why it does not deplete the practitioner.

Usui Reiki also encourages Reiki practitioners to use the Reiki ideals to aid spiritual balance in the practitioner. These are translated in various ways, but basically they state:

Just for today:
Do not anger.
Do not worry.
Be filled with gratitude
Devote yourself to your work.
Be kind to people.

Dr. Usui suggested that practitioners pray and chant these words twice a day. Sometimes, this is misconstrued as meaning that Reiki is a religion, but practitioners emphasize that it is merely an energy technique that can be used with any religion and with any other healing modality.

Reiki is characterized by always being helpful. As a means of restoring harmony and flow, it does not concentrate on what is wrong; instead, it concentrates on making things right. Therefore, the practitioner is not concentrating on anything bad and is not in danger of acquiring bad attitudes from the patient. Because it is a natural force, it will flow where it should flow and correct imbalances.

Most people teach that there are no side effects. However, William Rand states that some people will have a healing crisis, resulting in a headache, feeling of weakness, or stomach ache. In such a case, it is recommended that the person eat less and drink more fluid. This is basically a detoxification reaction. It has not been reported in animals.

There has not been much research on Reiki. However, a research project has shown interesting results. It tested three groups: one treated with Reiki and rest, a second with sham Reiki (given by those without any training) and rest, and a third with rest only. Those treated with Reiki and rest had significant reductions in diastolic blood pressure and heart rate compared with the other two groups (Mackay et al., 2004).

Also, a systematic review of touch therapy research articles showed its help in pain relief (So et al., 2008).

Veterinarian's Role

Some veterinarians are trained in Reiki and can administer a treatment themselves. However, this is rather time consuming and is an area in which a veterinary technician or nurse can play an effective part.

Technician's Role

The technician can use Reiki to good effect to calm patients before an office visit and when they are hospitalized. It is especially good for cats, who are very receptive to it.

Where to Learn How

Animal Reiki Source
https://animalreikisource.com/animal-reiki-source-academy/

Summary

What can the technician do?

1) Technicians can legally perform Reiki. Find a Reiki master whom you like and get your attunement. Attunement works best when you resonate with a practitioner.
2) Discuss how best to incorporate your training in the practice where you work. Reiki can be used in the hospital and at a client's home.

References

Conarton, L. 2019. Myofascial Trigger Points in Veterinary Patients. Accessed online on 6/27/2023 at https://todaysveterinarynurse.com/rehabilitation/myofascial-trigger-points-in-veterinary-patients/.

Halliday R.J. 1997. An outline of the history of acupuncture. In: Weber, V., ed. *Veterinary Acupuncture Course Notes*, 6th edition. Fort Collins, CO: IVAS.

Mackay N., et al. 2004. Autonomic nervous system changes during Reiki treatment: a preliminary study. *J Altern Complement Med* 10(6):1077–1081.

Shumway R. 2007. Rehabilitation in the first 48 hours after surgery. *Clin Tech Small Anim Pract* 22(4):166–170.

So P.S., et al. 2008. Touch therapies for pain relief in adults. *Cochrane Database Syst Rev* (4) CD006535.

Streich, M. 2007. How Hawayo Takata practiced and taught Reiki. *Reiki News Magazine* 6(1):10–18. Accessed online on 9/23/10 at https://www.reiki.org/sites/default/files/resource-files/TakataArticle.pdf

Ullmann G., et al. 2010. Effects of Feldenkrais exercises on balance, mobility, balance confidence, and gait performance in community-dwelling adults age 65 and older. *J Altern Complement Med* 16(1):97–105.

Usui, 1925. *Reiki Ryoho Handbook*. Handwritten for students, page 2 and 3. Translated by Richard Rivard and others, 2007. Karen Frazier. Accessed online on 9/24/2010 at https://threshold.ca/reiki/Handouts/Threshold-Reiki-Usui-Reiki-Hikkei.pdf.

Bibliography

General Massage

Horses

Blignault K. 2003. *Stretch Exercises for Your Horse: The Path to Perfect Suppleness*. North Pomfret, VT: Trafalgar Square Books.

Hourdebaigt J.-P. 2007. *Equine Massage: A Practical Guide*, 2nd edition. Ames, IA: Howell Book House.

Meagher J. 1985. *Beating Muscle Injuries for Horses: 25 Common Muscular Problems, their Cause, Correction, Prevention*. Port Townsend, WA: Hamilton Horse Associates.

Pailloux J.-P. 2001. *Physical Therapy and Massage for the Horse*. North Pomfret, VT: Trafalgar Square Books.

Dogs

Ballner M. 2001. *Dog Massage: A Whiskers-to-Tail Guide to Your Dog's Ultimate Petting Experience*. New York: St. Martin's Griffin.

Fox M.W. *The Healing Touch for Dogs: The Proven Massage Program for Dogs*, rev. edition. New York: Newmarket Press.

Hourdebaigt J.-P. 2003. *Canine Massage: A Complete Reference Manual*. Wenatchee, WA: Dogwise Publishing.

Acupressure

Schwartz C. 1996. *Four Paws, Five Directions*. Berkeley, CA: Celestial Arts.

Seem M. 1993. *A New American Acupuncture*. Boulder, CO: Blue Poppy Press.

Shiatsu

Meeus C. 2000. *Secrets of Shiatsu*. New York: Dorling Kindersley Publishing Inc.

Namikoshi T. 1981. *The Complete Book of Shiatsu Therapy*. Tokyo: Japan Publications, Inc.

Schultz W. 1976. *Shiatsu*. New York: Bell Publishing Co.

Trigger Point Therapy

Chaitow L. 1998. *Soft-tissue Manipulation: A Practitioner's Guide to the Diagnosis and Treatment of Soft Tissue Dysfunction and Reflex Activity*. Rochester, VT: Healing Arts Press.

Janssens L. 1991. Trigger points in 48 dogs with myofascial pain syndrome. *Vet Surgery* 20:274–278.

Janssens L. 2001. Trigger point therapy. In: Schoen A., *Veterinary Acupuncture, Ancient Art to Modern Medicine*, 2nd edition. St. Louis, MO: Mosby Publications.

Meagher J. 1985. *Beating Muscle Injuries for Horses*. New York: Dolphin Books.

Prudden B. 1980. *Pain Erasure: The Bonnie Prudden Way*. New York: M Evans.

Prudden B. 1984. *Myotherapy: Bonnie Prudden's Complete Guide to Pain Free Living*. New York: Dial Press.

Robinson N. 2001. Acupuncture and manipulative therapy: a perfect marriage. In: Schoen A., *Veterinary Acupuncture, Ancient Art to Modern Medicine*, 2nd edition. St. Louis, MO: Mosby Publications.

Travell J. and Simons D. 1983. *The Trigger Point Manual*. Baltimore, MD: Williams and Wilkins.

TTouch

Tellington-Jones L. 2000. *Improve Your Horse's Well-Being (A Step-by-Step Guide to TTouch and TTeam Training.)* North Pomfret, VT: Trafalgar Square Books.

Tellington-Jones L. 2001. *Getting in TTouch With your Dog*. North Pomfret, VT: Trafalgar Square Books.

Tellington-Jones L. 2003. *Getting in TTouch With your Cat*. North Pomfret, VT: Trafalgar Square Books.

Tellington-Jones L. 2007. *Getting in TTouch with Your Puppy: A Gentle Approach to Training and Influencing Behavior*. North Pomfret, VT: Trafalgar Square Books.

Tellington-Jones L. and Taylor S. 1995. *The Tellington TTouch: A Revolutionary Natural Method to Train and Care for Your Favorite Animal*. New York: Penguin.

Tellington-Jones L. and Taylor S. 1995. *Getting in Touch: Understand and Influence Your Horse's Personality*. North Pomfret, VT: Trafalgar Square Books.

Tui-Na

Mercati M. 1997. *The Handbook of Chinese Massage*. Rochester, VT: Healing Arts Press.

Reiki

Coates M. 2003. *Hands-On Healing for Pets: The Animal Lover's Essential Guide to Using Healing Energy*. United Kingdom: Random House UK.

Fulton E. and Prasad K. 2020. *Animal Reiki: Using Energy to Heal the Animals in Your Life*. Berkeley, CA: Ulysses Press.

Malone HR, Malone M. 2020. *Animal Reiki Master Teacher Manual: Everything You Need to Know to Practice Animal Reiki on Your Pets and Animals*. Independently Published

Prasad K. 2009. *The Animal Reiki Handbook—Finding Your Way With Reiki in Your Local Shelter, Sanctuary, or Rescue*. San Rafael, CA: Shelter Animal Reiki Association.

Rand W. 1991. *Reiki, The Healing Touch*. Southfield, MI: Vision Publications.

Webliography

International Association of Animal Massage & Bodywork
https://iaamb.org/about/
Association founded as a forum for animal massage and bodywork professionals to network and support each other.
https://www.youtube.com/watch?v=CeHMjfnfc_E
YouTube video on information about International Association of Animal Massage & Bodywork

Petmassage, Ltd.
https://www.petmassage.com/
Training, articles, and research on pet massage.

Trigger Point Therapy

(See also the sections on massage therapy and physical therapy.)
National Association of Myofascial Trigger Point Therapists
https://www.myofascialtherapy.org/
Web site specifically about myofascial release.

The Bodyworker.com
https://www.thebodyworker.com/triggerpoint.htm
Information for trigger points, but the site has other methods of bodywork in addition to trigger point therapy.

Reiki

National Center for Complementary and Alternative Medicine, a subsidiary of the National Institutes of Health
https://nccam.nih.gov/health/reiki/
The government's perspective on Reiki.

ReikiOne.com
https://www.reikione.com/
Information and resources for Reiki practitioners.

Reiki for Animals

Animal Reiki Source
https://www.animalreikisource.com/
Education in animal Reiki.

Margrit Coates, the Animal Healer
http://www.margritcoates.com/
Web site of an animal Reiki practitioner and animal communicator.

7

Detoxification and Fasting

Description

All beings accumulate waste products and toxic by-products in their systems as a consequence of what they eat and what they are exposed to. Even if we are never exposed to toxic chemicals, some of the breakdown products of foods (e.g., proteins) form potentially dangerous substances, such as ammonia and urea. The digestive system and urinary system are good at excreting water-soluble substances. If the waste products are the right size and shape, they will exit the body immediately, through the kidney or the bile. If not, they are broken down and transformed by the liver until they can leave.

We are used to looking at the kidney as the primary excreter of waste products. However, the liver is the organ responsible for removing and transforming most potentially harmful substances from the blood. The liver turns leftovers from body functions, such as cell waste products and unneeded hormones, into soluble substances that pass out of the body. The liver is also the organ that processes fat-soluble items.

If the liver can't immediately process waste products because it is overloaded by large concentrations of substances, these products are stored in the fat and in interstitial spaces in the body. Some livers are able to rapidly process the waste, and very little accumulates. Other livers are much less efficient, or they may be exposed to high concentrations of toxins, resulting in an excess of waste (toxins). When too many toxins accumulate, they will remain circulating in the bloodstream. If there is a high concentration in the bloodstream, these products can cause damage to cells and tissues, and may cause syndromes such as chronic fatigue disease. For example, for those exposed to the chemical Agent Orange, it may cause a number of separate diseases linked to that chemical exposure. The process of helping the body get rid of these products is called detoxification (detox). (See Figure 7.1.) A fast supported by supplements that help the liver deal with toxic substances is part of the detox process.

Currently, most natural diets tend to be high in protein, mimicking the diet of a wolf or wild cat on their best hunting days. However, especially in the case of wolves, this ignores normal periods of fasting after a big hunt or during the winter when prey is scarce. Fasting is a normal part of the canine diet and is a natural method of detoxification.

Complementary Medicine for Veterinary Technicians and Nurses, Second Edition. Nancy Scanlan.
© 2024 John Wiley & Sons, Inc. Published 2024 by John Wiley & Sons, Inc.

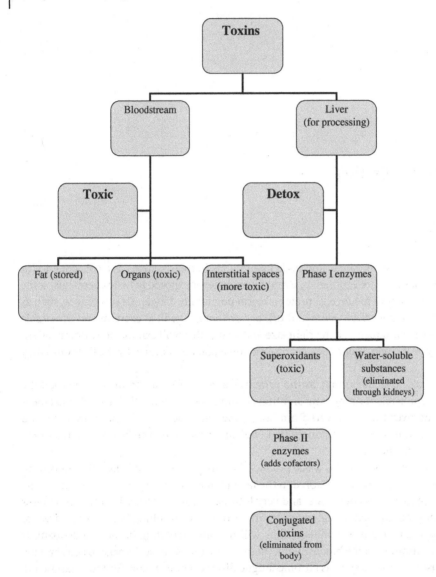

Figure 7.1 Detox occurs through the liver. When a body is toxic, there is a backup of toxins, either in the bloodstream or before or after a toxin is processed by phase I enzymes in the liver.

Purpose

Even if a patient is not drastically affected by high levels of toxins or metabolic by-products, detoxification can help get rid of substances that interfere with daily cellular reactions. At its best, it can cause dramatic changes in animals who have problems healing, who have low energy levels, who seem to be aging prematurely, or who get frequent infections.

Chronic conditions, including chronic fatigue, diarrhea, and skin problems, can often be helped by detoxification.

Detoxifying should be done no more than 3 days in a row if the patient's status is not known. Severely toxic patients may do best if they are treated for only one day, at intervals varying from once a week to once a month.

When to Detoxify

We can assume that there has been a toxin buildup in any animals on prolonged drug or antiparasite treatments, in those who have had chronic diarrhea, or as part of the aging process. To get rid of the toxins, we need to detoxify the body.

When a patient is toxic, fatigue is most noticeable. In addition, the animal can't fight off infections well. The skin looks bad. Digestion isn't normal. Bad breath is common, often accompanied by a lot of tartar on the teeth. Sometimes, there will be sores in the mouth.

The detoxification process, or "detox," is occurring at all times in the bodies of animal companions and their guardians. Detox consists of all the processes needed to neutralize toxins and waste products and pass them out of the body. In a perfect world, we wouldn't notice detoxification at all because there would never be a time when we have an excess of waste or toxins in our bloodstream. However, there is often a toxin buildup of which we are unaware. For most animals, inducing detoxification can be helpful in maintaining health. For some, it can be a primary key to restoring health.

Even though an animal companion may be getting all the recommended requirements of vitamins, minerals, antioxidants, amino acids, and other nutrients, there may still not be enough of these elements for all the toxins the liver needs to process.

There can be a natural detox overreaction, as well (called *toxic detox*). This can happen if nutrition is upgraded, especially by increasing antioxidants and decreasing fat and protein. A pet may react with diarrhea or, less commonly, vomiting, until the excess toxins have been eliminated from the body. If an animal is unhealthy, overloaded with toxins, or has lower than normal amounts of liver enzymes needed to process toxins, detox can be rather unpleasant and may even cause illness, including liver inflammation.

Avoiding Toxic Detox

By supplying everything the body needs as cofactors for detoxification, minimizing protein breakdown, minimizing the ingestion of anything that can turn toxic, and changing to a gentler detoxification method if a problem arises, one can minimize the chance of toxic detox.

History

The concept of fasting for purification appears in the Bible; the idea of detoxification is a more recent development. In 1993, the Institute for Functional Medicine was founded by Jeffrey Bland. The institute promotes research and seminars on degenerative diseases and their treatment, including specialized laboratory tests, detoxification, and nutraceuticals.

Currently, intermittent fasting and timed feeding have been promoted as an anti-aging method, and as a way to lose weight. For humans, intermittent fasting consists of spacing periods of very low caloric intake (400–500 kilocalories) with normal intake of food. A common proportion is 6 : 1 or 5 : 2 (6 days of a normal diet followed by 1 day of food supplying 400 calories, or 5 days of a normal diet followed by 2 days of food supplying 500 calories). Research has shown benefits for humans who have used intermittent fasting and timed feeding. Healthy participants have benefitted from increased SIRT3, the primary mitochondrial protein deacetylase in the mitochondria. Several studies have suggested a role for SIRT3 in protecting against oxidative stress. In mice, chronic low-calorie diets have increased lifespan, and intermittent fasting showed improvements in levels of adenosine triphosphate, nicotinamide adenine dinucleotide phosphate (NADP), reduced NADP and succinate, involved in the citric acid cycle and oxidative phosphorylation.

Detox combines low-calorie intake with supplements used by the liver when processing waste products.

How It Works

What Are Toxins and Where Do They Come From?

A toxin is anything that does not have a healthy function in the body. Toxins may simply slow down normal functions (causing headaches, sleepiness, lethargy, etc.) or they may actually cause cell damage. Strictly speaking, they are substances that have a bad effect on the body, although they may be part of normal metabolic processes. For example, ammonia is formed when protein is used for energy instead of for building muscles, cell walls, or enzymes. Lactic acid is formed during anaerobic exercise. Normally, the body can process these substances, but too much ammonia is poisonous and too much lactic acid can literally pickle muscles. (We see this problem in tying up syndrome in horses.) Toxins can be both internal (endotoxins in Table 7.1) and external (exotoxins in Table 7.2) and may come from many sources.

How do these substances cause trouble? It happens during the process of digestion. A few substances such as sugar can enter the bloodstream directly through the tissues of the mouth, but most food goes down to the stomach, where it mixes with hydrochloric acid and some stomach enzymes. In some animals, not enough acid is produced. This means the first enzymes don't work as well, and some proteins may not be broken down.

Table 7.1 Sources of endotoxins.

- From food (during normal metabolic processes)
- From metabolic processes (such as the production of ammonia and lactic acid and even as a result of part of the detoxification process)
- From bacteria in the intestinal tract, which may form some unhealthy waste products
- From substances absorbed by an unhealthy intestinal system (found with chronic diarrhea or IBD), usually partially digested food that would not normally cross the intestinal barrier into the blood. They may be present even if the stools look normal.

Table 7.2 Sources of exotoxins.

- From food (indirectly; fats and oils absorb toxic chemicals such as insecticides, which are carried into the body when we ingest them)
- From food additives (artificial flavors, colors, and preservatives, as well as other chemicals designed to improve perceived food qualities)
- From food containers (such as the plastic linings of some cans, which have goitrogenic chemicals)
- From insecticides (used to kill fleas and ticks)
- From drugs, including anesthetics (Many drugs are processed by the liver, and although they can be life-saving, they can have various side effects that reflect their actions in the body. We regularly see this as liver or kidney problems with certain drugs.)
- From other toxic substances (such as exposure to paint fumes, lawn and garden chemicals, cleaning supplies, etc.)
- From too much of some foods (The movie *Supersize Me* graphically illustrates this; a strict diet of fast food resulted in elevated liver enzymes in just a few weeks.)

Next, the food leaves the stomach and goes to the small intestine. If there aren't enough enzymes at this juncture, perhaps from an unhealthy pancreas or small intestine, food won't be broken down properly and the wrong breakdown products may be absorbed.

The normal intestine forms a barrier to undigested food, absorbing only the properly digested parts that the body can use. If the intestine is unhealthy, perhaps because of diarrhea or an overgrowth of abnormal bacteria, partly broken-down proteins can be absorbed, causing allergic reactions. Unusable bits can be absorbed, causing inflammation and an increased burden on the liver, which has to process these substances further.

One additional problem is enterohepatic circulation: processed substances leave the liver via the bile, which is dumped into the intestine. These substances may be reabsorbed, entering the bloodstream and then going to the liver and ending up in the recycling process again. This is another item that adds to the burden of the liver and the toxic load in the bloodstream.

Normal Liver Metabolism

The liver has many functions, which may be grouped into the following four categories:

1) Digestion (production of bile, processing lipids, production and breakdown of glycogen)
2) Nitrogen excretion (converting ammonia that comes from amino acid breakdown into urea)
3) Regulation of water distribution in the body (by producing albumin)
4) Detoxification of endogenous and exogenous toxins

Digestion, nitrogen excretion, and detoxification all use the same two detoxification enzyme systems: phase I and phase II enzymes. Detox is primarily concerned with the last function. In a healthy individual, the toxic products listed above are primarily processed by the two sets of enzymes and then passed out to the bile duct to be excreted in the feces or into the blood to be excreted by the kidneys. In addition, antioxidants are used by the body to help minimize side effects from the breakdown. As long as there are normal amounts and ratios of enzymes, antioxidants, and cofactors, and as long as the exposure to toxins is minimal, there is no toxic buildup and the individual and the liver stays healthy.

Because everything processed by the liver shares the same enzymes, an excess of food or an excess of normal body chemicals can act as toxins in the detox process. With so many different things using the same two procedures, it's easy to get a backup in the system.

As living beings get older, there comes a time sooner or later when there are so many things for the liver to process that it falls behind in its detoxification job. Toxins, garbage, and normal waste products all compete for the liver's attention.

How Toxins Are Normally Handled

Although some other parts of the body share some of the liver's enzymes, the liver is the main organ of detoxification. The two enzyme systems that act on toxic chemicals, called phase I and phase II systems, accomplish two steps in this process. Phase I is also known as the cytochrome p450 system, which is involved in oxidation–reduction reactions. There are a number of cytochrome P450 enzymes, each of which has an iron molecule in its active part. The enzymes act on a broad variety of substances, and they need various cofactors in order to function properly. The action of the enzymes is, generally, either to add a charged oxygen atom or to perform any other action that will create a free radical "handle" (such as removing hydrogen or methyl groups, adding epoxide rings or an alcoholic hydroxyl group, or by splitting or rear-ranging molecules).

These actions attack thousands of different types of toxic molecules and often render them less toxic. The resulting handle is highly reactive. Phase I transforms the substance so it will dissolve more easily in water or combine more easily with other substances. If it dissolves in water, it is flushed out of the kidneys. If not, the substance is processed further by phase II enzymes.

Induction (increased action) of phase I enzymes can occur if there is a toxic overload. Some natural substances that also increase phase I activity include the following:

- Antioxidants
- Iron
- Molybdenum
- Magnesium

This results in the overproduction of free radicals. There may not be enough phase II enzymes to handle the excess free radicals, and they can build up to a harmful level. Antioxidants are heavily used to stabilize free radicals produced in phase I, and they may be robbed from other parts of the body to help the liver (or vice versa). Any animal can become deficient in antioxidants if phase I is overstimulated.

Phase II is a conjugating system that uses the "handle" on products that have been through the phase I system to add other molecules or cofactors to the products to make them more water-soluble and less reactive. This makes these products even less toxic and helps them be eliminated through bile (which goes to the intestinal tract) and through urine (via the kidneys). Phase II enzymes *cannot* be induced to work at a higher level, so they can never catch up if phase I enzymes are induced to be more active.

Because the molecules from phase I are so highly reactive, if the phase II enzymes are too busy to handle them, or if there are not enough cofactors for phase II enzymes to add to them, the molecules may oxidize healthy tissue. This can result in damaged tissues and rancid fats in the body. In addition, sometimes the phase I reaction makes a product that is much worse than the original. I call these "supertoxins." For example, this happens with aflatoxin (found in moldy foods), which is transformed by phase I enzymes to a highly mutagenic form. Glutathione is the substance that phase II enzymes in most animals (but not the cat) add to it, but if the transformed aflatoxin escapes before glutathione is attached, the chemical attaches directly to the DNA of the liver. This can cause the cells to become cancerous. In humans, aflatoxin is one of the major causes of liver cancer.

Detoxification Problems

If either of the liver phases is slowed down or overloaded, toxic detox signs may appear. (See Table 7.3.) Not all animals are born with enough enzymes to easily process toxins. Some animals have an overabundance of phase I and phase II enzymes. These are the animals who can eat an incredible number of horrid things, including bird feathers, wool sweaters, tissues, and other pseudofood items and never feel a thing. (The human equivalents never get hangovers.)

Animals with low levels of both phase I and phase II enzymes will not be able to process toxins as quickly, and these toxins can build up in the body. Pets who are low on phase I enzymes, but normal on phase II enzymes often show the same signs as the animal companions who are low on both phase I and II enzymes.

Pets with high amounts of phase I enzymes and low amounts of phase II enzymes may become even more toxic as the pro-oxidant by-products of phase I reactions build up in their bodies.

Table 7.3 Causes of toxic detoxification.

	Quick detox		Slow detox			Toxic detox			
Low levels of toxins	X	X				X			
Moderate levels of toxins	X	X	X	X		X	X		
High levels of toxins					X	X	X		X
Low levels phase I enzymes		X	X						
Normal levels phase I enzymes				X	X		X		
High levels phase I enzymes	X					X			X
Low levels phase II enzymes		X		X			X	X	X
Normal levels phase II enzymes			X		X	X			X
High levels phase II enzymes	X								

Note: Lack of nutrients needed by the enzymes will have the same effect as a low level of those enzymes. Placement of the X indicates how much the substance contributes to the problem.

When they are deficient in both phase I and phase II enzymes, the whole process is slowed down. For instance, some kittens and puppies appear to be healthy as babies, but as they get older, they react to everything with lethargy and vomiting or diarrhea, whereas their littermates have no such reactions. These animals eventually process things through and feel better again. With enough time, they even get overloaded from their own bodily substances, reacting with a loss of energy and constant low-level infections such as respiratory diseases or diarrhea. At this stage, any extra toxins, such as insecticides or preservatives, can send them over the edge, creating a very sick pet. (Some people with all the signs of chronic fatigue syndrome actually have low levels of both phase I and phase II liver enzymes and an elevated toxin level.)

When the two systems are overloaded, the toxic chemicals pile up and make an animal sick. When there are more substances to be processed than there are enzymes to process them, a backup occurs and toxins flow into the bloodstream. At first, those toxins are stored in fat. Later, when fat depots are filled, these substances go into interstitial spaces, where they can damage neighboring cells. Finally, if these depots are filled, toxins stay in the bloodstream and circulate, continuing to damage body parts until they finally exit through the liver or kidney.

In addition, when there are enough toxins nearby or in the bloodstream and accelerating amounts of toxins spill into the blood, other parts of the body start breaking down. Mitochondria in the body's cells produce chemical fuel (ATP) on which animal cells operate. Mitochondria are six to seven times as sensitive to toxins and lack of antioxidants as cells as a whole. With antioxidants used up by excess phase I action and too many toxins floating around, the mitochondria produce less and less fuel. With less fuel, the liver and kidneys don't work as well, and toxins back up even faster.

Other tissues that need lots of fuel also suffer. This is when we start seeing signs relating to the heart, muscle, and brain, in addition to the liver, kidney, and intestine. Normally, when extra energy is needed, mitochondria multiply. The sick mitochondria try to do so but are so damaged that they don't multiply very rapidly, and when they do, their offspring are sick and damaged and can't do their job. The DNA of the mitochondria becomes defective and will produce only other defective mitochondria. Mitochondrial DNA is passed through mitochondria, not the nuclei of cells, so a cell with damaged mitochondrial DNA will always produce other cells with damaged mitochondrial DNA, even if the cell nucleus is undamaged. Affected mitochondria may die within the cell. Some nutrients can help prevent mitochondrial damage.

Nutrients needed by mitochondria include the following:

- Vitamin E
- CoQ 10
- Niacin
- B complex
- Carnitine

Overload can happen in a number of ways (see also Table 7.4):

- An animal is born with an insufficient level of both phase I and phase II enzymes (toxic items build up in the body).
- An animal is born with enough phase II, but not enough phase I enzymes (toxic items build up in the body).
- There is a higher level of phase I enzymes compared to phase II enzymes (either naturally or by induction of phase I enzymes, so toxic oxidized items build up in the body).
- There is an overload of toxic material, for example, from chocolate poisoning, in dogs who eat an entire bottle of liver-flavored NSAIDs, or in cats given Tylenol (all toxic items, and oxidized toxic items build up in the body).
- Liver disease decreases the ability of the liver to detoxify (both toxic items and oxidized toxic items build up in the body).
- There is an increased load on the liver from normal items in the diet.

When toxic overload occurs, eventually enough wastes can build up in the body to cause fatigue, skin problems, stomach problems, intestinal problems, or, at the worst, poisoning from overwhelming toxin buildup. From the mildest problems to the most severe, an animal may actually be in a toxic state, although this is not easy to determine from ordinary blood tests. If a blood panel shows normal values, the practitioner may assume everything is okay. The problem is that the panel is a static picture. It doesn't point out minor problems or how well organs are doing their jobs; it just indicates whether organs are severely damaged. To know how well they are working, functional tests are needed. There are very few functional tests available for animals and none is able to check phase I and phase II enzymes.

Almost anything an animal eats can contribute to the toxic state, though there are some foods that are worse than others: saturated fats from grain-finished animals and a very high-protein diet; some vitamins, especially niacin and riboflavin; some fruits, especially citrus and star fruit; and

Table 7.4 Liver enzyme overload and results in the body.

Overload Type	Result
Naturally low levels of both enzyme systems	Toxic items build up in the body.
Enough phase II, not enough phase I	Toxic items build up in the body.
Higher level of phase I vs. phase II enzymes	Toxic oxidized items build up.
Overload of toxic material	Both toxic items and oxidized toxic items build up.
Liver disease	Both toxic items and oxidized toxic items build up.

Table 7.5   Items that increase the load on the liver.

• Saturated fats	• Star fruit
• High protein diet	• Sassafras
• Niacin	• Pau d'arco
• Riboflavin	• Comfrey
• Citrus	• Pennyroyal

some herbs, such as sassafras. Any herb that is recommended for use in small amounts only or for short periods of time only, also has the potential to cause a toxic condition (see Table 7.5).

The feline liver itself engages in a little self-sabotage; cat livers are deficient in several phase II enzymes that dogs and humans use, including the one for the most important pathway: glucuronidation (using phenol UDP-glucuronosyltransferase (UGT) enzymes, including UGT1A6 and UGT1A9). That is why giving one whole acetaminophen tablet (such as Tylenol) to a 10-pound dog can make it a little sick, while doing the same for a 10-pound cat can kill the cat. This also explains why some drugs commonly given to dogs are either given to cats at a much lower dose and others are never given. Cats require saturated fats and a high-protein diet, which also stimulates the liver to increase their phase I enzymes. Complete fasts will decrease protein processing quite a bit for dogs and humans But feline livers never decrease phase I enzyme activities that deal with proteins. Thus, a complete fast in a cat will not decrease toxic by-products associated with protein breakdown, and it will increase protein loss from muscles. However, even dogs and humans need some protein in their diet daily, and to get it, their bodies will break down their own muscle tissue for protein if needed. Cats will do this even faster.

There are natural defenses against toxins. One way to minimize toxins is to make sure we keep ourselves and our companions healthy so they can use these defense systems. Another way is to minimize the number of chemicals we're exposed to. A natural diet without artificial flavors, colors, preservatives, or items that aren't easily digested, can obviously help. Vitamins, minerals, herbs, and other natural remedies can also help minimize the bad effects.

Lab Tests

How can we tell if an animal companion is a candidate for fasting? Unfortunately, normal lab tests show only when an organ has been damaged, not when it's in the very early stages of illness, overload, of dysfunction. Liver tests show elevated liver enzymes after liver cells die or become inflamed and release the enzymes into the bloodstream. They are useful when an animal has a high overload of toxins, but they will not show how a liver is working. To know about the phase enzymes, a test is needed to show how the liver is functioning.

For humans, the Great Smokies Diagnostic Laboratory has a test that measures SNPs to check gene phenotype and activity for the genes involved in Phase I and Phase II liver enzymes. This is the most direct way of seeing how a human liver is set up for these reactions. There is nothing similar for dogs or cats. (There are very few tests for any animal SNPs for any genetic problem.)

How Detoxification Works

There are three methods used to decrease toxin overload: fasting in some form, herbs (often with nutraceuticals), and homeopathy. If done properly, they will help the situation. If done improperly, they can make things worse. For example, if an relatively healthy obese cat fasts for more than

Table 7.6 Supplements and herbs used for liver support.

• Antioxidants in general	• Milk thistle
• Bioflavonoids	• Pycnogenol
• Carotenoids	• Selenium
• Copper	• Superoxide dismutase
• Co-Q10	• Vitamin A
• Cruciferous vegetables	• Vitamin C
• Lipotropic factors	• Vitamin E
• Manganese	• Zinc

Table 7.7 Items used by the liver in phase I.

Bioflavonoids
Cyanocobalamin (B_{12})
Folic acid
Glutathione
Niacin (B_3)
Pyridoxine (B_6)
Riboflavin (B_2)

3 days, there is a great danger that it will suffer from hepatic lipidosis (a type of liver toxicity in which much of the liver tissue is replaced by fat). This can be deadly, so it is important that detoxification be done correctly. For obese cats who also have other health problems, the risk is even greater, and they should not go through a full 3-day fast.

To get rid of toxins the fastest, we can minimize by-products of digestion and decrease waste products by fasting. This makes more "room" for toxins in the breakdown process. We can also speed up the phases by taking in more of certain nutrients. This processes toxins faster.

For the liver to be able to function properly, it requires a number of nutritional supplements, especially B vitamins (see Table 7.6). Without these substances, toxic materials can build up in the body. They keep the liver cells healthy and protected from inflammation and toxic products. Although most of these nutrients are present in pet food, it can be beneficial to supply any items that are not present in the food (such as vitamin C, cruciferous vegetables, and milk thistle), especially when planning a fast. Water-soluble vitamins are safe to add. When using vitamin A, the vitamin works best combined with carotenoids. When using vitamin C, the vitamin works best when combined with bioflavonoids. It is not wise to supplement with minerals unless the diet is extremely deficient. Even then, minerals are best added as part of a vitamin–mineral supplement rather than alone. (See Table 9.2 for recommended doses.)

For phase I to operate normally, there are a number of cofactors required (see Table 7.7). Although decreasing them can slow phase I reactions, it will not do so in a healthy manner.

For normal action of phase II enzymes, we need the cofactors that these enzymes add to free radicals from phase I (see Table 7.8). A deficiency of these materials will slow down the phase II process, so supplying them will help speed up this part of the process.

How Improper Fasting and Detoxification May Increase Toxicity

Extreme Fasts

A pure water fast will decrease the toxic load that comes from diet. It decreases the amount of ammonia that needs to be processed by the liver (from protein converted to carbohydrates). It eliminates any problems that come from any potentially toxic substances that are included in the food. Unfortunately, the body needs a certain amount of protein for normal processes. Part of cats' energy requirements must come from protein. All animals, and cats especially, will start converting some of their body's protein (from muscles, especially) in order to have enough protein to function. The longer the water fast, the greater the problem becomes. In addition, water-soluble vitamins are

Table 7.8 Phase II cofactors.

Acetates[a]

Acetyl-cysteine

Arginine

Glucuronic acid

Glutathione

Glycine (not used by cats; primary cofactor in dogs)

L-cysteine[a]

L-Glutamine

Ornithine

Sulfates

Taurine

[a] Cofactor can be supplied by *n*-acetyl cysteine, although in an animal that is sick, it is better to supply the cofactor itself. This puts less stress on the animal's metabolism.

Table 7.9 Detoxification side effects.

- Dandruff
- Diarrhea[a]
- Fatigue
- Foul breath
- Nausea
- Other skin problems
- Skin inflammation
- Vomiting[a]

[a] If severe, the detoxification process should be discontinued.

lost in the urine and, if not restored, will be quickly depleted in a prolonged fast. (There is a safer type of fast that will accomplish the benefits and minimize the risks, as discussed below.)

Toxins in the body pass back and forth across cell membranes, according to the amount on each side, until a steady state is reached and there is an equal amount on both sides.

If there is a lower concentration in the blood, toxins will start coming out of the tissues where they were stored and become available for the liver to start working on. There may be some toxins that cause more side effects than others. In humans, one common sign of detoxification is a headache, which may last for days, until the worst of the substances are eliminated from the system. Some animals may also suffer from headaches: we often see lethargy at the beginning of the process if an animal is very toxic. Later, the same animal will have increased energy. There are a number of other symptoms that are common during detoxification (see Table 7.9).

If these symptoms are mild and the animal seems to feel okay, otherwise, there is no problem. If the symptoms are severe, or the pet seems depressed, this is most likely a sign of toxic detox. The detox process should be discontinued immediately.

A pure water fast is the fastest way to eliminate toxins and is also the fastest way to see detox problems or toxicity, as discussed above. In addition, if a body's toxin load is large enough, toxic items may be released too fast, resulting in more damage to tissues. In cats, it can cause hepatic lipidosis, as quickly as 24 hours after the fast starts, if the cat is overweight or ill. Thus, this type of fast is not as beneficial for pets as some believe. There are better ways to accomplish detoxification.

Toxic Detox

For detoxification, the worst combination of abnormal liver enzymes occurs when a liver has normal or even worse, above normal amounts of phase I enzymes and below normal quantities of phase II enzymes. This is the worst case because phase I breakdown of toxins will proceed normally or even faster than usual, but there will be an accumulation of free radicals and the extra-toxic supertoxins. (A supertoxin is a toxin that has been transformed into an even more toxic form.)

The supertoxins remain in the liver until a spare phase II enzyme system is available to process them. If this takes too much time, they begin affecting cells in the liver, damaging them, knocking chemicals out of place, destroying cells, and eventually escaping into the bloodstream.

Once in the blood, the supertoxins travel to other parts of the body, especially fat, brain, and nerve cells. They may be stored in the fat for a while, but with weight loss, the fat disappears and they can emerge again and cause more signs of illness. If there is too high a level of toxins, there won't be enough room in the fat to store them, so some toxins will be forced to stay in the bloodstream, causing chronic disease symptoms because of their toxic effect on other tissues.

Excess supertoxins cause liver damage. Liver damage results in slower processing of toxins. This increases the amount of toxins, increasing damage and making everything worse. Free radicals, toxins, and supertoxins build up and can cause kidney damage, leading to kidney failure. If enough of certain toxin types are in brain tissue, you may see Alzheimer's-like symptoms. (For example, an older pet suddenly looking around like she forgot where she was.) Shaking or even convulsions may also appear.

Toxins can cause intestinal damage, leading to diarrhea, resulting in a leaky gut, which lets in more toxins, accelerating the process. A fast can make things even worse, especially if supported with single antioxidants. The fast accelerates the toxin production with the breakdown of extra protein. It brings toxins out of hiding by breakdown of body fat. Single antioxidants speed up phase I even more, causing more supertoxins to be produced. Diarrhea gets further out of control. To regain control, we need to replace fluids, nutritionally support the intestine, lower toxins in the intestine, and counter inflammation, but on a strict fast that doesn't happen.

Excess Phase I Enzymes

The most common cause of higher than normal phase I enzymes is increased exposure to toxins. When the liver is exposed to increased toxin levels, it increases the amount of phase I enzymes produced (see Table 7.10).

How Proper Detoxification and Fasting Can Decrease Toxicity

Detoxification Using Herbs, Nutraceuticals, and Homeopathy or Homotoxicology

Herbs can help detoxification in three ways: some (such as milk thistle) can protect the liver or even improve liver function, some (such as okra or slippery elm bark) can absorb toxins in the gut, and some (such as *uva ursi*) can speed up the excretion of toxins by stimulating urination or the

Table 7.10 Substances that can cause increased phase I enzymes.

- Barbiturates
- Charcoal-broiled meats
- Citrus fruits
- Cortisone
- Exhaust and paint fumes
- High-protein diet
- Male and female hormones
- Niacin
- Riboflavin
- Sassafras
- Saturated fats

flow of bile. Some herbalists also look for herbs that stimulate defecation (such as *cascara sagrada*) to the point of diarrhea. People who do not fully understand the process can get in trouble with the last group of herbs. Mild stimulants can help the process. Severe reactions can make things worse. A veterinarian who is familiar with herbs can recommend the correct ones and steer pet owners away from potentially harmful ones. A technician who is familiar with herbs can help alert the veterinarian about problems and help clients if they are using items that are harsh or dangerous.

Nutraceuticals are used to supply the cofactors needed for phase I and phase II enzymes to work at maximum capacity. Some speed up reactions, and others are used during phase II to make a chemical less harmful. Nutraceuticals can also decrease inflammation and other effects of toxic detox.

Homotoxicology theory is based on the premise that disease is based on the buildup of toxins in the matrix (which essentially consists of the interstitial spaces in the body). Part of treatment with homeopathic remedies emphasizes draining the matrix, using remedies that increase detoxification through the lymph system, the kidneys, the liver, and the intestines. Homeopathic concentrations of items such as mercury may be given, stimulating the body to excrete those items. In addition, there are remedies that are used to protect the liver as well as to help affected organs. This type of detoxification is mild, but some of the same effects seen in fasting, including diarrhea, dandruff, and sometimes vomiting or lethargy, can occur. Like other methods of detoxification, if the source of toxins is not eliminated or decreased, it is difficult to succeed in this process.

Detoxification Using a Modified Fast

Rather than a complete water fast, if we supply just enough protein for the body's needs, we will avoid the possibility of body tissue being broken down to supply the protein. By keeping the protein intake at a minimum during the detox process, we will also minimize the amount of ammonia the liver has to deal with.

If we supply the items that help the liver stay healthy (see Table 7.6), as well as cofactors for phase I (Table 7.7) and for phase II (Table 7.8), then the liver can process items at maximum speed. In addition, it is wise to add nutrients that will protect the body against any toxic effects of detoxification. First and foremost, we need to have items that protect against the free radicals produced by phase I enzymes (see Table 7.11). It is best to supply these factors rather than try to slow the phase I system. Slowing it down will result in an increase in the amount of unprocessed toxins.

If we think that the phase I process is a little sluggish, it may help to add supplements to stimulate it (see Table 7.12). Although certain toxins can increase the speed or activity of phase I enzymes, it is not wise to supply these if you are trying to induce more phase I actions. Instead,

Table 7.11 Antioxidants that help decrease the toxicity of phase I products (free radicals).	**Table 7.12** Nutritional supplements used to increase the activity of the phase I system without increasing toxicity.
• Bioflavonoids	• Bioflavonoids
• Carotenoids	• Carotenoids
• Copper	• Iron
• Manganese	• Magnesium
• Pycnogenol	• Molybdenum
• Selenium	• Pycnogenol
• Superoxide dismutase	• Selenium
• Vitamin A	• Superoxide dismutase
• Vitamin C	• Vitamin A
• Vitamin E	• Vitamin C
• Zinc	• Vitamin E

Table 7.13 Supplements for nutritional support of the intestinal tract.

- Antioxidants:
  Beta carotene and other carotenoids
  Selenium
  Superoxide dismutase
  Vitamin A (carefully)
  Vitamin C
  Vitamin E
  Zinc
- Butyric acid
- Insoluble fiber (wheat bran or canned pumpkin)
- L-arginine
- L-glutamine
- Pantothenic acid
- Soluble fiber (FOS or pectin or slippery elm bark or psyllium husk)

many supplements that help the liver or that decrease the toxicity of free radicals can also speed the action of phase I enzymes. Note that these include a number of antioxidants, so we are not stimulating it in a toxic way.

In addition, we can give supplements to help mitochondria, listed above (and to minimize the chance of diarrhea with subsequent uptake of toxins) (Table 7.13). We can also give supplements to help lower toxins that are already in the intestine (Table 7.14).

If an animal fasts with just enough protein for its minimum needs and is taking in extra antioxidants (to protect against phase I reactions) and extra cofactors (to help phase II do its job), then there are a minimum of toxic products produced in the body. This allows the liver to work primarily on products that have been stored in the body. In addition, without the buffer of extra products in the blood (which push back on toxins that would otherwise enter into the bloodstream), large amounts of toxins may suddenly emerge into the bloodstream, making an animal even worse. Thus, fasting must be done very carefully. Because the functional tests available for humans that determine the level of phase I and phase II enzymes are not available for animals, we can't judge how fast or slow to detoxify. We have to guess, and the best way to guess is to assume that we need to be conservative with all animals. The longest that we can safely perform a modified fast for an extremely toxic animal with minimal enzyme levels is 3 days, and if an animal is very ill, it is better to start with only 1 day of fasting per week.

Table 7.14 Supplements to lower toxins in intestine.

- Bentonite clay
- *Bifidobacteria* species, especially *B. bifidus*
- Digestive enzymes
- Inulin
- *Lactobacillus* species, especially *L. acidophilus*
- Pantothenic acid (vitamin B5)
- Soluble fiber (oat bran or rice bran or pectin)
- White rice

A big part of detoxification is avoiding toxins, including those taken in as food or treats (or by rooting in the garbage can). To minimize the possibility that a pet will raid the trash when on a detox program, white (not brown) rice is recommended as part of the modified fast. White rice will help with any problems related to intestinal irritation or diarrhea caused by toxic products being eliminated through the intestines. White rice is basically starch (which does not play a role in the toxic process), and a very small amount of rice protein is not enough to contribute to the protein load of the diet.

Detoxification can cause diarrhea, vomiting, or skin changes if too many substances are being excreted at once. At times, this can be debilitating, so detoxification should not be rushed. Some clients who have read about detoxification may use a harmful method and believe that the resulting dehydration and intestinal damage are part of the normal process. A technician can help enlighten them as to the proper way to detoxify, as well as the possible need for hospitalization if dehydration is severe enough.

Putting It All Together

If we know an animal has been exposed to a particular toxin (such as mercury), a homeopathic form of it (such as Mercurius) can be administered to help the animal expel the toxin. If the animal has chronic diarrhea, a homeopathic or homotoxicological remedy can help, as well as using Chinese or Western herbs to control diarrhea and soluble fiber to help improve the health of the intestinal tract. To start, the animal's body should be as healthy as possible.

If an animal is reasonably healthy with symptoms such as lethargy, dandruff, etc., or if they just need a little help to detoxify, then the use of a modified fast with supporting nutrients will accomplish the goal.

For the fast, they should eat the following: Enough protein to meet their basic needs, and no more (Table 7.15); a very small amount of liver (1/10 as much as the meat); as much easily digestible carbohydrate as needed to meet energy and hunger needs (such as white rice or potato as desired); and supplements to support the liver and intestinal tract.

Chicken broth can be added to the carbohydrate source to make it more palatable. It's best to assume the worst and give full support of supplements throughout the fast and never go longer than 3 days at a time (to prevent toxic detox). The fast can be repeated with 1 week to 1 month between fasts. If an animal is especially toxic, the fast should only last 1 day.

Table 7.15 Ounces of protein per day for a fast.

Cats	
All sizes	2 2/3 ounces meat per day
	Very small piece of liver (half the size of the last joint of your little finger)
Dogs	
11 pound	1 ounces meat per day
22 pound	2 2/3 ounces meat per day
33 pound	3 1/3 ounces meat per day
66 pound	5.6 ounces meat per day

Enough supplements should be given to keep both phases working at top speed, with extra antioxidants given to make up for excesses used in a speeded-up phase I. Animals, especially cats, should eat enough protein to prevent the breakdown of muscle tissue. Unless rapid weight loss is desired, animals should eat a source of energy that is easily digested and that won't add toxins. Supplements are needed to prevent damage to mitochondria, and if diarrhea occurs, lost nutrients must be replaced, and the veterinarian must guard against toxins absorbed. Fortunately, not every single supplement used by the liver is needed.

The easiest way to provide most of the nutrients is to use a supplement designed for this purpose. One is Ultra Clear Plus, from Metagenics, and the other is MediClear from Thorne. Add a dose of one of these to each meal, proportional to the human dose. In addition, because all the substances a liver needs are in the liver, a small piece of liver can be added to provide any extra vitamins or cofactors missing in the supplement. (A small piece is between the size of the last joint of the little finger and the size of half a golf ball, depending on the size of the animal—about 1/10 of the amount of meat given.) Too much liver will cause diarrhea.

The fast can be repeated as often as once a week for a 1-day fast, or every 2–4 weeks, for a 3-day fast. The aim is to achieve the maximum benefit with the minimum harm. The fast is repeated until the animal has regained strength. For animals that seem to have problems all the time, a 1-day fast once a month may help them retain their balance.

Veterinarian's Role

When veterinarians suspect some kind of toxicity, they will usually perform a complete blood test, and look especially at possible abnormalities with kidney and liver. Some veterinarians include various aspects of detoxification in their practice treatment, with or without fasting. Herbs and/or supplements may be prescribed. The diagnosis and specific treatment plan must be made by the veterinarian.

Technician's Role

If the veterinarian has recommended fasting, it is especially important that the owner understand the type of fast, including what is and is not allowed, any supplements needed, and how long a fast or special diet is to be continued. Technicians can answer questions and call the owner daily to make sure that the animal is responding properly.

Where to Learn How

Currently, there is no training specifically for detoxification for animals. There are some books for humans (see the bibliography), and there are occasionally lectures on the subject at the annual AHVMA meeting, and in the *AHVMA Journal*. The companies who sell MediClear and UltraClear have handouts and brochures for their use in humans, which can be adapted for use in dogs.

USING A FAST FOR CHRONIC INFECTION AND LETHARGY

Shortly after I had learned about the benefits of fasting when properly done, and how to do it properly, a golden retriever was brought to me. The dog had been a field trial champion and had the misfortune to acquire a foxtail that entered at his shoulder and gradually moved down the left side of his body over the course of a year. During this time, every so often a hole would open up in the vicinity of the foxtail. The dog's veterinarian probed the holes (a standard procedure for trying to find foxtails). As time went on, he anesthetized the dog several times, and cut open the tracts (tunnels) where the foxtail had been traveling (also a normal procedure). The dog was put on antibiotics several times.

During this time, the dog became more and more lethargic until he finally had to be retired from the field. Finally, a hole formed on his rump near his tail, and the veterinarian was able to find the foxtail and remove it. The hole healed immediately, and everyone was happy until it opened again a month later and the veterinarian once again could not find anything. At that point, the owner decided to try a different approach.

When I examined the dog, he looked normal except that he moved like an old man and he had a small, draining hole near his tail. I could not find a foxtail in it, either. Going by the theory that repeated antibiotics and anesthetics, as well as repeated infections from the foxtail itself, had caused a toxic overload, we started the dog on a detox program, using a modified fast with the supplement powder for 2 days every weekend. First, the hole closed up. Then the dog began to regain energy. His coat became shinier. Finally, he felt so well that the owner started him back in field trial work, where he went back to winning matches again.

Summary

What can the technician do?

1) Be sure to understand all the ramifications of detoxification, including the right way, the wrong way, and the problems associated with each.
2) Be sure to call a client 24 hours after starting detox for the first time to be sure their pet is not having problems. (Question them specifically about vomiting, diarrhea, and lethargy. Not all owners fully realize that there might be problems associated with these signs.)
3) Be sure the veterinarian gets in touch with the client if a client calls in with concerns about signs of detoxification. Something that sounds mild can turn out to be more severe than it appears at first.
4) Be familiar with the diet, with acceptable substitutes, and with items the owner should not use at all. Be prepared to explain the diet again if the owner calls.
5) Be able to explain why detoxification has been recommended in the first place.

Bibliography

Bailey D.G. and Dresser G.K. 2004. Interactions between grapefruit juice and cardiovascular drugs. *Am J Cardiovasc Drugs* 4(5):281–297.

Baker S.M., et al. 2005. *Textbook of Functional Medicine*. Gig Harbor, WA: Institute for Functional Medicine.

Bland J. 1999. *Genetic Nutritioneering*. New York: McGraw-Hill.

Bland J. 1999. *The 20-Day Rejuvenation Diet Program*. New York: McGraw-Hill.

Bland J.S., et al. 2004. *Clinical Nutrition: A Functional Approach*. Gig Harbor, WA: Institute for Functional Medicine.

Chaudhary A. and Willett K.L. 2006. Inhibition of human cytochrome CYP 1 enzymes by flavonoids of St. John's wort. *Toxicology* 217(2–3):194–205. doi: 10.1016/j.tox.2005.09.010.

Goodsell D.S. 2001. The molecular perspective: Cytochrome P450. *Oncologist* 6(2):205–206.

Strandell J., et al. 2004. An approach to the *in vitro* evaluation of potential for cytochrome P450 enzyme inhibition from herbals and other natural remedies. *Phytomedicine* 11(2–3):98–104.

Wannemacher R.W. and McCoy J.R. 1966. Determination of optimal dietary protein requirements of young and old dogs. *J Nutr* 88(1):66–174.

Zeratsky K. 2008. Grapefruit Juice: Can It Cause Drug Interactions? Ask a Food & Nutrition Specialist. Accessed online 2/9/2009 at https://www.mayoclinic.com/health/food-and-nutrition/AN00413.

Zhang J.W., et al. 2007. Inhibition of human liver cytochrome P450 by star fruit juice. *J Pharm Pharm Sci* 10(4):496–503.

Webliography

Institute for Functional Medicine
https://www.ifm.org/
Information and resources for human functional medicine; useful for animals also.

8

Holistic Diet and Nutrition

Description

If you want to hold the attention of holistic clients, you must understand their concerns about conventional pet foods. Clients want a "natural" product, with whole foods and without artificial flavors, colors, or preservatives. They want to feed their pets a diet that is as close to a wild diet as possible. (Although their idea of a wild diet might not match nature's idea.)

Why "Natural"?

Artificial flavors, colors, and preservatives have been linked to both allergic reactions and to cancer. The inclusion of highly processed items such as corn gluten meal, meat meal, and the dry form of by-products can result in a product that has a lower amount of volatile amino acids and decreased digestibility of cross-linked amino acids. Some items (such as corn gluten meal) may be relatively deficient in certain amino acids (such as lysine). Although this can be remedied by adding a higher quality protein, those who follow the holistic viewpoint prefer to use better quality protein sources in the first place. In addition, gluten intolerance is well recognized in human medicine as celiac disease, and holistic owners and practitioners are cognizant of its presence in animals, also. The presence of melamine (and possibly other adulterants from China in the future) in pet foods that were not derived from all-natural sources is another instance of concern for pet owners, since it is easier to adulterate gluten with a chemical than to hide a chemical in meat. Finally, the by-products of gluten digestion can add to a body's toxic load, increasing the need for detoxification.

Human nutritionists recognize that natural sources of substances such as bioflavonoids and carotenoids have a more beneficial effect than a single source, such as beta carotene. High amounts of beta carotene, when used as the sole antioxidant at the megadose level, have actually been associated with an increase in several types of lung cancer in humans. Using high levels of vitamin E as the only source of additional antioxidants has also been linked to an increased incidence of cancer in humans. Irradiation of cat food as a method of sterilization in Australia has resulted in the destruction of antioxidants, especially vitamin A, to the point of rapidly causing vitamin A deficiency. Using natural sources instead of purified vitamins avoids these problems. The best natural sources combine antioxidants. (For example, vitamin C plus bioflavonoids – both are present in an orange, and not separated out as they are in many pills.)

Complementary Medicine for Veterinary Technicians and Nurses, Second Edition. Nancy Scanlan.
© 2024 John Wiley & Sons, Inc. Published 2024 by John Wiley & Sons, Inc.

Many clients are interested in a raw diet because it is much closer to the diet of a wild carnivore than a canned or dry product. Many available raw diets are not balanced and have not been tested in a food trial (feeding a dog or cat long term to be sure they maintain health, can grow, and reproduce on the diet). The same is true for many published recipes. Many veterinarians are concerned about possible bacterial contamination in raw meat. There is at least a little bacteria in all meat. Animals that are immune compromised (including the elderly) may be more likely to suffer from diarrhea or worse when eating these foods. Some animals do better on slightly cooked diets – genetic manipulation to create pure breeds can result in the loss of genes involved in the best ways to digest raw foods. In addition, clients may stop adding supplements, including calcium, needed to maintain good health. However, if done properly, we often see benefits from feeding a raw diet.

Other clients may not want a raw diet for their pet, but they still believe that a home-cooked diet is healthier than anything from a can or bag. Home cooking is certainly a way to avoid cross-linked proteins. However, these pet owners may also be guided by misinformation when preparing their pet's food.

OWNER'S MISUNDERSTANDING CAUSES SEVERE CALCIUM DEFICIENCY

A 1-year-old cat was referred to me because he could not walk and his veterinarian had recommended euthanasia. Ever since he was a kitten, the owner had fed him boiled breast of chicken (without the skin because she had heard that the skin was not healthy). She did not feed the kitten cat food or anything else besides the chicken breast. A radiograph revealed folding fractures of most joints, and the bones were difficult to visualize because they did not have much calcium. I treated him with calcium for his bones and acupuncture for his pain, and within a month, he was running and chasing birds, although he had the appearance of the feline version of Quasimodo.

Good nutrition is a lifetime commitment. Some clients, when they hear all the work involved in a healthy homemade diet, prefer to buy a top-quality pet food. Others are dedicated to feeding a homemade diet for the life of their pet.

Because cheap pet food is made from cheap ingredients, the best quality pet foods always cost more. This is even more true of homemade diets. The cost may influence the choice of what type of natural diet to feed.

There are two parts to veterinary nutrition that are somewhat different in the holistic world: the actual diets themselves and the use of nutritional supplements for various disease processes. This chapter will discuss specific diets, and the next chapter will discuss nutritional supplements.

History

James Spratt invented the first "dog cake," a combination of wheat meals, vegetables, beetroot, and meat, in London in 1860. Not only was this the first commercial dog food, but it also was the first one delegated to another company (Walker, Harrison, and Garthwaite) for production. English country gentlemen fed Spratt's food to their hunting dogs.

Spratt's Patent (America) Ltd. began in New York City, but the growth of his company soon required a move to Newark, NJ.

In 1907, F. H. Bennet Biscuits Company was organized in New York City, and started producing Bennet's Milk-Bone Dog and Puppy Foods. (At that time, most dog foods were basically made from waste products, but Bennet's food included meat, cereals, milk, cod liver oil, wheat germ, yeast, and minerals.) Milk-Bone was acquired by the National Biscuit Co. (now Nabisco) in 1931, and thus is the oldest American dog food or treat still sold in the United States. Because Nabisco sold their products in grocery stores, their sales force was able to convince these stores to start stocking dog food. Nabisco overcame the reluctance of both grocery store owners (appalled at selling any-thing that wasn't for humans) and of dog owners (reluctant to spend money on dog food) to con-sider the idea of food for dogs to be comparable to food for humans.

In the late 1920s, Dr. Leon Whitney, a veterinarian in Orange, CT, created Bal-O-Ration, based on the idea that dogs needed a scientifically balanced ration for optimum health. This brand was sold to Tioga Mills, evolved into a Pampa brand, and finally was sold to the Quaker Oats Company.

During the Great Depression, dog food companies flourished. One report showed 221 brands of dog food. However, 200 of them were produced at six plants, which would have the same formula for various companies that supplied empty cans and labels. Dry dog food was similarly limited, although a large number of brands hid this fact (Pet Food Institute, 2009).

In 1943, Dr. Mark Morris became interested in the idea that special diets could help treat some diseases in pets. He developed a recipe for a low-protein, low-salt diet for dogs with kidney disease. Morris Frank, whose Seeing Eye dog, Buddy, was suffering from renal failure, asked Dr. Morris for his help. Originally Mr. Frank had to mix the diet himself, but because he traveled so much, he persuaded Dr. Morris to can the food for him. This became the first Hill's Pet Nutrition Prescription Diet product, Canine k/d, the world's first prescription pet food designed for dogs with kidney disease.

AAFCO (The Association of American Feed Control Officials, Inc.) was formed in 1909 to deter-mine the legality of items in pet food in the United States. That role has continued to the present. If an item is not listed in their handbook, it may not be included in pet food. Labels must conform to the AAFCO standards to minimize misleading statements. Despite these standards, there are still label items that can be confusing when owners compare different brands.

Definition

A holistic diet does not have any artificial flavors, colors, preservatives, or other additives. In addition, the contents are real food, not food derivatives such as gluten or by-products. The ideal diet comes from plants that are organic and animals that are raised in a free-range environment, with access to pasture, good water, and outside air and sunshine, and that are handled and killed in a humane fashion. (Note that organic plants are never GMO plants.) Vitamins and minerals are added to ensure that a diet meets the minimal standards set by the government, but additional nutritional substances may also be added to accomplish specific purposes. For example, glucosamine or other glycosaminoglycans may be added to a diet formulated for older animals.

There are several categories of natural-sounding labels that can be confusing. In the United States, "100% organic" means just what it says: all items are grown in a method that is classified as organic. "USDA Organic" (without the "100%") means that the contents are at least 95% organic, and the remaining ingredients are approved for use in an organic product. Products that have at least 70% organic ingredients may state "made with organic ingredients" and list up to three of the organic ingredients or food groups on the label. If the product contains less than

70% organic ingredients, ingredients may be identified as being organic in the list of ingredients, but there can be no organic claims on the main panel of the label. In all cases, the company that certified the ingredients as organic must be listed on the label (USDA Agricultural Marketing Service, 2009).

Brand names such as Newman's Own Organics that were registered before this labeling law was in effect may contain the word *organic* in the name without meeting the USDA definition of "organic" (Crane, 2009).

As for "natural" food, AAFCO states that, except for added vitamins and minerals, all the ingredients in a food labeled "natural" must meet these requirements:

> A feed or ingredient derived solely from plant, animal, or mined sources, either in its unprocessed state or having been subjected to physical processing, heat processing, rendering, purification extraction, hydrolysis, enzymolysis, or fermentation, but not having been produced by or subject to a chemically synthetic process and not containing any additives or processing aids that are chemically synthetic except in amounts as might occur unavoidably in good manufacturing practices.

Thus, "natural" ingredients may still include substances such as by-products and corn gluten meal. They can't include anything such as ethoxyquin (a preservative), which is strictly chemical and not derived from a food source. Finally, there are "human-grade" foods. This term has not been officially defined and is not generally recognized (Nestle and Nesheim, 2008).

By-Products: Why Are They Unacceptable?

The term "by-products," as used by the holistic community, was originally defined by AAFCO (until 2008) as a rendered product, including all parts of diseased, dead (before they arrived at the processing plant), dying, and "downer" (can no longer get up from a down position) animals, except for hair, horn, hoof, hide, or gut contents. Generally, there is minimal to no meat or bone included. Dead and dying animals are considered permissible because these parts are sterilized by pressure cooking at high heat and long processing times so that disease organisms are no longer present. All liquid is evaporated, and the result is ground into a powder. The holistic community objects to the inclusion of diseased and dead animals and to the fact that a small amount of pentobarbital has been found in some dog and cat foods (from animals that were euthanized). (DNA was analyzed from these samples, and no dog or cat DNA was found, which indicates that the samples were from euthanized large animals, not pets (FDA, 2002; Syverson, 2009).)

In addition, the length of cooking time at high heat and pressure results in the loss of some volatile amino acids, as well as cross-linkages of other amino acids. An analysis will show a better amino acid balance than is actually available to the pet because it is more difficult for an animal to digest and absorb cross-linked amino acids (Achinewhu and Hewitt, 1979; Ashes et al., 1999; Friedman, 1999; Hurrell and Carpenter, 1978).

This is an old AAFCO definition, and does not match their definition since 2008: "Secondary products produced in addition to the principal product" (2008 AAFCO Official Publication, p. 240). (*Principal product* refers to products for human consumption.) Technically, by-products include all organ meats, intestines, and even plant products such as beet pulp and tomato pomace. State regulators contend that poultry meal (made of flesh, skin, and bones, only) is also technically a by-product, because it is made of parts discarded during the processing of chicken meat for human food (Dzanis, 2009). For the past decade, the pet food industry has been in discussion with AAFCO to allow them to add other descriptive terms rather than *by-products*. AAFCO does allow the use of *liver* as a separate item on ingredient labels, contrary to the wishes of some state regulators, partly because of a court case in which a judge noted that liver is generally considered to be meat by most consumers (Dzanis, 2009).

There are companies that use organ meats rather than the rendered product and they include such meats on the label as by-products. This also falls under the AAFCO definition of by-products. Unfortunately, it isn't possible to determine from the label if organ meats or rendered products are being used unless the organs are specifically listed on the labels. Less-expensive pet foods usually use the rendered by-products exclusively.

In addition, the various types of by-products vary in percentage of protein, amino acid balance, and digestibility, so some pet foods with by-products have much higher quality protein than others. It isn't possible to determine which companies are using these higher-quality proteins just by looking at the labels. Reputable companies may choose their by-products by analyzing the percentage of protein in a sample (personal communication, Steve Crane, PhD, Hills Pet Nutrition, March 2009) or by using only specific fresh organs, tripe, or intestines. The only way to know for sure is to talk to the specific companies.

Other Ingredients

Besides the drive for more natural ingredients, there are a number of different theories about the best ingredients for dog and cat foods. Some believe that dogs should never have grains and should primarily eat meat with ground bones and possibly some fruits and vegetables (Billinghurst, 2001; Lonsdale, 2005). Lonsdale recommends that all dogs regularly get raw, meaty bones as part of their diets. Billinghurst is the proponent of the "BARF" diet, which stands for biologically appropriate raw food. He recommends that dog food be prepared from raw meats, raw fruits, raw vegetables, and no grains.

This comes from a belief that dogs are carnivores, not omnivores or even carno-omnivores. It ignores the fact that dogs' molars are more adapted to grinding than are cats' molars. It also ignores the fact that DNA evidence shows that dogs began their developmental split from wolves as long as 125,000 years ago, with adaptation to being scavengers and/or companions of humans along with corresponding changes to their diets (Vila et al., 1997).

Wolves also have been observed scavenging old carcasses and eating rodents and vegetation, although ungulates are usually their prey of choice. They first eat internal organ meats (including intestines), then meat, and eventually bones and hides. Note that bones are usually eaten with the hair on the accompanying hide (Stahler et al., 2006). There are statements that wolves do not eat bones—they eat only muscle meat. Besides the fact that, without bones, wolves would not have enough calcium in their diet to form their own bones, let alone supply milk to their cubs, statements such as these tend to be based on reports of initial wolf behavior at kills and do not consider that wolves eventually consume bones and hide.

Omega-3 fatty acids are higher in game meat, and the total percentage of fat content is lower. This is also not addressed by the BARF group (Mann, 2000). To get a fat profile that is as close to nature as possible, it is best to use pasture-finished ruminants (which eat only grass, no grain) and omnivores (pigs and chickens) that are both pastured and fed organic grains. These animals have a higher percentage of omega-3 fatty acids in the carcass, and the fat content more closely matches that of wild game (Enser et al., 1998).

As for calcium, some believe animals should get their calcium in the form of ground poultry bones, chicken and turkey necks, and raw, meaty bones (especially the ends of cattle femurs). They believe dogs and cats can easily digest bones because of their stomach acid's high level of acidity and that there is no problem with bones injuring the intestinal tract (Billinghurst, 2001; Lonsdale, 2005). However, animals with problems such as renal insufficiency or inflammatory bowel disease may be on drugs designed to decrease the amount of stomach acid. These animals may not have enough acid to do the job properly. There are also breeds, such as the Boston terrier, that have genes that decrease the amount of stomach acid available (Clark and Stainer, 1994). For these breeds, ground bones can also constitute a problem. Small rodents, the primary prey of cats' ancestors, consist of 5% bone (Prange et al., 1979). Diets that consist of whole, ground chicken carcasses may differ from this proportion.

Others believe that calcium should be given only as a supplement because small ground bones may puncture intestines and large bones may cause slab fractures of the teeth. In 2010, the FDA came out with a statement agreeing with this view, stating that all bones are unsafe for dogs (Food and Drug Administration, 2010).

There are recommendations that all vitamins come from natural sources such as vegetables. In the wild, gut contents of rodents and lagomorphs are consumed by canines and felines; plant material, including sprouts and berries in season, are also eaten by canines. They may also eat herbivore feces (Stahler et al., 2006). No company has reproduced this combination in their pet food, and it is difficult to reproduce the same effects by feeding cooked mature vegetables. Therefore, it is wise to advise all owners to add a vitamin supplement to the pet's diet if they plan on feeding home-prepared meals, even if they include vegetables. See also the analysis of several home diet recipes in Appendix 10, including items found to be deficient (analysis done by BalanceIT®).

Diet and Dilated Cardiomyopathy (DCM)

Taurine deficiency has been linked to DCM in cats, and the recommended minimum value in cat food has been increased twice. In dogs, DCM used to be considered an inherited disease, with greater incidence in specific breeds, including Dobermans. More recently, they found that in some breeds such as the Golden Retriever, the DCM responded to taurine—perhaps a breed-specific increased requirement for taurine.

In 2019, the FDA responded to increasing concerns about a possible connection between grain-free diets and DCM and even some deaths in breeds that had not previously been reported to have any inherited problems with DCM. This had not been reported with some of the older grain-free diets based on animal protein and potatoes. Subsequent research zeroed in on pulses (legumes, especially peas) that were included in the newer grain-free diets. As of 2023, there have not been enough studies with enough dogs for long enough periods of time to completely establish the connection, but most veterinarians (both conventional and holistic) are trying to stay away from grain-free diets which include pulses (Quilliam et al., 2021, 2023). The FDA is still collecting information from concerned owners and veterinarians, and testing any grain-free foods being fed dogs that developed DCM while on those diets. The FDA still believes that additional taurine is not required by dogs because dogs can produce enough of their own (FDA, 2022), even though veterinarians have recognized DCM cases that respond to taurine supplementation (Bakke et al., 2022; Kaplan et al., 2018; McCauley et al., 2020).

There is also a concern about the use of GMO (genetically modified organism) products. Currently, almost all GMO food crops in the US are "Roundup Ready" crops. Roundup is glyphosate, a weed killer made by Monsanto, which was originally designed to kill all the weeds in a field before it was planted with a crop. After it had disappeared from the field, the farmer could plant crops in a weed-free environment. Before this, weeds had to be plowed under to get rid of them. Because the weeds can grow again, and conventional plants are also killed by weedkiller, Monsanto found a way to insert a gene that made plants able to withstand the effect of glyphosate. Research has shown that pigs fed on GMO corn developed ulcerations along their intestinal tract. Animals fed glyphosate also become ill. GMO corn has been shown to retain some glyphosate after it has been harvested.

Human and pet foods that are Organic do not have any GMO content. The main GMO crops currently grown in the US that are most likely to be included in pet food include corn, soybeans, canola oil, and sugar beets (in the form of beet pulp as a form of fiber). Pet foods created in the US that contain any of these, including beet pulp added as fiber, contain GMOs and possibly some glyphosate. Companies are not required to identify their human foods as containing GMOs, except in Vermont. (Other states may follow this in the future.) Some companies, such as Kellogg, have begun inserting a notice (in small print) on their labels stating "produced with genetic engineering." Another term you may also see is BE, for bioengineered.

Due in large part to the fact that large corporations lobbied successfully against any federal requirement to label their products as GMO products at the time, in 2007, the Non-GMO Project was created by The Natural Grocery Company in Berkeley, California, and The Big Carrot Natural Food Market in Toronto, Ontario as a way to identify and promote non-GMO foods. Companies can apply to have their products verified, and then feature the Non-GMO verification label on their foods. The first products with the Non GMO product label appeared in 2010, and the list is steadily growing. The Non GMO Project is committed to preserving the Non GMO food supply by educating consumers, supporting manufacturers, and educating retailers. They offer North America's most trusted certification for GMO avoidance (Figure 8.1) (Non-GMO Project, 2023).

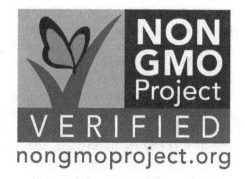

Figure 8.1 Non GMO project label.

Raw or Cooked?

Some believe that all meat should be fed raw (Billinghurst, 2001; Frazier and Eckroate, 2008; Lonsdale, 2005; McKay, 1992; Pitcairn and Pitcairn, 2005). Others cite problems with meats sold for human consumption and recalls for salmonella and *Escherichia coli* contamination, as well as the possibility of contracting toxoplasmosis and other parasites from raw meat (Crane, 2009). Carcasses of pasture-finished animals have a much lower coliform and salmonella count than feedlot-finished animals, so it is safer to feed this type of meat in a raw diet. Many believe that home-cooked meals are better than commercial diets. There is also a small contingent that believes that animals, as well as people, should be vegetarians.

Raw and home-cooked diets have improved skin conditions and chronic intestinal problems when commercial diets have been unable to do so (Pitcairn and Pitcairn, 2005; Remillard et al., 2000). Whatever the preferences of the owner or veterinarian, it is important to choose a diet that is balanced and that meets the needs of the patient.

In summary, there is no real definition of a natural or holistic diet for dogs or cats. The one thing everyone agrees on is that there should be no artificial flavors, colors, preservatives, or ingredients in the diet.

Description of Natural Diets

There are two main groups of diets: commercial and homemade. These can be divided further in a number of ways. This book will briefly discuss canned, dried, fresh, and frozen diets, with the pros and cons of each. The biggest benefit of commercial diets is that they are balanced for vitamins and minerals. If owners are conscientious, they will do the same; however, in the experience of many veterinarians, the first items in a homemade diet to be discarded or changed are vitamins and minerals. Therefore, for many owners, the best method of feeding may be a commercial diet, possibly supplemented with fresh foods. If you are advising an owner who wants to start making their own food, take the time to determine how realistic it is for them to properly measure and mix all the items needed for a truly balanced diet.

The most highly processed diets are dry foods. The least processed diets are raw foods. Even if a dry food does not contain by-products, it does contain meat or poultry meal. Meat meal is created by cooking meat under pressure at a high temperature until it turns dry, then grinding it. The cooking and drying processes produce cross-linkages in amino acids, rendering them less digestible and some volatile amino acids are lost. Canned products are not subjected to heat for as long a time; thus, their proteins are not as denatured. Most pet foods from large companies such as Friskies, Purina, Iams, and Hills Pet Nutrition contain by-products and other ingredients such as corn gluten meal. Less expensive diets contain artificial flavors, colors, and preservatives; premium pet foods have less or none of these (depending on the brand). Holistic dry diets emphasize products free from chemicals, by-products, and food derivatives. They usually contain meat and grain (except for dehydrated diets) and often contain vegetables and perhaps some fruit. Holistic canned foods are processed in a way that ensures no bacteria will be present in the final product.

Because they contain protein sources that are from meat, dairy, and fish rather than gluten meals, holistic items usually are not prone to contamination such as the melamine contamination seen from contaminated ingredients from China. However, if a company sources any of its products from outside the United States, their food may still be exposed to contamination. For example, in 2008 melamine was found in powdered milk that originated in China. Throughout 2008, the FDA issued multiple warnings about salmonella in dehydrated chicken meat originating from China. Although a meat product is considered "natural," it is not necessarily safe. Items with imported ingredients may say "packaged in the U.S.A." but may also state "made in China." It is important to read the label to determine the true origin of an item.

Labels can be misleading if you don't know how to read them. For example, to compare the percentage of protein or the total percentage of fat in two foods, it isn't useful to compare a dry formula to a wet formula. If they are compared, almost every time, the wet food will appear to contain less protein than the dry food because water is counted as one of the ingredients, diluting all the others. In terms of how the body uses the carbohydrates, fat, and protein, the effects are best seen by comparing only the dry parts of the meal.

In a tablespoon of oil, 100% of the calories are supplied by fat. A tablespoon of water will measure no calories, including 0% from fat. No argument there. If you look at whole milk, the label will usually tell you it is around 3.7% fat. The skim milk label will read "0% fat." However, when you drink whole milk, your body knows that whole milk is actually mostly water and that almost 50%

of the calories in the solid part of whole milk are from fat. This is a lot more than you would think when reading "4% fat."

This is why canned must be compared to canned and dry to dry. In addition, if the canned food has a lot of gravy (as milk has a lot of water), the analysis is even more misleading. The best way to judge is on a "dry matter basis," but nobody requires this analysis on a label. If a pet needs a low-protein diet, then the veterinary staff needs to give a separate recommendation for canned products and dry products.

One other problem for pet owners is that once they start reading labels, they may become mistakenly alarmed by ingredients that don't sound natural. They think that the vitamins and minerals listed sound like chemicals. Minerals are often supplied in the form of mineral complexes, which *are* a kind of chemical. *All* life is based on chemical processes. The difference is natural versus artificial chemicals. For example, here is a list of vitamins and minerals similar to many you will see on bags of natural dry dog and cat food: Dicalcium phosphate, calcium carbonate, potassium chloride, zinc sulfate, zinc proteinate, iron proteinate, ferrous sulfate, copper proteinate, copper sulfate, manganese proteinate, manganese sulfate, sodium selenite, beta-carotene, alpha tocopherol, ascorbic acid, retinoic acid, niacin, calcium pantothenate, riboflavin, vitamin D-3 supplement, pyridoxine hydrochloride, thiamine mononitrate, folic acid, biotin, cyanocobalamin, choline chloride, taurine, mixed tocopherols. Other than the vitamin D-3, how many vitamins do you recognize?

Labels list ingredients starting with the ingredient that is present in the highest amount, continuing down to the last, which is the ingredient with the lowest amount in the food. If more than one type of carbohydrate is used, then you may see some type of protein listed first (such as chicken), followed by several grains (such as corn, barley, and rice), implying that there is more of the protein ingredient than grain. However, if the total weight of the grains exceeds the total weight of the chicken, then the protein content is not as high as the label implies.

Something that is labeled "limited ingredients" may only have one item that is limited. There may be only one type of protein but many types of carbohydrates or vice versa. A truly limited-ingredient food, for allergy purposes, should contain a single type of protein and a single type of carbohydrate. In addition, not everyone may realize that there is protein in many carbohydrates in the form of gluten. Thus, one single animal protein in a product does not mean that there is only one type of protein present.

The name of the food itself may also be misleading in terms of ingredients. A product that is labeled as, for instance, "Fish and Potato" may have the actual ingredients listed as follows.

Main Ingredients—
Fish, barley, rye flour, fish meal, sweet potatoes, canola oil (*followed by a list of other items in lower quantities, vitamins, and minerals*).

If your veterinarian has recommended that a pet be fed a limited-ingredient diet, it is usually because that animal has problems with either allergic dermatitis or with gastrointestinal disease. They need a truly limited diet, with only one carbohydrate source and one protein source. Note the number of carbohydrate sources (three) in the product labeled "Fish and Potato": barley, rye flour, and sweet potatoes. If an animal is sensitive to barley or rye, this diet is not suitable.

Compare this to the ingredients of a truly limited-ingredient formula (often prescribed by conventional veterinarians, for these problems).

Potato, herring meal (source of fish oil), catfish, animal fat (*followed by a list of items with lesser quantities, vitamins and minerals*), ethoxyquin.

This diet has one carbohydrate source (potato) and one protein source (fish). It is truly limited.

For the purpose of allergic dermatitis or chronic diarrhea, which can only be controlled with a fish and potato diet, the second food described is the better formula. Why don't all holistic veterinarians use it as part of their regular recommended diets? Note the last ingredient: ethoxyquin. This is an artificial preservative. Some holistic veterinarians may never recommend a brand with ethoxyquin listed in the ingredients or may only recommend it if there are no other alternatives. Sometimes we have to remember that holistic is "whole-istic," or all encompassing, and use some of these other diets. In addition, sometimes we have to compromise in order to have the best outcome for our patients.

Fortunately, there are some canned and dry items that are truly limited and more holistic. In the United States, the Natural Balance Allergy Formulas (and only their allergy formulas) and Instinct Raw Boost Mixers are brands that are truly limited to one protein and one carbohydrate source, without ethoxyquin. (These are not the only brands, but they are readily available ones.)

Another thing to be aware of: flavorings that are sprayed on dry foods may not be the same limited ingredient protein as the protein in the list of ingredients. The government does not require pet food companies to declare what meat is in those flavorings. Some veterinary dermatologists never use dry food—not even the prescription ones—when they are testing a novel protein diet on a dog suspected of having food allergies.

In addition, a homemade or raw diet can also be truly limited. The owner is the one who mixes the ingredients. Homemade diets can be either cooked or raw. One thing to be aware of is that many published recipes are not balanced nutritionally. There is more to balancing a diet than mixing together the things that sound good to a human. If your clients are mixing their own pets' food, be sure to ask them about all the ingredients they are using. Often they have no idea that calcium is so important. It is usually the first thing they leave out because there is so little of it compared to the rest of the diet. People who use ground bone to supply enough calcium are depending on having an animal with a normal digestive tract and on bone that is ground finely enough to be easily digested. Elderly animals, animals with a compromised immune system, and breeds (such as the Boston terrier) that are known to have an inadequate amount of stomach acid may not be able to properly digest the bone or to absorb enough calcium. For these animals, a diet with a calcium supplement will often work better.

Another problem can exist when an owner relies on a single vegetable, without any organ meats, to supply all needed vitamins and minerals. It is best (and safest) for most owners to add a vitamin supplement to the diet. A recent independent evaluation of published home-cooked recipes for dogs and cats showed that over half of these recipes are deficient in one or more essential nutrients (Lauten, SD, ACVIM Proceedings, 2005). A final problem is that "one cup of ground (fill in the blank)" can vary, depending on how finely ground the item is. "Ground fat" does not state what species of fat. "Ground broccoli" does not state how much is florets and how much is stem. This is important because there is a great deal of difference between nutrients in florets and the stem. Stacey Perea, DVM, MS, DACVN, from BalanceIT (www.balanceit.com) says that although they give both common measurements and amounts in grams, they recommend that pet owners buy a gram scale for the most accurate and balanced diets.

The websites www.balance.it, and www.petdiets.com will help owners (or their veterinarians or technicians) to formulate a homemade diet for their pet that is truly balanced. There is a charge for this, and both of the websites recommend supplements to add to the diet to make it truly balanced.

Finally, commercial diets can be approved in two ways: they can be chemically analyzed to meet AAFCO standards, including approved ingredients from the AAFCO list, or they can be approved by actual feeding trials in which they are fed to animals for 6 months during which time the animals are given regular physical exams and blood tests to show that they are healthy. All the veterinary prescription diets undergo feeding trials before they are released. Many, but not all, premium diets undergo feeding trials. Feeding trials are expensive; thus, companies may prefer to just submit their food for chemical testing. In the 1970s, generic dog food that met AAFCO's label requirements was sold in supermarkets as a super-cheap substitute for other brands. It was easy to spot dogs that were fed this food from the way they smelled and the scruffiness of their coats. Purina did feeding trials with this food, compared to Purina Dog Chow, and showed that puppies fed with the generic food were thin and stunted, and puppies fed Purina Dog Chow looked normal. So when comparing diets, look for companies that are doing their best to determine what really works for an animal, not what matches a formula or idea.

How Much to Feed?

A number of books (and not just holistic ones) recommend that pets choose their own food (free feeding) and say that pets will choose the correct amount if the diet is healthy. This attitude contributes to the obesity epidemic we see in our pets, as well as humans. Some do self-regulate and lose weight on a raw diet. However, others are a little too enthusiastic about the food; pets can gain weight on raw diets, including those without any grains. The amount to feed depends on the pet's appetite and metabolism; the owner must keep an eye on the weight to know how to properly adjust the diet.

Changing the Diet

If an owner asks about changing to a raw diet, before expressing any concerns about raw meat (which can result in their tuning you out), make sure they know about the necessity for properly following a balanced recipe. The most common problem with homemade diets is that the owner starts omitting calcium. (They run out, there isn't that much added, they drop it, and they see no change in their pet so they figure no problem.) The next concern is, what do they do if they have to leave the pet? Do they premake food? Is their significant other willing to take on the burden? The third problem is the cost. Homemade diets, with their emphasis on large amounts of meat, can be costly.

If an owner is feeding a raw diet, there are four concerns: Is it balanced? Are they adding calcium? Are they adding a vitamin/mineral supplement? Is the pet immune-compromised? Some published diets for pets are balanced, but many are not. Susan Wynn's website or the BalanceIT website are the best places for pet owners to go to get a truly balanced diet. Their recommendations include items that can be substituted in their basic diet, and they sell the supplements needed for the diet to be truly balanced.

When changing to a new diet, it is important to do it very slowly. It is common to see a client who heard about a great new diet, changed their pet to it overnight (resulting in diarrhea), changed to a different diet (instead of going back to the old diet), and made things worse. They then bring the animal to your practice. A good rule of thumb when changing diets is to increase the amount of the new diet, and decrease the amount of the old diet by one-fourth every 3 days. For example, when feeding 1 cup of food per meal,

- for the first 3 days, feed ¼ cup new food and ¾ cup old food;
- for the next 3 days, feed ½ cup new food and ½ cup old food;
- for the next 3 days, feed ¾ cup new food and ¼ cup old food;
- on the 10th day, feed only the new food.

At any time, if the diarrhea gets worse instead of better, owners should retreat to the previous mixture for 2 or 3 more days, then try again.

For a pet with diarrhea, the best thing temporarily is a very bland diet. This consists of an equal ratio of boiled nonfatty meat (breast of chicken or turkey, or low-fat hamburger) to boiled white rice. The meat should be shredded so that the pet can't pick it out of the rice. The rice should be white rice, not brown rice. If the pet doesn't like the rice, cream of white rice boiled in chicken or beef broth can be used. At this point there should be no fiber, including FOS (fructo-oligosaccharide). Unfortunately, many "intestinal" diets and an increasing number of probiotics are adding FOS, which often does not help this type of diarrhea and sometimes makes it worse. A few diets are now adding ground cellulose, an insoluble fiber, which can compound the problem.

This is not a balanced diet. However, it is being used to get the diarrhea under control, not as a long-term diet. Once the diarrhea stops, their regular diet can be slowly added in.

Prescribing Specific Diets

Nutritional knowledge varies greatly from one veterinarian to another and holistic veterinarians are no different from conventional ones. Most veterinarians have at least some knowledge of the changes in diet that are recommended for specific diseases. Most holistic veterinarians are very interested in the ideas behind natural or holistic diets, commercial versus homemade, cooked or raw foods, etc. Many have specific ideas about the best diets to feed and will tend to want everyone to recommend the same items. Some veterinarians prefer to discuss this with clients themselves, and others will make recommendations but prefer that the technician discuss the fine details.

There are some specific conditions that can be helped by specific diets. For any problems involving food sensitivity (especially skin problems, vomiting, or diarrhea), a home-cooked diet may also be preferable (Remillard et al., 2000), especially if all commercially available diets for the condition have been tried without success. The diet chosen will depend on the pet's condition and how the pet responds to that diet. The veterinarian will recommend diets depending on his or her experience with them.

Specific Diets for Specific Conditions

The aim of allergic conditions is to give food containing ingredients that the pet has not been exposed to before and to omit chemicals that may make the condition worse. Even if food allergy has not been identified as a source of itching, a change in diet can often help. Years ago, neither lamb nor rice was used in pet food. Thus, a lamb and rice diet was available for an allergic pet, and owners could easily make their own. Today, lamb and rice are common ingredients, so lamb and rice diets are often not suitable. More exotic ingredients such as venison, duck, fish, and potato are currently used for these pets. If owners have already fed these (because they are becoming more available in holistic pet foods), we are often forced into using items such as quinoa for a grain and ostrich or buffalo for a protein source. Another option is to use a hydrolyzed protein product, such as Hills z/d. This turns the protein into a type that is novel again.

Irritable or inflammatory bowel disease (IBD) is another problem that may be helped by diet. There are many factors that figure into this problem, so that there are several approaches to this disease complex. Novel diets can help sometimes, so the same diets that help allergic dermatitis can also help some cases of IBD. Some pets do best on a high-fiber diet, so a weight-control diet such as Hills w/d can also help them, although this can cause problems with weight loss in an animal that is already having problems. Another option is to add canned pumpkin to the diet as an insoluble fiber, but sometimes a more soluble fiber such as beet pulp or even pectin is preferable. Others do best on a low-fiber diet, so if a homemade diet is being used, be sure that only low-fiber ingredients are used. This means white rice, not brown rice, if the owner is using rice. It may be necessary to explain that although brown rice is preferable for its nutrient content, white rice is best for this particular pet because of its low fiber content. Another low-fiber carbohydrate is potato. Prescription diets such as Hills i/d are low in fiber, but the FOSs that are found in i/d may cause a problem for some pets. Again, in this case, a homemade diet may give better results.

With diabetes in cats, two different approaches are used. Many diabetic cats are obese, and a high-fiber weight control diet can help them and also help stabilize blood sugar levels. Hills w/d or even r/d are used for obese diabetic cats. If this does not work, another diet that is closer to a wild cat's diet may be preferable. The prescription version is Hills m/d, but a homemade diet with meat, vegetables, and little to no grain may be the one that works best. Be sure owners always add calcium and taurine (as well as vitamins) to any homemade diet, and that the quantities they add are the those recommended for the recipe they are using.

There are also two approaches to renal disease. First, a high-protein diet does not cause kidney disease. However, once an animal has renal disease, research has shown that a lower protein diet will reduce symptoms and prolong life. There is some argument between prescription diet companies regarding how much lower the protein content has to be. It is important to note that, while people argue about the level of decrease necessary, everyone is in agreement that some decrease in protein can be helpful. A meat and vegetable diet that does not contain any carbohydrates is not suitable for canine patients.

In addition, restricting phosphorus also prolongs life. Even those companies that do not agree on extreme restriction of protein, do agree that lower phosphorus levels are important for the control of this disease. The biggest source of phosphorus is meat. This is another reason for some restriction on meat and the addition of carbohydrates in canine renal diets.

Animals with liver disease require good-quality protein. This is not a problem for homemade diets using meat, poultry, or fish. Overweight cats with hepatic lipidosis need enough calories to maintain their daily needs (often in a form that can be fed through a feeding tube) without causing weight gain. In fact, a slight weight loss can be beneficial. Animals with end-stage liver disease may need less total protein, because at that point, the liver may not be able to handle the ammonia that is generated by protein digestion.

For animals with bladder stones, a diet should help make the urine more dilute. Salt can help dogs with this problem, but cats do not have a good thirst mechanism, and salting a cat's food can lead to dehydration. Homemade or canned food is usually better at increasing water intake than dry food, even though owners will see their pets drinking more water with dry food. There are two groups of stones: those that form in alkaline urine and those that form in acidic urine. Some commercial diets make urine more acid or alkaline, whereas others make it more neutral. When discussing diets for bladder stones, it is important to know which type of stone is the issue in order to recommend the proper diet and to discuss the pros and cons of various supplements with the owners.

Other conditions are more straightforward. Obesity is a growing problem, and low-calorie, high-fiber diets are the best for weight control. Obesity contributes to joint pain, and sometimes losing a lot of weight can help an animal decrease or even stop some arthritis medications.

Congestive heart failure is helped by a low-sodium diet (although this is not always a very palatable approach). Animals with cognitive dysfunction can be helped by adding foods high in antioxidants and flavonoids (such as berries). Tartar control diets usually are harder than regular diets and may have fiber added to keep them from shattering. Bones may be fed for the same purpose, but be careful never to give cooked bones or a bone that can splinter (such as pork chop bones or lamb bones). If a dog bites off large pieces and swallows the pieces whole, bones are not suitable for him. Diets for arthritis usually have supplements added that help joint disease (see Chapter 9). Animals on prescription diets may benefit from ingredients that are not in the food, but they usually don't need any additional amounts of any substance that is already in the diet. Commercial holistic diets may or may not have enough of these supplements added, so owners may need to be warned that they need to add glucosamine, fish oil, or other ingredients in addition to the items listed on the package. For homemade diets, these supplements may be added to the diet itself or given separately.

In the United States, there are four main companies that make prescription diets: Hills Pet Nutrition, Purina, Iams, and Royal Canin. See Appendix 9 for a list of disease problems, the reasons for each special diet, and the prescription diets that may be used for them.

Veterinarian's Role

The veterinarian sets the standards for what type of food the practice recommends. He or she may encourage only raw food; only homemade food, but raw or cooked; only cooked food; or only commercial food. The veterinarian may sell natural foods in the office or send clients to a local holistic pet store or to online services. Discuss pet diets with your veterinarian, and see what their views are. There are valid arguments for and against all methods of feeding, so become acquainted with your veterinarian's point of view so that you can help explain it and make recommendations to your clients.

Technician's Role

Veterinary technicians have a large and often primary role in the client education process when it comes to discussion of the holistic diet, tips and tricks for switching diets, getting animals to eat what we want them to, weight-loss programs, and feeding for specific life stages and diseases. Clients are also curious about diet fads as well as holistic ideas about diets that are not always recognized by conventional medicine. They will want to know about the latest supplement fad or fact. You can take a big load off your employer's shoulders if you can explain the basics. Clients often relate better to technicians than to their veterinarian when discussing the need for a special diet and problems they may have in converting an animal to a new type of diet.

There are times when a conventional prescription diet is the best thing for a pet with a chronic disease. The technician can be helpful here, too, explaining why a diet that appears to be less than ideal, not meeting all the specifications of a holistic diet, can actually be better for specific diseases. In addition, when a technician is conversant with all research findings, she has an answer to statements that are based only on opinion.

For a new client, it can be very helpful to know what a pet is being fed. Often people are more forthcoming to a technician than to a veterinarian. Technicians may be viewed as being less judgmental. With your veterinarian's permission, you can note in the chart, not only the diet itself, but treats and supplements. Don't forget to ask "what else?" at the end. You'd be surprised at how many people have something else to add.

Often, clients have questions about canned food versus dry food, homemade versus commercial, holistic brands versus regular brands, where to get the food, and where to get recipes. Again, the technician can be an invaluable source of knowledge regarding answers to these questions.

The technician should know which stores in their area carry the various items. If the veterinarian carries special diets and supplements, the technician should also be prepared to answer questions and give recommendations about them. For recipes, some may be found in the book, *Small Animal Clinical Nutrition*, but the best option is to direct the clients to one of websites devoted to helping pet owners create a homemade diet. This way, they can find a recipe that includes the ingredients they want to use, that will allow for substitutions, and that will recommend the correct supplements.

Clients will also ask how much to feed their pets. Most companies will have recommendations, and if they do not, the technician can make recommendations based on a similar product from a company that does. Keep in mind two factors: when looking at two dogs that look the same, one may require up to four times as many calories as the other (Burkholder and Toll, 2000), and many manufacturers tend to recommend the top of this range. It is best to recommend about three-fourths (or even one-half, if the breed is known to gain weight easily) of the manufacturer's recommendation, to start.

Where to Learn How

Certification in Small Animal Natural Nutrition (2-year course)
College of Integrative Veterinary Therapies
PO BOX 352
Yeppoon 4703
QLD, Australia
collegeoffice@civtedu.org
https://civtedu.org/courses/certification-small-animal-natural-nutrition

Natural Animal Nutrition (5 month course, not as extensive)
College of Integrative Veterinary Therapies
PO BOX 352
Yeppoon 4703
QLD, Australia
collegeoffice@civtedu.org
https://civtedu.org/courses/natural-animal-nutrition

Summary

What can a technician do?

1) Learn the controversies surrounding conventional pet food and holistic pet food. To give information to clients, you need to know why your practice uses the food it does. There are reasons for and against every food on the market. And remember, something that started as a good food may not stay that way if the company changes ownership. Keep up to date on changes.
2) Learn the characteristics of prescription pet foods and why each is prescribed. This is important, even if your practice does not dispense them. Sooner or later, someone will come to your practice whose pet is eating one of these, and you should know the reason for it.
3) Learn the philosophy of your practice concerning pet foods. Some practices are dedicated to feeding raw food only, whereas others may only use prescription diets. Know why your practice makes its recommendations so you can discuss the reasons with the pet owners who come in.

4) Be knowledgeable enough to be the primary person describing and recommending a pet food, after the veterinarian has determined what is best for the pet. Owners often have many questions, usually after they have left and had time to think things over. Technicians can also help by making sure the owner understands the concept of *slowly* changing from one food to another or that snacks might not be allowed on strict diets for certain diseases.

5) Call the client 3–5 days after a new diet is started to see how the change is going. If there are problems, the technician may be able to help before they escalate without having to call in the veterinarian.

6) Be prepared to answer the question "I thought you were holistic! Why are you recommending XXX diet!" This may be asked even if the diet you recommend is considered by most to be holistic.

7) Be knowledgeable enough to be the point person for ordering, dispensing, recommending flavors, and learning about new diets and their advantages and disadvantages.

8) Be knowledgeable and able to discuss common facets of holistic diets. The field of nutrition engenders a lot of conversation and the technician can save a lot of time for busy veterinarians.

References

Achinewhu S.C. and Hewitt D. 1979. Assessment of the nutritional quality of proteins: the use of "ileal" digestibilities of amino acids as measures of their availabilities. *Br J Nutr* 41:559–571.

Ashes J.R., et al. 1999. Nutritional availability of amino acids from protein cross-linked to protect against degradation in the rumen. *Adv Exp Med Biol* 459:145–159.

Bakke AM, et al. 2022. Responses in randomised groups of healthy, adult Labrador retrievers fed grain-free diets with high legume inclusion for 30 days display commonalities with dogs with suspected dilated cardiomyopathy. *BMC Vet Res* 18(1):157.

Billinghurst I. 2001. *The Barf Diet (Raw Feeding for Dogs and Cats Using Evolutionary Principles)*. Bathurst, NSW: Ian Gregory Billinghurst.

Burkholder W.J. and Toll P.W. 2000. Obesity. In: Hand M.S., et al. *Small Animal Clinical Nutrition*, p. 409. Topeka, KS: Mark Morris Institute.

Clark R. and Stainer J. 1994. *Medical and Genetic Aspects of Purebred Dogs*, p. 118. Fairway, KS: Forum Publications.

Crane S., 2009. *Hills Symposium Proceedings*. Topeka, KS: Hill's Pet Nutrition.

Dzanis D.A. 2009. Petfood Insights: No By-products' No More? Accessed online 3/22/2009 at https://www.petfoodindustry.com/ViewArticle.aspx?id=23578

Enser M., et al. 1998. Fatty acid content and composition of UK beef and lamb muscle in relation to production system and implications for human nutrition. *J Meat Sci* 49:329–341.

Food and Drug Administration/Center for Veterinary Medicine. 2002. Report on the Risk from Pentobarbital in Dog Food. Accessed online at https://www.fda.gov/cvm/FOI/DFreport.htm.

Food and Drug Administration/Consumer Health Information. 2010. No Bones About It: Bones Are Unsafe for Your Dog. Accessed online 5/8/2010 at https://www.fda.gov/downloads/ForConsumers/ConsumerUpdates/UCM209196.pdf.

Food and Drug Administration 2022 FDA Investigation – Potential Link Between Certain Diets and Canine Dilated Cardiomyopathy. Accessed online 5/15/2023 at https://www.fda.gov/animal-veterinary/outbreaks-and-advisories/fda-investigation-potential-link-between-certain-diets-and-canine-dilated-cardiomyopathy

Frazier A. and Eckroate N. 2008. *The Natural Cat: The Comprehensive Guide to Optimum Care*, p. 71–75. New York: Penguin Group.

Hurrell R.F. and Carpenter K.J. 1978. Digestibility and lysine values of proteins heated with formaldehyde or glucose. *J Agri Food Chem* 26:796–802.

Kaplan JL, et al. 2018. Taurine deficiency and dilated cardiomyopathy in golden retrievers fed commercial diets. *PLoS One* 13(12):e0209112.

Lonsdale T. 2005. *Work Wonders: Feed Your Dog Raw Meaty Bones*. Wenatchee, WA: Dogwise Publishing.

Mann N. 2000. Dietary lean red meat and human evolution. *Eur J Nutr* 39(2):71–79.

McCauley SR, et al. 2020. Review of canine dilated cardiomyopathy in the wake of diet-associated concerns. *J Anim Sci* 98(6):skaa155.

McKay P. 1992. *Reigning Cats & Dogs: Good Nutrition Healthy Happy Animals*. Delhi, India: Oscar Publications.

Nestle M. and Nesheim M. 2008. Natural, human grade, organic dog food: really? *The Bark*: 50.

Non-GMO Project. 2023. What Is the Non-GMO Project Standard? Accessed online 6/28/23 at https://www.nongmoproject.org/the-standard/

Pet Food Institute. 2009. *Pet Food Industry Magazine.* The history of the pet food industry. Accessed online 3/22/2009 at https://www.petfoodinstitute.org/petfoodhistory.htm.

Pitcairn R. and Pitcairn S. 2005. *Dr. Pitcairn's New Complete Guide to Natural Health for Dogs and Cats*, 3rd edition, p. 20–21. Emmaus, PA: Rodale Books.

Prange H., et al. 1979. Scaling of skeletal mass to body mass in birds and mammals. *Am Nat* 113(1):103–122.

Quilliam C, et al. 2021. The effects of 7 days of feeding pulse-based diets on digestibility, glycemic response and taurine levels in domestic dogs. *Front Vet Sci* 8:654223. doi: https://doi.org/10.3389/fvets.2021.654223. PMID: 34026892; PMCID: PMC8131660.

Quilliam C, et al. 2023. Effects of a 28-day feeding trial of grain-containing versus pulse-based diets on cardiac function, taurine levels and digestibility in domestic dogs. *PLoS One* 18(5):e0285381.

Remillard R., et al. 2000. Making pet foods at home. In: Hand M.S. *Small Animal Clinical Nutrition*, 4th edition, p. 168. Topeka, KS: Mark Morris Institute.

Stahler D.R., et al. 2006. Foraging and feeding ecology of the gray wolf (*Canis lupus*): lessons from Yellowstone National Park, Wyoming, USA. *J Nutr* 136(7 Suppl):1923S–1926S.

Syverson D. 2009. AAFCO Pet Food Committee Questions and Answers Concerning Pet Food Regulations. Accessed online 3/19/2009 at https://www.aafco.org/Portals/0/Public/Q-AND-A-REGARDING-PETFOODREGS.PDF.

USDA. 2009. Agricultural Marketing Service/Natural Organic Program/Organic Labeling and Marketing Information. Accessed online 3/5/2009 at https://www.ams.usda.gov/AMSv1.0/getfile?d DocName=STELDEV3004446&acct=nopgeninfo.

Vila C., et al. 1997. Multiple and ancient origins of the domestic dog. *Science* 276:1687–1689.

Webliography

College of Integrative Veterinary Therapies
PO BOX 352
Yeppoon 4703
QLD, Australia
collegeoffice@civtedu.org
https://civtedu.org/

9

Nutraceuticals

Definition

If your practice uses some form of glycosaminoglycans, you are already using nutritional supplements. SAM-e, lysine, zinc, choline, and fish oil are other supplements readily available to conventional veterinary medicine, which are already in common use. In addition to glycosaminoglycans and omega-3 fatty acids (in the form of fish oil, not flaxseed oil), most older animals can benefit from antioxidants. Vitamin C, in combination with bioflavonoids, vitamin E, selenium, and coenzyme Q10, is a good basic combination. Carotenoids and flavonoids from berries are also helpful. Vitamin E should never be given without vitamin C because it cycles from antioxidant to pro-oxidant when it is used and needs C as a cofactor to cycle back to an antioxidant. B complex is also useful, especially for animals that have polyuria or decreased appetite.

Additional useful supplements are taurine for heart disease (both canine and feline), L-carnitine for geriatric muscle weakness, L-lysine for feline herpes, DL-methionine as a urinary acidifier (it can help cystitis as well as struvite crystals), and DL-phenylalanine for arthritis. These supplements are discussed further below.

How They Work

Some nutritional supplements are given because the substance may not be at high enough levels in a regular diet. A vitamin–mineral supplement and taurine are examples of this type of supplement. Most nutritional supplements are substances that are used in higher-than-required amounts to help a specific disease or diseases. Nutritional supplements can be used to prevent and help treat almost any problem seen in a veterinary practice. In addition, they are used to maintain optimum health in a pet.

Supplements that are sold by companies directly to veterinarians and that are unavailable to the public are generally high quality. Supplements sold over the counter are often less expensive; however, in a number of studies, some samples have shown little to none of the ingredients listed on the label. Technicians and nurses should be aware of which companies sell legitimate products. The website www.consumerlabs.com is a good resource to help find this out. You can also talk to the companies and ask about their quality control methods.

Complementary Medicine for Veterinary Technicians and Nurses, Second Edition. Nancy Scanlan.
© 2024 John Wiley & Sons, Inc. Published 2024 by John Wiley & Sons, Inc.

Purpose

Nutraceuticals are nutritional supplements that are used to treat diseases or disease symptoms. You will sometimes see this practice called "orthomolecular medicine." It generally does not include deficiency diseases, although veterinarians do see and treat nutritional deficiencies (sometimes previously unrecognized, as in the case of taurine).

History

About 3500 years ago, Egyptians recognized that night blindness could be treated with specific foods. (We now know the problem is a lack of vitamin A.) This knowledge was later lost. In 1747, Sir James Lind, a Scottish surgeon, found that scurvy was treatable with citrus fruit. However, because others still believed it was caused by a lack of cleanliness, among other things, people continued to die from scurvy for decades. (Now we know it is caused by a lack of vitamin C.) After Koch and Pasteur found that bacteria caused many diseases, many people thought some deficiency diseases were infectious diseases. In the late 1800s, studies on beriberi, a thiamine (B$_1$) deficiency, revealed that it could be produced by a diet high in polished (white) rice and cured by brown rice or meat. Before that time, it was thought to be caused by a fungus or possibly a toxin in white rice.

In the early 1900s, specific vitamins were gradually isolated. Originally, they were called *vitamines* from "vita" (life) and "amine" (amino acids) because it was believed they all contained nitrogen. The *e* was later dropped in the United States when it was found that they belonged to various chemical categories other than amines.

Rickets (calcium deficiency) had a history similar to scurvy. Romans, Greeks, and Egyptians recognized rickets as a disease connected with mothers who did not properly care for their infants. In Europe, lack of vitamin D was originally identified as the main problem, but later, it was recognized that calcium also played a part.

Other mineral deficiencies took longer to recognize. For example, selenium toxicity was recognized in the early 1800s, but selenium deficiency was not proven as a problem in the United States until 1957 (Schwarz and Foltz, 1957). Minerals in conventionally farmed soils are gradually depleted and the mineral content of crops has gradually decreased, as seen by comparing USDA information from the 1940s with USDA information from the 1990s. Among other things, minerals act as cofactors that increase the efficiency of various reactions. Deficiencies of microminerals may not be recognized as such, but they may contribute to ill health, slow healing, and a weak immune system. When sources of these minerals are added to the diet, health may improve.

Amino acid deficiencies in pets have not always been recognized. The recommended amount for taurine in cat food has so far been revised upward twice because initial studies with purified diets did not last long enough for long-term deficiency symptoms to appear. An additional change may be forthcoming.

Description

All dietary supplements fall into the nutraceutical category. Broad groups include vitamins, vitamin-like substances, cofactors, minerals, amino acids, trace fatty acids, dietary fiber, and other substances such as glucosamine.

Originally, the discovery of the actions of these factors resulted in the recognition of their role in deficiency diseases and in recommended minimum amounts for pet food. Over time, it has been recognized that nutritional supplements can also be used to treat certain disease symptoms when used in amounts much larger than that recommended for normal health. Some, such as vitamin C, can be used in large amounts with nothing worse than diarrhea as a side effect. Others, such as selenium, are toxic in large doses and must be carefully monitored. Excess minerals are often excreted through the kidneys; thus, owners who enthusiastically supply their pets with overdoses of mineral supplements may inadvertently end up contributing to the formation of kidney stones or bladder stones. Finally, these supplements, especially minerals, may interfere with each other or with certain drugs. Pet owners should be questioned about any supplements they are giving (the amount as well as the type), and the alert technician can help avoid overdoses, as well as interference with chemotherapy, cardiac drugs, or other drugs that a pet may be taking.

The following is a discussion of the primary nutritional supplements, their use, suggested dose, possible side effects, and interference with drugs and with each other. Deficiency disease will be discussed only when it is common. Often, recommended doses are based on human studies or laboratory animal studies because there are few published dog and cat studies on the use of these substances as nutraceuticals. Recommended doses are from Hand's *Small Animal Clinical Nutrition* or (if not available from Hand) extrapolated from human or laboratory studies unless otherwise indicated (Hand et al., 2000).

Antioxidants in General

Antioxidants should be given as a group, not singly. Vitamins E and C are synergistic, and C helps keep vitamin E from turning into a pro-oxidant (see the section on Vitamin E below). Carotenoids as a group are beneficial, whereas beta carotene, when used alone as the only carotenoid, has been associated with an increased incidence of lung cancer in humans. Bioflavonoids have subtly different effects, so no single bioflavonoid will do the whole job. Some antioxidants are water soluble, whereas others are fat soluble, so they obviously have their effects in different parts of the body.

When working with cancer patients, you need to know if they are also dealing with an oncologist and, if so, what the oncologist is doing. Oncologists who use radiation therapy may rely on a certain amount of skin redness (inflammation) to indicate if an animal is especially sensitive or resistant to radiation and, thus, how to adjust the dose of radiation accordingly. High doses of antioxidants will hide this redness because they decrease inflammation and thus may lead to a level of radiation that the oncologist had not intended. Some types of chemotherapy rely on the effects of free radicals to kill cancer. Antioxidants counteract or "quench" free radicals. Oncologists who use this type of chemotherapy will usually not want antioxidants used, unless they are working with the veterinarian to establish an appropriate dose and time schedule.

Finally, clients may read a claim such as "pycnogenol has 10 times the antioxidant effect of vitamin E." This means that 1 gram of pycnogenol can give up 10 times as many electrons to free radicals as can 1 gram of vitamin E. It does not tell us in which chemical reaction this occurs or in what part of the body. If all antioxidants were equal, then the same deficiency disease would be caused by a deficiency of any antioxidant, and it would not matter if an antioxidant is fat soluble or water soluble. Caution any pet owner who is excited about the latest "wonder nutrient" that it is only part of the picture and cannot be used to the exclusion of everything else.

Vitamins and Vitamin-Like Substances

Vitamin A and Carotenoids

Cats are carnivores and need an animal source of vitamin A. Cats can't convert beta carotene into vitamin A, although to a certain extent, dogs can. (Dogs may not be able to do this as well as people, however.) If your veterinarian has recommended vitamin A, caution owners to read the label of any vitamin A supplements they buy. Some say "Vitamin A" and then, in smaller print "in the form of beta carotene." This means there is no real vitamin A in the supplement, and a cat can't use it.

Do not give beta carotene in isolation. Several studies have shown high doses of beta carotene to increase the incidence and severity of three types of lung cancer in human smokers and those exposed to asbestos. For the few studies using mixed carotenoids, this effect was not seen. Vitamins C and E did not mitigate the effect (Goralczyk, 2009). As part of its chemical reaction when it acts as an antioxidant, beta carotene, like vitamin E, may temporarily turn into a pro-oxidant. There is some suggestion that in heavy smokers, there may be such a high concentration of pro-oxidants that large amounts of beta carotene also turn into a pro-oxidant, which increases the risk of cancer (Truscott, 1996). Although pets are not heavy smokers, the effect of being exposed to smog can be the same as smoking, and cats are closer to dust and dirt, which they might inhale.

When giving vitamin A topically, keep in mind that, for cats especially, the topical dose often turns into an oral dose as the pet licks it off. Too much vitamin A is toxic. Tretinoin (Retin-A) is a metabolite of vitamin A that is used for acne and for some types of skin cancer, and it can have similar harmful effects.

Use
Acne (especially topically)
Candidiasis
Gastrointestinal disease (including inflammatory bowel disease)
Some skin conditions (both topically and orally)
Cancer (including topically, on skin cancer)

Suggested Dose
Orally: 2500 IU/35 pounds bodyweight, daily
Topically: 2500 IU daily on the skin

Possible Side Effects
Excess vitamin A is toxic to the liver and can cause calcification of joints.
Excess carotenoids can turn pink skin orange. Vitamin A can irritate some forms of skin disease when applied topically. High doses of vitamin A should not be given to pregnant animals.

Interference
If an oncologist is using some form of retinoic acid to treat a skin cancer, vitamin A will add to the effect and may increase irritation.

Vitamin D

Use
Renal disease (in the form of calcitriol)
Rickets or diet-induced osteoporosis (especially from homemade diets)

Suggested Dose

Give 2.5–3.5 ng/kg/day, or 12 ng/kg twice a week for renal disease, as long as blood phosphorus levels are normal.

Possible Side Effects

Excess vitamin D can cause calcification of soft tissues. If vitamin D is used when the phosphorus level is elevated in renal failure, it may increase the speed of decalcification of bones.

Interference

Calcitriol is a form of vitamin D. Do not use the two together. It should not be used with Epakitin or calcium carbonate. (Epakitin contains calcium carbonate.) If given together, it will elevate blood calcium levels.

Vitamin E

Vitamin E and selenium are synergistic. Often if the two are used together, the result is better than if either is used alone. Selenium is much more toxic than vitamin E, so owners must be cautioned that more is not better.

When vitamin E acts as an antioxidant, it turns into a pro-oxidant. Vitamin C helps it cycle back to an antioxidant. Without additional vitamin C, the pro-oxidant form of vitamin E will continue to increase, and it will no longer have an antioxidant effect. High doses of vitamin E should never be given without additional vitamin C. Even though dogs and cats make their own vitamin C, they do not make enough to counteract the effects of megadoses of vitamin E.

Use

Cardiac failure
Dermatitis
Cancer

Suggested Dose

Cardiac failure: 2 IU/lb, once a day at the closest dose available. For example, liquid vitamin E is available, and this dose can be closely followed. For a 45-pounds dog, 90 IU is recommended, but 100 IU is the most commonly available size for that dose. Therefore, you would use 100 IU.
Dermatitis: 10 IU/lb once a day
Cancer: 20 IU/lb once a day

Possible Side Effects

Diarrhea
May turn a tri-colored collie or Shetland sheepdog into a merle.
When large doses are given without extra vitamin C, it will act as a pro-oxidant and increase inflammation.
Has an anticoagulant effect.

Interferences

Vitamin E increases the effect of digoxin, thus can cause digitalis toxicity in any animal that is taking that drug; it should be used only at low doses in those patients. Oncologists may object to its use with some of their chemotherapy protocols.

B Complex

The B vitamins are often best used together as B complex, rather than as individual vitamins. The exception is B_{12}, especially in the case of inappetence or chronic diarrhea, when it is best given as an injection (see below). B vitamins are lost when there is excess urination, such as from diuretics, renal disease, or Cushing's disease.

Use
Inappetence
Cushing's disease
With diuretics
Renal disease

Suggested Dose
B complex is usually available from veterinarians in tablets or liquid or over the counter as "B-50," which is a capsule in which all of the B vitamins are present in 50 milligram or microgram amounts. B-50 is the form most likely to cause inappetence.

Possible Side Effects
When given orally, high doses of B complex can cause nausea and inappetence. If an owner has suddenly become enamored of supplements, and their pet has stopped eating, question the owner to find out if they have suddenly started giving large doses of B vitamins or other supplements. Excess B complex can be one of the causes. On the other hand, lower amounts of B complex vitamins can stimulate appetite. For this general purpose, twice the amount available in a pet vitamin is usually sufficient.

Interferences
Not applicable

Vitamin B_1 (Thiamine)

Use
Anemia
Cancer
Pain
Wound healing
Ethylene glycol toxicity (antifreeze poisoning)

Suggested Dose
Cats: 25 milligram daily
Dogs: 1 mg/lb, daily by mouth. For antifreeze poisoning, 10–100 milligram IM

Possible Side Effects (Mainly From Injection)
When injected, it can cause allergic symptoms, especially edema, urticaria, dyspnea, and anaphylactic shock.

Interference
Digoxin, dilantin, and diuretics may reduce the blood level or availability of thiamine.

Vitamin B$_2$ (Riboflavin)

Use
Best used as part of B complex, except for lipid storage disease.
Acne
Cancer
GI disease
Lipid storage disease

Suggested Dose
Dog: 10–20 milligram daily
Cat: 5–10 milligram daily

Possible Side Effects
None found.

Interferences
None found.

Vitamin B$_3$ (Niacin)

Use
Cancer
Hypercholesterolemia (very carefully)

Suggested Dose
Use 2.5 mg/lb, twice a day. Start lower and build up to this dose. Decrease if the pet is uncomfortable.

Possible Side Effects (High Doses)
Liver damage
Stomach ulcers
Skin rashes
Pruritis
Low blood pressure
In humans, headaches and skin flushing (which can be seen as lethargy and panting in animals)

Vitamin B$_6$ (Pyridoxine)

Use
Asthma and allergic bronchitis (antihistamine effect)
Cushing's disease
Doxorubicin-induced "hand-foot syndrome"
When giving alcohol for antifreeze poisoning

Suggested Dose
Give 1 mg/lb daily (maximum, 100 milligram)

Possible Side Effects
High doses for long periods of time (over 200 mg/day in humans) can damage sensory nerves and cause ataxia.

Interference
Unlikely

Vitamin B$_{12}$ (Cobalamin)

Use
Chronic diarrhea
Inflammatory bowel disease
Anemia

Suggested Dose
Note that animals with chronic diarrhea are not absorbing this properly from the ileum (first part of the small intestine), so an oral dose will not help. In addition, excess bacteria that may be causing the diarrhea will absorb large amounts of cobalamin, making it unavailable for the patient.

Doses below are given once a week for 6 weeks, then every 2 weeks for 6 weeks, then once a month. It is stored in the liver for a short period of time.

Small dog or cat: 250 microgram subcutaneously
Medium dog: 500 microgram subcutaneously
Large dog: 1000 microgram subcutaneously

Possible Side Effects
Very benign

Interference
Unlikely

Folic Acid

Use
anemia
hepatitis
gingivitis
periodontal disease

Dose
Give 1.5 mcg/lb orally.

Possible Side Effects
Toxicity has been seen in mice on high doses, but not in dogs or cats.

Interference
Normal doses of folic acid can mask B$_{12}$ deficiency, resulting in nerve damage without anemia. It is best to give it with vitamin B$_{12}$.

Choline

Use
Canine and feline cognitive syndrome
Hearing loss

Suggested Dose
Give 10 mg/lb orally twice a day

Possible Side Effects
Excess nervousness
Pacing
Diarrhea (reducing the dose usually stops this problem)

Interference
None found

Biotin

Use
Weak nails and hooves
Biotin deficiency (caused by excess raw egg whites; has been seen when dried egg whites have been used as a protein source. This has happened in foxes grown for their fur and in cats fed a purified diet for experimental purposes.)

Suggested Dose
Give 12.5 mcg/lb daily

Possible Side Effects
Not seen

Interference
Unlikely

Vitamin C and Bioflavonoids (Such as Quercetin and Rutin)

Use
Autoimmune disease
Cancer
Cystitis
Degenerative myelopathy
Distemper (best before nervous system signs show up)
Respiratory disease
Arthritis
Vestibular disease

Dose
Dosage is adopted from Bellfield (1967) for sodium ascorbate orally, not ascorbic acid:
Give 10 mg/lb once to twice daily by mouth to bowel tolerance (usually between 1.5 and 6 grams total).

For ascorbic acid: Give 1000 mg IV, diluted, slowly, for cats and small dogs and 2000 mg IV for medium to large dogs, 3 days in a row for viral diseases. (Caustic to veins; so it should always be diluted and given slowly.)

For cancer: Use a ratio of 100 parts vitamin C to 1 part vitamin K3. Use 1 cc of McGuff Pharmaceuticals Vitamin C (500 mg) in 5 cc of 0.9% saline for small volumes (administered slowly); for larger doses, in 200–300 cc of saline. 500 mg/lb for dogs is a good starting dose for IV use.

The veterinary uses are adapted from the human data. Be sure to use a preservative-free vitamin C source (McGuff makes a good one) and mix it with 0.9% saline (other solutions can cause precipitation). The diluted solution should be administered over a 2-hour period. The first day, a half dose should be administered. For the second and third days, full doses should be administered.

Possible Side Effects
Diarrhea
Kidney or bladder stones

Interference
Can interfere with treatment for oxalate stones

Minerals

Calcium

Use
Use with caution in patients with renal or cardiac disease. *Be sure owners are using a source of calcium if they are feeding a homemade or raw diet.*

Eclampsia (hypocalcemia in bitches)

Suggested Dose
Should be added to homemade diets at the rate of 500 mg per cup of meat. Other doses for problems such as eclampsia should be determined by the veterinarian.

Possible Side Effects
Constipation
Excess calcium in concentrated urine can lead to bladder or kidney stones.
Large-breed puppies exhibit developmental bone problems when oversupplemented with calcium (also seen in Friesian horses).
Excess can leach calcium from bones and cause hypercalcemia.

ALWAYS ASK ABOUT SUPPLEMENTS

A canine patient was referred to me because no matter which diet he was on, he developed bladder stones. At first, he had struvite stones. When the diet was changed to make his urine more acid in order to dissolve struvite crystals, he developed oxalate stones. When I asked the owner what supplements she was feeding, she showed me three different calcium supplements. The dog was being given over three times the maximum recommended daily dose of calcium. When the supplements were stopped, the dog had no further problems.

Interference
Strontium

Phosphorus

Use
Phosphorus is not lacking in a meat-based diet. Phosphorus binders are needed for animals with renal disease. (Excess phosphorus can accelerate the progression of renal failure.) A natural phosphorus binder is calcium carbonate. There is a commercial natural substance (Epakitin) that also binds phosphorus, as does calcium carbonate.

Dose
Not applicable: Phosphorus is not needed in a normal diet. Excess phosphorus is the most common problem.

Possible Side Effects
Excess phosphorus in the diet will leach calcium out of the bones, eventually resulting in osteoporosis. Rather than adding more calcium to the diet, the better remedy is to reduce the phosphorus.

Interference
Not applicable

Sodium

Use (In the Form of Sodium Chloride)
Large animals and rabbits can become dehydrated if there is a lack of sodium in their diet. Some horses eat salt blocks like candy, which is not healthy. They should instead be given loose salt in their feed.

Dogs and cats more often suffer from excess sodium in the diet, especially if they have heart disease. For them, salt should be restricted.

Possible Side Effects
Edema is possible if an animal is not able to excrete sodium properly.

Potassium

Use
Heart patients being given furosemide
Chronic diarrhea

Suggested Dose
Using potassium gluconate (such as Tumil-K) give 1/4 teaspoonful (2 mEq) per 4.5 kg body weight orally in food twice daily.

Possible Side Effects
Excess potassium can cause gastritis
IV potassium chloride is irritating to veins
Contraindicated with renal failure and untreated Addison's disease
Enalapril can cause increased retention
Contraindicated with potassium-sparing diuretics (such as spironolactone)

Selenium

Use
Heart disease
Arthritis
Selenium deficiency (in livestock or horses pastured on selenium-deficient soil)

Dose
Give 1 mcg/10 IU vitamin E.

Possible Side Effects
Selenium toxicity

Magnesium

Use
In small animals, ventricular arrhythmias 0.15–0.3 mEq/kg/day
Muscle relaxant in large animals with grass tetany
Critically ill pets (54% in one study were found to have hypomagnesemia) (Martin et al., 1994)
Pets with hypokalemia (hypokalemia was found in one study to be a significant predictor of hypomagnesemia) (Khanna et al., 1998)

Suggested Dose
For small animals with life-threatening ventricular arrhythmias or other critical care patients: 0.75–1 mEq/kg/day in 5% dextrose (Fascetti, 2003)
For large animals: use with calcium borogluconate. For cattle, up to 500 mL given slowly IV

Possible Side Effects
Diarrhea
CNS depression
Bradycardia
Hypotension (from overdose)
Hypocalcemia

Manganese

Use
Trace mineral

Suggested Dose
Give 0.11 mg/kg/day total. This is present in dog foods and should not be supplemented.

Possible Side Effects
Diarrhea
Interferes with iron absorption at high doses
Ataxia, tremors, and possible pancreatitis at high doses

Iron

Use
Chronic blood loss anemia
When giving erythropoietin

Suggested Dose
For cats treated with erythropoietin: 50–100 mg by mouth once a day
For dogs: 60–300 mg by mouth once a day for 2 weeks

Possible Side Effects
Gastritis

Interference
Fats with iron form soaps
Antacids, eggs, milk reduce absorption
Binds to tetracycline
Chloramphenicol delays its effects.

Copper

Use
Skin disease
Anemia

Dose
Not applicable: Copper is present in vitamin–mineral mixes. Copper deficiency is not seen when feeding normally, but excess copper is a problem in copper storage disease.

Possible Side Effects
Liver toxicity. Some dogs (especially Bedlington terriers) have an inherited disease (copper storage disease) that allows buildup of copper in the liver. *Do not* give copper to these dogs or in a case where it is possible a dog may have this disease.

Interference
Zinc

Zinc

Use
Skin disease
Treat copper poisoning
Treat copper accumulation in liver disease

Dose
Give 10 mg/kg daily of zinc sulfate or zinc gluconate

Possible Side Effects
Copper deficiency. Do not treat this by giving more copper. Treat it by decreasing the dose of zinc.

Interference
Copper

Iodine

Use
Actinomycosis and actinobacillosis (cattle and sheep), sporotrichosis (horses, dogs, cats)
Hypothyroidism
Hyperthyroidism, in early stages (but effects wear off rapidly and higher doses cause iodine poisoning)
Skin disease, especially pigmented skin

Suggested Dose
For kelp (source of iodine and can also be a source of arsenic, so be careful of the source): 6 mg/lb once to twice daily
For potassium iodide: 0.4 mg/lb for dogs for skin disease and hypothyroidism
20 mg/lb for sporotrichosis in dogs
70 mg/kg for cattle with actinomycosis and actinobacillosis

Possible Side Effects
Iodine poisoning

Chromium

Use
As a trace mineral

Dose
Not applicable

Possible Side Effects
Gastroenteritis

Trace Fatty Acids

Omega-3 (Eicosapentaenoic Acid and Docosahexaenoic Acid)

The most common sources of omega-3 are fish oil and flax oil. Cats lack the enzyme to convert the alpha-linolenic acid in flax oil into eicosapentaenoic acid (EPA). Fifteen grams of flaxseed oil has about 8 grams of alpha-linolenic acid. In humans, about 5% of this is converted into EPA, and dogs may be less efficient than this. Thus, fish oil or an algal source of the oil may be the best sources for pets. The current protocol for atypical Cushing's disease calls for flax oil because the lignans in flax oil can inhibit the conversion of adrenal androgens to estrogens. There are no lignans in fish oil, so flax is the better oil to use for Cushing's disease.

Fish oil contains both EPA and docosahexaenoic acid (DHA).

Use

Cancer (DHA)

Skin disease (EPA)

Arthritis (EPA)

Suggested Dose

For atopy and arthritis: 1000 mg of fish oil twice daily in large breed dogs; 22–50 mg/kg of EPA/day.

Flax oil for atypical Cushing's: 1 teaspoonful/25 lb/day

For cancer: 3 : 1 ratio of total omega-3 to omega-6 fatty acids, or 1000 milligram DHA/m^2/day for dogs and 200 milligram DHA/day/cat

Possible Side Effects

May increase the need for vitamin E

Can increase clotting time of blood

Diarrhea and vomiting

Omega-6 (Linoleic and Arachidonic Acids, and Gamma-Linolenic Acid)

Although omega-6 fatty acids are essential, especially for skin health, it is rare to see omega-6 fatty acid deficiency in the United States. This was not always the case, so many skin supplement products still contain omega-6 oils (mostly linoleic and arachidonic acids). Because an excess of these two omega-6 fatty acids can make some skin conditions worse and may increase the chance of cancer, it may be better to avoid supplements with linoleic and arachidonic acid.

GLA (gamma-linolenic acid) is another type of omega-6 fatty acid that increases tryptase activity and decreases histamine release. Sources of GLA include borage oil, evening primrose oil, black currant seed oil, hemp seed oil, and spirulina.

Use

Skin disease

GLA: autoimmune disease, cancer, and arthritis

Suggested Dose

GLA: 100 mg/kg/day black currant oil

Possible Side Effects

For all: nausea, vomiting, diarrhea

For linoleic and arachidonic acids: can make skin disease worse, increase the need for vitamin E, and increase the chance of cancer

Omega-9

Olive oil has the highest amount of omega-9. The body can produce omega-9 oils from omega-3 and omega-6.

Use

Skin problems

Type 2 diabetes

Suggested Dose
Give 1/4 tsp olive oil twice a day for large dogs

Possible Side Effects
Diarrhea (although the expense of this product makes it unlikely that pets will get that much)

Dietary Fiber

Fiber has been divided into soluble and insoluble types, but there is actually a spectrum ranging from very insoluble to very soluble. Some animals do better with more fermentable (more soluble) fiber, whereas others do better with less fermentable (more insoluble) fiber. An owner may have to experiment to determine the type and amount that work best.

Some natural sources of fiber include insoluble canned pumpkin (without spices), soluble apple pectin, soluble slippery elm bark, intermediate flaxseed, and intermediate psyllium husks. (See Table 9.1 for a summary of fiber types.)

Table 9.1 Dietary fiber (from least to most soluble).

LEAST SOLUBLE FIBERS
Fibers with primarily cellulose, hemicellulose, lignan:
Powdered cellulose
Wheat bran
Oat fiber (husk, hulls)
Soy fiber
Pea fiber
Carrot fiber
Potato fiber
Beet pulp
Fibers with beta-glucans
Oat bran, barley
Psyllium husk 75% soluble fiber
Psyllium (extracted from the husk)
Pectin
Fructooligosaccharides
Gums: guar gum (from guar seeds), carrageenan (from seaweed), agar (from seaweed)
Inulin
Fibers with gums, mucilages, polyfructoses, pectins
MOST SOLUBLE FIBERS

Source: Adapted from Linus Pauling Institute's (2023) and Tarte (2009).

Use
Diarrhea
Constipation

IBD
Megacolon
Weight loss

Suggested Dose
Depends on the type of fiber and the problem
For canned pumpkin: 1 tbsp or more for a large breed dog
For pectin: 1/4 teaspoonful for a large breed dog

Possible Side Effects
It can make diarrhea or constipation worse, as well as better, so use carefully.

Amino Acids

DL-Methionine

Use
To acidify urine

Suggested Dose
Give 5 mg/lb twice daily

Possible Side Effects
Excess acidification of the urine, increased chance of oxalate stones, occasional nausea (evidenced by drooling, decreased appetite).

L-Taurine

Use
Cardiomyopathy

Suggested Dose
Give 50 mg/lb per day

Possible Side Effects
Nausea

Interference
None found

L-Carnitine (Formed From Lysine and Methionine)

Use
Muscle weakness
Heart disease

Suggested Dose
Give 50 mg/lb/day

Possible Side Effects
Nausea
Diarrhea

Interference
None found

L-Tryptophan

Use
Insomnia (but insomnia can be from a number of things, including Cushing's disease, hyperthyroidism, and sundowner syndrome. L-tryptophan should be used after all other possibilities have been explored and corrected).

Suggested Dose
Give 10 mg/lb/day (possibly best given at night before bedtime)

Possible Side Effects
Original side effects (eosinophilia-myalgia syndrome) reported in the news in 1989 were from contamination. Current sources have not had any reported contamination.
  Serotonin syndrome is possible if given with DLPA, Tramadol, or SSRIs such as Prozac. Do not use together.

L-Lysine

Use
Chronic feline herpes (works best in adult cats, given long-term)

Suggested Dose
Give 300–500 mg/day, up to 500 milligram twice daily

Possible Side Effects
Nausea
Vomiting

DL-Phenylalanine (DLPA)

The L form of phenylalanine, although a more natural form, has no pain-relieving property. It does help anxiety. There is no pure D form, so for an analgesic effect, the DL form must be used. Occasionally, those who work in health food stores may convince your clients that they should not use the D form because it is not natural or because they believe all the research was done on the L form. This is not true.

Use
Arthritis (as a pain reliever)
Anxiety

Suggested Dose
Give 500 milligram twice daily for a large breed dog

Possible Side Effects
Side effects are nausea and vomiting. *Reduce or eliminate the dose if giving with tramadol or SSRIs such as Prozac.* Dextromethorphan can also be a problem, although usually not as severe. Otherwise, serotonin syndrome is possible. Serotonin syndrome is potentially fatal. Symptoms of serotonin syndrome include the following:

Agitation, confusion, or restlessness
Nausea, vomiting, or diarrhea
Tachycardia
Hyperthermia
Ataxia and muscle stiffness
Hyperreflexia
High blood pressure
Shivering or tremors

Treatment of serotonin syndrome includes the following:

Diazepam for anxiety and muscle stiffness
Cyproheptadine (which blocks serotonin production)
IV fluids

In severe cases, assisted breathing and nerve blockers (to decrease muscle spasm) may be required.

L-Arginine

Use
Heart failure
Wound healing
Muscle building (in senior animals)
Metabolic alkalosis
High blood pressure

Suggested Dose
Give 500 mg once a day in a large dog

Possible Side Effects
Nausea

Interference
Lysine

L-Glutamine

Use
Promotes cell growth (both normal and possibly cancer)
Promotes GI cell growth and regeneration with severe trauma or severe diarrhea
Acute and chronic diarrhea
Increases muscle mass in seniors

Suggested Dose
Give 1–15 g/day in divided doses

Possible Side Effects
Nausea
Vomiting
Diarrhea
Skin rash

Interference
Use low doses with hepatic or renal impairment
Probably best to avoid in cancer patients

Glycine

Use
Insomnia
Hypoglycemia

Suggested Dose
Give 500–1000 milligram twice daily for a large breed dog

Possible Side Effects
GI signs
Rash

Cofactors—CoQ 10

Use
CoQ 10 is a cofactor in the production of ATP. It is used for the following:
Heart disease

Decreased tear formation
Cancer

Suggested Dose
Give 30–60 mg twice daily for a large breed dog. More to treat cancer.

Possible Side Effects
Nausea
Diarrhea

Other

Inositol, IP6 (Inositol Hexaphosphate)

Use
Depression
Anxiety
Cancer

Suggested Dose
Give 400–800 mg twice daily for a large breed dog

Possible Side Effects
Flushing (seen as panting) for IP6

PABA

Use
Pemphigus
IBD

Suggested Dose
Give 25 mg/lb four times a day

Possible Side Effects
Vomiting
Skin rash

Probiotics

Probiotics should contain the species that inhabit both the small intestine (such as *Lactobacillus* spp.) and the large intestine (such as *Bifidobacter* spp.). *Saccharomyces* is a probiotic that is a beneficial yeast. It is not affected by antibiotics.

Use
After antibiotics
Chronic diarrhea

Inflammatory bowel disease
Yeast infections

Suggested Dose
Add small pinch of the powder to the food twice daily

Possible Side Effects
Occasionally, diarrhea

Interference
Antibiotics kill the probiotic bacteria. A beneficial enteric yeast (*Saccharomyces boulardii*), not affected by the antibiotics, is often included in probiotic formulas.

Glycosaminoglycans

Glucosamine, chondroitin, green-lipped mussels, gelatin, sea cucumber, and cartilage all contain glycosaminoglycans.

Use
Arthritis
Diarrhea

Suggested Dose
For glucosamine, 500–750 milligram twice daily for a large dog

Possible Side Effects
Diarrhea
Allergic reactions for animals allergic to shellfish (most glucosamine is made from crab shells. However, there is a vegetarian formula that avoids this problem.)

Interference
Can prolong clotting time. Decrease 5 days before surgery.

MSM (Methyl Sulfono-Methane)

MSM has been touted as the dry form of DMSO. Although related, it does not have the same properties (ability to penetrate skin, for example).

Use
Arthritis

Suggested Dose
Give 10 mg/lb twice a day

Possible Side Effects
Diarrhea
Nausea

N-Acetyl-Cysteine

Use
Respiratory disease
Acetaminophen poisoning
Hepatitis
Cancer

Suggested Dose
Give 500 milligram once daily for a large breed dog
For acetaminophen toxicity: 140 mg/kg by mouth or intravenously as initial dose, then 70 mg/kg by mouth every 4–6 hours for 3–5 treatments

Possible Side Effects
Nausea, allergic reaction

N-Acetylcarnosine

Use
Cataracts

Suggested Dose
Use topically, 1% solution. Takes at least 2 months to see results.

Possible Side Effects
Stinging

Caprylic Acid (From Coconut Oil)

Use
May help yeast infections (Papavassilis et al., 1999)

Suggested Dose
Full-strength topically, or up to 5 cc (1 tsp) twice daily for a large breed dog

Possible Side Effects
Diarrhea

DMG (Dimethyl Glycine)

Use
Liver disease

Dose
Give 4 mg/lb per day

Possible Side Effects
Nausea

Pycnogenol (Extract From the Bark of the Maritime Pine)

Use
Arthritis
Skin disease
Heart disease
Allergies

Suggested Dose
Give 0.5 mg/kg twice daily

Possible Side Effects
Nausea

Undecylenic Acid (Derived From Castor Oil)

Use (Topically Only)
Fungicidal
Bactericidal
Virucidal
Psoriasis

Suggested Dose
Topical 10% solution, applied daily

Possible Side Effects
Can burn skin

SAM-e (s-Adenosyl Methionine)

Use
Liver disease
May help arthritis

Suggested Dose
Give 9 mg/lb/day; may be divided into two doses

Possible Side Effects
Diarrhea
Nausea

Diatomaceous Earth (DE)

There are several forms of diatomaceous earth. The form used for swimming pool filters has been heated and is not appropriate for animals. DE that is designed to be used in gardens as a pesticide may also have pyrethrins or other insecticides added. The only type of diatomaceous earth that should be used on or in pets is the type that is pure and that has come straight out of the ground.

Use

Insecticide

Parasiticide

Mineral supplement (especially for microminerals)

Suggested Dose

For flea control: Sprinkle lightly over the skin and work in, as you would a flea powder. (Do not inhale.)

For food supplement: 1 tsp daily per 50 lb body weight

Possible Side Effects

If inhaled, can cause lung damage, similar to silicosis

Lactose

Lactose is made of two simple sugars: glucose and galactose. It is not digested or absorbed by most adult mammals. It is fermented by bacteria, and lactose and fermentation products in the intestinal lumen draw liquid into the intestinal tract. This liquid helps softens stools. It can be used the same way as lactulose, which is made of fructose and galactose, and works the same way.

Lactose can be given in the form of milk. It works best in conjunction with a fiber supplement and can be given in place of lactulose.

Use

Megacolon

Constipation

Suggested Dose

For a cat, start with 10 mg of lactose, or ½ teaspoonful of milk, and gradually increase until the pet is defecating properly. If excess gas and cramping occur before the desired effect is reached, stop.

Possible Side Effects

Cramping

Diarrhea

Interference

Lactose and lactulose work in similar ways, but milk tastes better than lactulose. When using them together, the dose of lactulose must often be decreased. Owners often like this, since most cats prefer milk to lactulose.

Melatonin

Use

Cushing's disease (hyperadrenocorticism)

Atypical Cushing's disease

Alopecia X

Reversed sleep-wake cycle (especially in elderly dogs)

Suggested Dose

1–3 milligram at night, ½ hour before bedtime

For atypical Cushing's disease: 1 mg/20 lb bodyweight (maximum dose 5 milligram), once a day at night. (Many recommend that it be given twice daily, but better results are possible when using it as the body does: one big dose at night.) It is even better when given with flaxseed.

Possible Side Effects

Sleepiness

Phosphatidyl Serine

Use

Canine cognitive syndrome

Dose

Give 2 mg/lb once a day

Side Effects

Unlikely; nausea and vomiting possible

Phosphatidylcholine

In lecithin, pure lecithin may be less effective and often causes nausea.

Use

Canine cognitive syndrome

Liver disease

Topically for acne and psoriasis

Dose

Give 25–50 mg/kg/day

Alpha Lipoic Acid (for Dogs Only)

Do not use in cats. It can be toxic, even in doses as low as 13 mg/kg.

Use

Liver disease

Peripheral neuropathy

Cognitive dysfunction

Dose

Up to 300 mg/day for a large breed dog

Side Effects

May decrease the amount of insulin needed in diabetic dogs

These supplements are summarized in Table 9.2.

Table 9.2 Nutraceuticals: indications, doses, and interactions.

Category	Subcat	Nutraceutical	Indication	Dietary source	Dose	Possible adverse effects	Interactions	Comments
Vitamins								
	Fat-soluble							
		Vitamin A	Some skin conditions (topically and orally–topically for acne), GI disease including IBD, candidiasis, cancer (topically)	Liver, fish oil	Oral: 2500 IU per lb body weight, daily; Topical: 2500 IU daily on skin	Excess dose is toxic to liver; calcification of joints; irritates some forms of skin disease when used topically. Avoid in pregnant animals.	Adds to the effect of retinoic acid (for skin cancer) and can increase irritation	
		Beta carotene				High doses of beta carotene have increased the incidence of three types of breast cancer in humans		Cats can't convert it to vitamin A
		Carotenoids				High doses can turn pink skin orange		
		Vitamin D	Renal disease (used as calcitriol), rickets, or diet-induced osteopenia or osteoporosis	Sunshine, liver, fish oil	2.5–3.5 ng/kg/day, or 12 ng/kg twice a week for renal disease as long as blood calcium levels are normal	High doses can cause calcification of soft tissues. If used in renal failure with elevated phosphorus level, can increase the speed of decalcification of bones	Calcitriol is a form of vitamin D. Do not used the two together.	

(Continued)

Table 9.2 (Continued)

Category	Subcat	Nutraceutical	Indication	Dietary source	Dose	Possible adverse effects	Interactions	Comments
		Vitamin E	Cardiac failure, dermatitis, cancer	Cardiac failure: 2 IU per pound SID (at the closest dose available); Dermatitis: 10 IU/lb SID; Cancer: 20 IU/lb SID	Increases clotting time; high doses of vitamin E without additional vitamin C can cause increased risk of cancer. Diarrhea. High doses can turn a tri-colored collie or shetland sheepdog into a merle	Synergistic with selenium. Increases the effect of digoxin and can cause digitalis toxicity in pets taking a normal dose of digoxin. Vitamin C required as co-factor to cycle the pro-oxidant form of vitamin E back to its anti-oxidant form		
		Vitamin K						
Water-soluble		B complex	Inappetence, renal disease, Cushing's disease, diuretics			Large doses can cause nausea and inappetence		
		B_1 (thiamine)	Anemia, cancer, pain, wound healing, ethylene glycol toxicity		Cats: 25 mg/day; Dogs: 1 mg/lb daily. Antifreeze poisoning: 10–100 mg IM	When injected can cause edema, urticaria, dyspnea, anaphylactic shock	Digoxin, dilantin, and diuretics can reduce blood level or availability	
		B_2 (riboflavin)	Lipid storage disease		Cats: 5–10 mg/day; Dogs: 10–20 mg/day 2/5 mg/lb BID			

Vitamin	Uses	Dose	Side effects	Comments
B_3 (niacin)	Cancer, hypercholesterolemia (carefully)		Liver damage, stomach ulcers, pruritis, skin rashes, low blood pressure, lethargy, panting	
B_6 (pyridoxine)	Asthma, allergic bronchitis, Cushing's disease, when giving alcohol for antifreeze poisoning, doxorubicin side effects	1 mg/lb, maximum of 100 mg	High doses for long periods of time: damaged sensory nerves, ataxia	
B_{12} (cobalamin)	Chronic diarrhea, IBD, anemia	Cats and small dogs: 250 mcg SQ; medium dogs: 500 mcg SQ; large dogs 1000 mcg SQ (see schedule under comments)		Must be injected if used for chronic diarrhea. Give once a week for 6 weeks then every 2 weeks for 6 weeks, then once a month
Folic acid	Anemia, hepatitis, gingivitis, periodontal disease	1.5 mcg/lb	Toxicity from high doses seen in mice, not reported in dogs or cats	Can mask B12 deficiency, resulting in nerve damage without anemia; Best given with Vitamin B_{12}
Choline	Canine and feline cognitive syndrome, hearing loss	10 mg/lb orally BID	Excess nervousness, pacing, diarrhea (resolves with decreased dose)	
Biotin	Weak, brittle nails and hooves; excess raw egg whites in diet	12.5 mcg/lb/day		Raw egg whites destroy biotin

(Continued)

Table 9.2 (Continued)

Category	Subcat	Nutraceutical	Indication	Dietary source	Dose	Possible adverse effects	Interactions	Comments
		Vitamin C	Autoimmune disease, cancer, cystitis (carefully), degenerative myelopathy, distemper (before nervous systems signs appear), respiratory disease, arthritis, vestibular disease			Diarrhea, kidney or bladder stones	Can interfere with treatment for oxalate stones	Use sodium ascorbate orally, ascorbic acid IV; for cancer use 100 parts vitamin C to 1 part vitamin K3
		Bioflavonoids	Use with vitamin C	Rose hips, citrus peel			Improves effectiveness of vitamin C	
Minerals		Calcium	Homemade or raw diet without bones		Calcium gluconate: 94–140 mg/kg IV slowly to effect	High doses: Constipation, bladder or kidney stones, developmental bone problems in large breed puppies and Friesian horses (possibly also draft breeds); Injectable form: Do not use with ventricular fibrillation; use with caution with renal or cardiac disease	Strontium blocks uptake when fed together; strontium and boron increase bone strength when fed separately; vitamin D increases absorption; excess phosphorus causes calcium excretion	

Phosphorus	Meat					Excess phosphorus leaches calcium from bones and speeds deterioration of kidneys in renal patients
Sodium		Required by large animals and rabbits		Fluid retention, especially in animals with heart disease		
Potassium		Pets given furosemide	Potassium gluconate (Tumil-K) 1/4 tsp (2 mEq)/4.5 kg PO BID	Gastritis; IV is irritating to veins; contraindicated with renal failure and untreated Addison's disease	Increased retention with enalapril	
Selenium		Selenium deficiency (large animals); heart disease, arthritis	1 mcg for every 10 IU vitamin E given	Selenium poisoning		
Magnesium		Muscle relaxant		Diarrhea		
Manganese		Trace mineral		Diarrhea		
Iron		Anemia		Gastritis	Fats form soaps with iron	
Copper		Skin disease, anemia		Liver toxicity	Zinc blocks uptake of copper	Copper storage disease, seen in breeds such as the Bedlington terrier, causes accumulation of copper

(Continued)

Table 9.2 (Continued)

Category	Subcat	Nutraceutical	Indication	Dietary source	Dose	Possible adverse effects	Interactions	Comments
		Zinc	Skin disease			Copper deficiency	Interferes with copper absorption	
		Iodine		Kelp, potassium iodide	Kelp: 6 mg/lb SID-BID; KI: Dogs: 4 mg/lb for skin diseases 20 mg/lb for sporotrichosis; Cats: not recommended; Cattle: 70 mg/kg	Injectable form: Do not use with ventricular fibrillation; use with caution with renal or cardiac disease; Iodine poisoning possible, especially in cats		
Trace fatty acids		Chromium	Trace mineral			Gastroenteritis		
		Omega-3 fatty acids (EPA and DHA)	Cancer, skin disease, arthritis, atypical Cushing's disease	Fish oil, flax oil, some algae	Fish oil: 1000 mg BID for large dogs; EPA: 22 mg/kg/day; flax oil for atypical Cushing's disease: 1 tsp/25 lb/day	May increase need for vitamin E, increased clotting time, diarrhea, vomiting		Cats require fish oil; in dogs flax oil is poorly converted to omega-3 and large quantities are needed
		Omega-6 fatty acids (linoleic and arachidonic acids)	Some skin diseases	Canola oil		Excess can increase inflammation, worsen some skin conditions, may increase chance of cancer; caution in dogs with pancreatitis, chronic diarrhea, type 2 diabetes		

	Supplement	Indication	Sources	Dose	Side effects		
	GLA (the other omega-3 fatty acid)	Autoimmune disease, cancer, arthritis	Borage oil, evening primrose oil, black currant seed oil, hemp seed oil, spirulina				
	Omega-9	Skin disease, type 2 diabetes	Olives, avocados, almonds				
Amino acids							
	DL-methionine	Alkaline urine		5 mg/lb BID	Excess acidification of urine, oxalate stones, nausea		
	L-taurine	Homemade cat diets; cardiomyopathy		50 mg/lb/day	Nausea		
	L-tryptophan	Insomnia		10 mg/lb/day	Side effects originally reported were from contaminants, not the L-tryptophan		
	L-lysine	Feline herpes		300–500 mg/day	Nausea, vomiting		
	DL-phenylalanine (DLPA)	Pain and anxiety		500 mg BID for a large dog	Nausea, vomiting, serotonin syndrome if used with tramadol	Decrease or stop when using tramadol or else may cause serotonin syndrome; may also occur with SSRIs such as Prozac	D-form helps pain, L-form helps anxiety

(Continued)

Table 9.2 (Continued)

Category	Subcat	Nutraceutical	Indication	Dietary source	Dose	Possible adverse effects	Interactions	Comments
		L-arginine	Heart failure, wound healing, metabolic alkalosis, hypertension, muscle building		500 mg BID for a Nausea large dog		Lysine interferes with its actions	
		L-glutamine	Diarrhea, increasing muscle mass in seniors		1–15 g/day in divided doses	Nausea, vomiting, diarrhea, skin rash	Use low doses with hepatic or renal impairment	
		Glycine	Insomnia, hypoglycemia		500–1000 mg BID for a large breed dog	GI signs, rash		
	Combination: lysine plus methionine							
Cofactor		L-carnitine	Muscle weakness, heart disease		50 mg/lb/day	Nausea, diarrhea		
		Coenzyme Q10	Heart disease, cancer, decreased tear formation		30–60 mg BID for a large dog; higher for cancer	Nausea, diarrhea		
Other		Alpha lipoic acid	Dogs: liver disease, cognitive dysfunction, peripheral neuropathy. NOT FOR CATS		Dogs: up to 300 mg/day for large dogs		Can decrease the amount of insulin needed for diabetic dogs	Do not use cats
		Caprylic acid	*Malassezia* infections	Coconut oil	Topically: full strength; orally: up to 1 tsp BID for large dogs	Diarrhea		

Diatomaceous earth (oral form)	Insecticide, mineral supplement	.	1 tsp BID orally for mineral supplement	Inhalation causes lung damage	
DMG (dimethyl glycine)	Liver disease		4 mg/lb/day	Nausea	
Glycosaminoglycans	Arthritis, diarrhea		Glucosamine: 500–750 mg BID for a large dog	Diarrhea, allergic reactions (especially if allergic to shellfish), can prolong clotting time	
Inositol, IP6	Depression, anxiety, cancer		400–800 mg BID for a large breed dog	Flushing (panting) for IP6	
Lactose	Megacolon	Milk	Cats: 10 mg lactose or 1/2 tsp milk BID and increase to desired effect	Gas and cramping, diarrhea	Decrease lactulose if using lactose/milk
Melatonin	Cushing's disease, alopecia X, reversed sleep–wake cycle		1 mg/20 lb, in pm 1/2 h before bedtime	Sleepiness	
MSM	Arthritis		10 mg/lb BID	Nausea, diarrhea	
N-Acetyl cysteine	Respiratory disease, acetaminophen poisoning, hepatitis		500 mg SID for a large breed dog for acetaminophen poisoning; 150 mg/kg loading dose then 50 mg/kg q4h for 17 doses (dog) or 3–5 doses (cat)	Nausea, allergic reaction	
N-Acetyl carnosine	Cataracts		1% solution in eye SID-BID for at least 2 months	Stings	

(Continued)

Table 9.2 (Continued)

Category	Subcat	Nutraceutical	Indication	Dietary source	Dose	Possible adverse effects	Interactions	Comments
		PABA	Pemphigus	Liver, kidney, brewer's yeast	25 mg/lb QID	Vomiting, skin rash		Can interfere with actions of sulfonamides
		Phosphatidylcholine	Canine cognitive syndrome, liver disease, topically for acne and psoriasis	Lecithin	25–50 mg/kg/day			
		Phosphatidyl serine	Canine cognitive syndrome		2 mg/lb daily		Best effects when given with phosphatidyl choline	
		Probiotics	When giving antibiotics, diarrhea, IBD, yeast infections		Small pinch of powder on food BID (at least 1/2 h after antibiotics, if they are being given)		Antibiotics kill most probiotics, with the exception of Saccharomyces	
		Pycnogenol	Arthritis, skin disease, heart disease, allergies	Bark of the maritime pine	0.5 mg/kg BID	Nausea		
		SAM-e	Liver disease		9 mg/lb/day			
		Undecylenic acid	Topical fungicide, bactericide, virucide, psoriasis	Castor oil	Topical 10% solution applied daily	Nausea, diarrhea		

Veterinarian's Role

A veterinarian may be well versed in supplementation, may know a few supplements beyond the traditional veterinarian's armamentarium, or may just follow the crowd. As of the writing of this book, the following nutraceuticals are commonly presented to traditional veterinarians by veterinary drug companies:

Glycosaminoglycans (glucosamine and chondroitin, as well as perna canaliculus and sea cucumber)
L-lysine
DL-methionine
SAM-e (in combination with the herb milk thistle)
Choline
Injectable vitamin E with selenium
Zinc
Probiotics (often with prebiotics)

As veterinarians become more aware of the benefits of supplements, this list will continue to grow. Only two of these items were being marketed to veterinarians in 1970.

A veterinarian must diagnose the condition for which supplements may be helpful. Your veterinarian may prefer to recommend the initial program or prefer that the technician explain it. In addition, a veterinarian may prefer to stock all supplements or send a client to a nearby vitamin store or holistic pet store to buy them.

Technician's Role

A good technician will be aware of any drugs that may be affected by supplements. When in doubt, look it up. A technician can help clear up any confusion the client may have about dosage, storage, and giving with or without food or other medication. The technician can keep track of items that are especially popular or come from companies that might be a little slow to deliver so that enough items are ordered far enough in advance to avoid running out. Be aware of which over-the-counter supplements are acceptable and which may not be a good substitute for the veterinary version.

Where to Learn How

There are no easy, short courses in nutraceuticals; their potential medicinal use must be teased out of books on nutrition. Seminars sponsored by pet food companies are often good sources of information, although you will not always be told actual doses of substances. Meetings that have sessions that include complementary medicine often will have items relating to nutraceuticals.

Summary

What can a technician do?

1) Ensure that nutraceuticals are properly stocked and items are rotated by date so the oldest gets used first. Keep track of popular and less-popular items to avoid running out of the popular ones and over-ordering those that are used less often.

2) Watch websites such as consumerlabs.com. They keep track of which items have the amount and potency of the ingredients claimed on the bottle. Also watch for news of contamination or of companies going out of business. This can impact the items your clinic carries. Let your veterinarian know of any potential supply problems and help them decide what to do next, before you run out of the item in question.

3) Answer clients' questions about nutraceuticals.

4) Be aware of potential drug interactions, possible toxicities, or items that should not be used with certain diseases. Clients tend to think that if it is a vitamin, it is harmless.

5) Get a list of all supplements a pet is taking and put it at the front of the chart.

References

Bellfield W. 1967. Vitamin C in treatment of canine and feline distemper complex. *Vet Med Small Anim Clin* 62:345.

Fascetti A. 2003. Magnesium: pathophysiological, clinical and therapeutic aspects. *Proceedings of ACVIM 2003 meeting*, 6–8th June 2003. Charlotte, North Carolina: ACVIM.

Goralczyk R. 2009. Beta-carotene and lung cancer in smokers: review of hypotheses and status of research. *Nutr Cancer* 61(6):767–774.

Hand M.S., et al. 2000. *Small Animal Clinical Nutrition*, 4th edition Topeka, KS: Mark Morris Institute.

Khanna C., et al. 1998. Hypomagnesemia in 188 dogs: a hospital population-based prevalence study. *J Vet Intern Med* 12:304–309.

Linus Pauling Institute Micronutrient Information Center. 2023. Fiber. Accessed online 07/20/2023 at https://lpi.oregonstate.edu/infocenter/phytochemicals/fiber/#intro;

Martin L.G., et al. 1994. Abnormalities of serum magnesium in critically ill dogs: incidence and implications. *J Vet Emerg Crit Care* 4(1):15–20.

Papavassilis C., et al. 1999. Medium-chain triglycerides inhibit growth of *Malassezia*: implications for prevention of systemic infection. *Crit Care Med* 27(9):1781–1786.

Schwarz K. and Foltz C.M. 1957. Selenium as an integral part of factor 3 against dietary necrotic liver degeneration. *J Am Chem Soc* 79:3292–3293.

Tarte R. ed. 2009. *Ingredients in Meat Products*. New York: Springer, pp. 85–90.

Truscott T.G. 1996. Beta-carotene and disease: a suggested pro-oxidant and antioxidant mechanism and speculations concerning its role in cigarette smoking. *J Photochem Photobiol B* 35(3):233–235.

Bibliography

Jamison J.M., et al. 2002. Autoschizis: A novel cell death. Department of Urology, Summa Health System/Northeastern Ohio Universities College of Medicine. Accessed online 05/05/2023 at jmj@neoucom.edu.

Lim-Sylianco C., et al. 1992. Antigenotoxicity of dietary coconut oil. *Sci Diliman* 4(1):1–24.

Mandelker L. 2004. Nutraceuticals and other biological therapies. *Vet Clin NA* 34(1):xi–xii.

Michaud D.S., et al. 2000. Intake of specific carotenoids and risk of lung cancer in 2 prospective US cohorts. *Am J Clin Nutr* 72(4):990–997.

Ogbolu D.O., et al. 2007. *In vitro* antimicrobial properties of coconut oil on *Candida* species in Ibadan, Nigeria, *J Med Food* 10(2):384–387.

Padayatty S.J., et al. Intravenously administered vitamin C as cancer therapy: Three cases. Molecular and Clinical Nutrition Section, Digestive Diseases Branch, National Institute of Diabetes and Digestive and Kidney Diseases, Bethesda, MD 208921372, USA.

Ruaux C. 2002. *Cobalamin and Gastrointestinal Disease*, 7–9th June 2002. Conference Proceedings. Lakewood, CO: ACVIM.

Thorne Research. 2002. Undecylenic acid monograph. *Altern Med Rev* 7(1):68–70.

Werbach M.R. 1996. *Nutritional Influences on Illness*, 2nd edition Tarzana, CA: Third Line Press.

Webliography

EBSCO Publishing
https://www.ebsco.com/products
Their health library is a subscription-based library accessible online, including alternative medicine sources.

Mayo Clinic Herb and Drug Guide
https://www.mayoclinic.org/drugs-supplements
One of the best online references for herbs including interactions with drugs, from a physician's point of view. Information for humans, but applicable to animals.

10

More Treatments with a Certification Program

The following chapter provides an introduction to additional types of holistic practices that have certification programs. The first ones Chinese food therapy, Western herbal medicine, aromatherapy, and Veterinary Orthopedic Manipulation (VOM) are available for veterinary technicians. The next modality in this chapter, homeopathy, has a veterinarian-only certification course, but certification in homeopathy for humans is available to technicians.

After that, equine osteopathy taught by the Vluggen Institute, occasionally accepts non-veterinarians on a case-by-case basis. The last three, acupuncture, Chinese herbal medicine, and Ayurvedic medicine do not have certification courses for technicians. An explanation of the theory behind these is included so that technicians can better explain these to clients, if any of them are included in their practice. In addition, since technicians can become certified in acupressure, the section on acupuncture gives a little deeper dive into the theory behind it. The only online training in Ayurveda that is available is very oriented toward mind, body, and spirit practice in humans. There are three levels, so the first can give a better idea of what it is all about, but at this point, the other two levels are not appropriate for someone who just wants to know about some herbs for animals.

Traditional Chinese Medicine Theory

Definition

Traditional Chinese medicine (TCM) is a medical system used in China for thousands of years. This system includes acupuncture; Chinese herbal therapy; food therapy; Tui-Na, and for humans, Qi Gong and other spiritual elements. Many of the terms used in TCM sound unusual or strange and can be hard for the Western mind to grasp. Some view the concepts as ancient superstition. However, TCM is another way of diagnosing and treating diseases and can give insight into conditions that we don't always fully comprehend in Western medicine.

Traditional Chinese Veterinary Medicine (TCVM) is TCM as it is applied to animals. There are some differences, especially when related to anatomy. For example, the number of thoracic vertebrae in humans is 12, but in animals, it ranges from 13 (dogs and cats) to 17 (horses) to many more (snakes). Horses have one toe, not 5. Dogs have 5 in front and (usually) 4 on the back feet. They also have a tail with a tail point at the end. So acupuncture points vary a little. Tongue diagnosis also varies

Complementary Medicine for Veterinary Technicians and Nurses, Second Edition. Nancy Scanlan.
© 2024 John Wiley & Sons, Inc. Published 2024 by John Wiley & Sons, Inc.

a little, since tongue color and moistness can vary with species. Mental state can be a little harder to discern, depending on the patient. Even with these differences, the basic principles remain the same.

Description

TCM is used to treat illness. It works especially well for chronic disease. TCM looks at disease patterns and attempts to bring the body back to a balance, treating only the part that is unbalanced. Western medicine narrows the cause of a disease down to a single item and then tries to control that single item. This can work especially well for emergency situations, acute disease, and anything that requires surgery. TCM is best for chronic conditions such as arthritis and skin disease.

When discussing Chinese food therapy and Chinese herbs, it is good to know a little bit about TCM theory because the method of choosing diet ingredients or Chinese herbs can be a little different when TCM theory is used. For example, if a dog has a runny nose, the conventional veterinary diagnosis is rhinitis (inflammation of the nose). A common treatment would be antibiotics to treat any bacterial infection that is present or, in the case of a viral disease, bacteria that might invade tissues inflamed and weakened by the virus. If there is too much congestion, some type of decongestant or even anti-inflammatory agent might be given. Using TCM theory, the treatment would be different for a nose that has a clear discharge than for a nose with a yellowish or greenish discharge. Clear mucus is considered to be a "cold" condition, whereas yellow mucus is considered to be a "heat" condition. Herbs, food, and acupressure points would be different for each one.

In TCM theory, there are a number of types of signs and symptoms that are considered when diagnosing a disease: internal, external, heat, cold, wind, dampness, yin, and yang. Some of these types seem like polar opposites, yet in Chinese medicine, they are considered to be different sides of the same coin. Sometimes a body swings too far one way, and the object of Chinese medicine is to bring the body back to the middle.

The easiest to understand are the concepts of external and internal. External problems are acute, and internal problems are chronic. Most of the things we see in holistic veterinary medicine are chronic (internal) problems because, currently, most pet owners come to see us for those problems.

Next, heat, cold, wind, and damp are used to characterize the symptoms. Anything that is red, hot, or inflamed is showing heat signs. Discharges that are bloody or colored also indicate heat signs. A clear discharge is a cold sign, and a pet who lies curled up or even shivering when it is warm is also showing cold signs. Dampness is retained fluid, so edema shows dampness. An extreme form of dampness is arthritis; the theory is that the dampness thickened so much that it finally turned bony. Dampness can be hot or cold: a skin infection that is red and oozing is a damp heat problem. Finally, wind problems come and go: spasms, pounding headache, off-and-on lameness, itching, etc. Wind problems are often made worse by actual wind: arthritis is usually worse in windy weather—even hot wind. Migraines may be worsened by drafts. Again, skin problems may be wind heat problems, with redness and itching that comes and goes and is worse when wind blows more pollen around.

The reason we go through all the trouble of identifying these signs is so that we can use the correct herbal formula, food, or acupuncture points. For example, a spasm in the back is a wind problem, but along with acupressure points in the back, we would also want to apply pressure to two points at the base of the skull (known as "wind pond"), even though they are far from the problem. This is because the wind pond points are especially good at relieving spasms. The initial session for a veterinarian who uses a lot of TCM theory in his or her practice will often be much longer than the first exam done by a conventional veterinarian because of the extra questions the veterinarian will be asking. A good veterinary technician can help by preparing a client for the extra time and even by asking them to observe their pet more closely for some of these signs in preparation for talking to the doctor.

Chinese Food Therapy

Get an idea of whether or not an animal is in balance. If they have a problem that causes inflammation, such as arthritis or hot itchy skin, or are always panting, or drink more than normal, they are basically too hot and need something that will cool them down. The best protein for them is fish, duck, or rabbit. (Rabbit is a little low in taurine, so if you use rabbit, it would also be good to add some taurine.) Barley, quinoa, or millet are good grains to add. The owner can use melon or banana for treats. They need moisture in their diet, so they will do better on canned or home-made diets.

If the dog sleeps curled up all the time, likes to burrow under the covers, sleep in the sun, and gets cold easily in the winter, he needs warming foods. Chicken, lamb, or venison are good protein sources for him. Oatmeal, especially with cinnamon, is a good way to warm them up also. Some spices also fit into the Food Therapy diet. Turmeric, black pepper, and cinnamon are warming and can also help with cold problems. There is a formula called "Golden Paste" that combines these with coconut oil, which can be used with the food.

Old, weak dogs with tongues that are a little pale will also do well if you add sweet potato and Shitake mushrooms for an energy boost (also known as a "Qi tonic").

One other problem that can be seen is "dampness." One giveaway is when you notice the sides of their tongue have slight indentations where the tongue contacts the teeth. Soft stools with mucus or even diarrhea, especially with mucus, can indicate dampness. Lamb, pork, and dairy products can promote dampness, so even though cottage cheese is often recommended to help with diarrhea, remove it from the diet.

Veterinarian's Role

Many veterinarians do not know about food therapy, even if they use some other form of Chinese medicine. So usually the main role of the veterinarian is to establish a Chinese diagnosis. If they are familiar with food therapy, they can also recommend the proper diet, from a Chinese standpoint.

Technician's Role

This is where the technician can shine. You can get some suggestions from the Four Paws Five Directions book, but even better, become certified in Chinese Food Therapy. You can learn more at Chi University, and from the book "Integrative and Traditional Chinese Veterinary Medicine Food Therapy Small Animal and Equine" published by Chi University (Fowler 2020) (see bibliography at the end of this chapter).

Where to Learn How

Certified Food Therapy for Veterinary Technicians
Chi University
9700 West Hwy 318
Reddick, FL 32686
(800) 860-1543
https://chiu.edu/courses/vtec130_usa

Summary

What can the technician do?

1) A veterinary technician can become certified in Chinese food therapy.
2) A veterinary technician certified in Chinese food therapy can give advice about proper diet after a veterinarian has made a Chinese diagnosis.
3) A veterinary technician certified in Chinese food therapy can formulate diets using Chinese food therapy and a food formulator or a website such as Balance It.

Herbal Medicine

Description

There are two main groups of herbal supplements used most commonly by holistic veterinarians: Chinese herbs and Western herbs.

Some other herbal systems, such as Ayurvedic and South American, are also beginning to be used. Ayurvedic herbs depend upon another ancient medical theory, whereas South American herbs are used more like Western herbs.

Unless your veterinarian is very familiar with Chinese medicine, Chinese herbs should always be used in a balanced formula, not as individual items. They are best used if someone in the practice has a basic knowledge of Chinese medical theory. However, there are some formulas that are general enough to be used by a beginner. Western herbs are used more like conventional drugs: either alone or in combination, for various disease problems. If the veterinarian uses Denamarin, he or she is already using milk thistle, for example. Chinese and Western herbs have their own sections in this book.

There are some herbs that are commonly known by the general public, and because they are so common, they are found in any herb or health food store. Even if your practice does not dispense them, it is good to have some familiarity with them and their use.

Anyone who is discussing herbs should be aware that comfrey (*Symphytum officinale*) is hepatotoxic because of its pyrrolizidine alkaloid content; thus, it is not recommended for internal use. (In some countries, it is still used internally for ulcers and arthritis, but not for more than 1 month at a time.) Comfrey applied externally also helps speed the healing of wounds, but because animal patients cannot be relied upon not to ingest ointments, its use is not recommended.

You should know the Latin names of herbs, as well as the common names. Both *Symphytum officinale* and *Eupatorium perfoliatum* are known as boneset, among other names, so when discussing "boneset" be sure you know which one you are referring to. *E. perfoliatum* is much less likely to cause liver problems (although it can be toxic). A discussion with a knowledgeable client can backfire if you aren't talking about the same plant.

Pennyroyal (*Mentha pulegium*) is also toxic and has been used as a flea repellant. Most herbalists have recognized its toxicity and have stopped recommending it, but you may run across it occasionally in herbal flea sprays.

Like nutritional supplements, herbs vary in quality and shelf life. The highest quality are more expensive to produce, and a knowledgeable herbalist will help his or her herb company to determine the best form for each herb. Again, there are some companies that sell only to licensed individuals, whereas others sell to the general public. Herbal products that are especially inexpensive often do not have enough of the active herbs to do much good. They may also have combinations of herbs that do not make sense, especially in the case of Chinese herbs. Herbs that are available through multilevel marketing are usually expensive, and the expertise of their sales force may be in question.

Western herbs will be discussed next because there is a certification course available for veterinary technicians and nurses. Chinese herbs and Ayurvedic herbs will be discussed later in this chapter because although there are some short courses that veterinary technicians can take, there are no certifications available for technicians as of 2023.

Western Herbal Medicine

Definition

For this book, Western herbal medicine is defined as the use of herbs based on European tradition, using both European and American herbs (which include indigenous herbs from North and Central America and information from native Americans). This does not include most South American or Polynesian herbs, although a few of these are gradually being brought to the United States each year. Animal Herbology is plant-based therapy for animals, utilizing the natural power of plants to support animal health and wellbeing.

Purpose

Western herbs are used in the same way that we use drugs: singly or in combination, for various diseases.

History

Herbs have been found in prehistoric graves dating back more than 60,000 years. Writings about herbs have been found in ancient Greek, Roman, and Anglo-Saxon texts. The first veterinary school, which opened in Lyons, France in 1762, included the use of medicinal herbs to treat conditions in animals.

Juliette de Bairacli Levy is the herbalist who did the most to promote herbal medicine for animals in modern times. She bred and showed Afghan hounds, and in the late 1930s, she treated dogs for distemper by fasting, a natural diet, and the use of herbs.

In the late 1940s, she traveled through Spain, France, North Africa, Turkey, and the United States, gathering information about herbs wherever she went. Juliette wrote books about herbs for dogs, cats, and farm animals that formed the foundation of veterinary herbal medicine for many of us.

Description

Herbal medicine is one of the more misunderstood modalities. You often see warnings that herbs are unsafe or contaminated, that they interfere with drugs, or that they do not work at all. You may see statements that there is no research for herbal medicine. Actually, there is a growing body of research, and herbal medicine is recognized by a number of European countries.

In 1978, the German Commission E was formed. This is a German governmental regulatory agency composed of scientists, toxicologists, physicians, and pharmacists who review herbs for the German government. They initially reviewed over 300 herbs and found good evidence that about 200 have value. The commission published monographs on the herbs, listing their use, dosage, side effects, and interactions with drugs. These monographs have been translated and published by the American Botanical Council as the *German Commission E Monographs.*

The *Physicians Drug Reference (PDR)* has compiled a summary of references on over 600 herbs. The summary includes scientific and common names, a description, physical properties, intended usage and expected pharmacological effects, precautions and adverse reactions, recommended dosage and methods of administration, and references for additional reading, including the latest Commission E findings. One of the most helpful features is the book's multiple indexes: alphabetical, therapeutic category, indications, homeopathic use, Asian indications, and side effects. It also has a section on drug/herb interactions. The authors' first effort was rather limited, but the latest volume is a worthwhile reference. The book also includes full-color pictures of hundreds of herbs.

When choosing herbs, one must be sure that the company that manufactures them is ethical and that the capsules actually contain the herbs listed on the label. Companies that sell to veterinarians only can generally be trusted to do this, whereas companies that sell their products in health food stores don't necessarily all follow this rule. The web site www.consumerlab.com reviews and tests herbs and supplements from up to 35 different companies (depending on the herb or supplement) to see whether the contents match the label. You can get a partial report of companies that passed their tests, but for a full report, you must subscribe to their service.

Table 10.1 briefly lists some common herbs and their uses.

Table 10.1 Western herbs and their uses.

Name	Latin Name	Common Uses
Aloe vera	*Aloe vera*	Soothing to skin and GI tract
Bilberry	*Vaccinium myrtillus*	Eye problems (e.g., PRA, cataracts)
Black walnut	*Juglans nigra*	Anthelminthic; topically for dermatitis
Calendula	*Calendula officinalis*	Soothing to skin and GI tract
Chamomile	*Matricaria recutita*	Anxiolytic, eyewash, dermatitis
Cranberry	*Vaccinium macrocarpon*	Cystitis
Garlic	*Allium sativum*	Anthelminthic, flea repellant, hyperlipidemia
Ginger	*Zingiber officinalis*	Antiemetic, arthritis
Gingko	*Gingko biloba*	Cognitive dysfunction
[a]Ginseng, American	*Panax quinquefolius*	Adaptogen, diabetes
[a]Goldenseal	*Hydrastis canadensis*	Infections, stomatitis
Hawthorn	*Crataegus oxycantha*	Congestive heart failure
Lavender	*Lavandula* spp.	Topical: mites, dermatitis; Internal: anxiolytic
Milk thistle	*Silybum marianum*	Liver disorders
Neem	*Azadirachta indica*	Ectoparasites, wound healing
Saw palmetto	*Serenoa repens*	Prostatitis
Slippery elm	*Ulmus fulva*	Diarrhea
Tea tree oil	*Melaleuca alternifolia*	Dermatitis (toxic to cats)
Valerian root	*Valeriana officinalis*	Sedative, anxiolytic
White willow bark	*Salix alba*	Use like aspirin; same side effects
Yucca	*Yucca schidigera*	Arthritis

[a] Endangered species.

Veterinarian's Role

A veterinarian can gain training in Western herbal medicine in a number of different ways. Veterinarians must diagnose problems in an animal, and their training can give them a slightly different way of looking at things. They may add mild diuretics or herbs that have detoxification action. They may rely on their own knowledge, but delegate preparation and dispensing of herbs to a veterinary technician. If the technician is also certified in Western herbal medicine, the veterinarian may leave it up to the technician to answer common questions, as well as to call owners to see how well the patient is doing.

Technician's Role

Without certification or experience with Western herbal medicine, the role of a technician in a practice using herbal medicine is similar to the role of a technician in a conventional practice using pharmaceuticals. There might be a few differences: the veterinarian might teach the technician how to make tinctures and ointments, and some special storage techniques if they buy herbs in bulk.

Technicians who are certified in Western herbal medicine are on a more equal footing with a veterinarian. Animal herbalists are proficient in herbal medicines and a holistic approach to animal health. They also know how herbal medicines integrate with regular veterinary care to avoid negative herb–drug interactions. They can have a bigger input on the herbal portion of treatment for an animal, and play a bigger part in client education on the use of herbs.

Where to Learn How

Certification in Small Animal Herbology
College of Integrative Veterinary Therapies
PO BOX 352
Yeppoon 4703
QLD, Australia
collegeoffice@civtedu.org
https://civtedu.o0rg/courses/certification-small-animal-herbology

Summary

What can the technician do?

1) A technician can become certified in small animal herbology.
2) A certified technician can be a significant asset to a practice using Western herbs, actively contributing their knowledge in cases where herbs are used.
3) A technician is usually the one responsible for the herbal portion of a pharmacy, and their knowledge about storage and preparation of herbal tinctures and ointments is more than the conventional technician can add to dispensing herbal products.
4) A technician with a broad knowledge of herbs can also act as a consultant to companies that sell herbs for animals.
5) A technician with a broad knowledge of herbs and an entrepreneurial background can create their own herbal company, join a holistic pet shop, or serve as a consultant to holistic pet shops.

Aromatherapy

Definition

In holistic medicine, aromatherapy refers to the use of volatile plant oils, called essential oils, for both mental and physical health. The oils are concentrated mostly by steam distillation of whole flowers (most often) or other plant parts (such as leaves).

Purpose

In veterinary medicine, aromatherapy is used to help muscle problems, for relaxation, for fleas, and for certain medical problems.

History

The ancient Egyptians invented an apparatus to distill cedarwood oil. They also used clove, cinnamon, nutmeg, and myrrh oils, probably as infusions. They were used medicinally as fragrances and for cosmetic use, as well as to embalm the dead.

Hippocrates, the Greek "father of medicine," used fragrances both for their perfume and for medicinal purposes. The Roman doctor, Discorides, in his *De Materia Medica*, described the properties of plants, including the use of aromatic floral waters (not distilled). In the 11th century, Avicenna from Persia invented a coiled pipe that made the steam distillation process more effective and enabled a more effective means of producing essential oils. In the 12th century, Hildegard, an Abbess from Germany, grew lavender, distilled lavender oil, and used it for medicinal purposes.

By the 15th century, oils were distilled from an increasing number of plants. Paracelsus is credited with coining the term *essence* and focused on the use of plants as medicines. In the 16th century, plant oils became available at apothecaries, and the art of perfumery came into its own. The 20th century saw the rise of synthetic fragrances and a decline in the use of natural oils. However, a French chemist named René-Maurice Gattefossé became focused upon the medicinal use of aromatic oils when he accidentally burned his arm. There are two versions of what happened next: he plunged his arm into lavender oil, and although the burn was severe, it healed quickly and left no scar, or he developed gas gangrene and treated it successfully without losing his arm.

Either way, lavender oil helped heal his arm. Gattefossé created the term *aromatherapy*, and in 1937 wrote *Aromathérapie: Les Huiles Essentielles Hormones Végétales*, which was translated into English and remains widely read to this day. A French surgeon, Jean Valnet, used the antiseptic properties of essential oils to treat soldiers during World War I and later wrote his own book titled *Aromathérapie*. Robert B. Tisserand, an English aromatherapist, was one of the first people to spread the knowledge of aromatherapy to Great Britain and other English-speaking nations.

The healing and calming properties of lavender have been tentatively verified by research (Cavanagh and Wilkinson, 2002), but more is needed to establish the best plant species and concentration for these purposes.

Description

Although true aromatherapy uses plant oils, products at the store that use synthetic fragrances or ingredients may also be labeled "aromatherapy." You may like their scent, but they are not true examples of aromatherapy oils. There are no laws in the United States regulating the labeling of these products. Claims of "made with essential oils" or "made with natural ingredients" are similar to the "all-natural" claims for food: they might be in the product, they may be of natural origin, but that does not mean that they are truly aromatherapy products. In addition, perfume oils are not essential oils.

Essential oils are distilled from plants and are extremely concentrated. Used in their pure state they may have harmful effects, especially in cats, so they are generally diluted in carrier oils or other substances. They should be diluted only in natural oils such as almond oil, never in manmade oils such as mineral oil.

Essential oils are either diffused into the air, directly inhaled, or the oils may be applied topically. To diffuse an oil, a few drops are placed on a tissue or on a glass or ceramic surface to gradually diffuse through the room, or an aromatherapy diffuser can be used. Direct inhalation (by smelling the oil) can cause problems in susceptible or allergic individuals; thus, it should be recommended only by those who have studied aromatherapy. A safer method for direct inhalation is to put two cups of boiling water into a bowl and add about four drops of the essential oil, then place it near the pet. Do not just leave it under their nose—it can cause respiratory problems. Again, this is to be done on the advice of experienced people only. For topical use, the oils must be added to a carrier oil (up to 20 drops per ounce of oil) and applied sparingly to the skin. Read the safety data on any essential oils you use.

The oils should be stored in dark glass bottles, in a cool, dark place. Aromatherapy oils should not be stored in bottles with a rubber top or rubber stopper. The oils will make the rubber gummy.

In general, because of their strength, the oils should never be used undiluted, especially in cats. Undiluted, they can cause contact dermatitis or other allergic responses, as well as asthmatic reactions. They should be avoided during pregnancy and by asthmatics and epileptics. (There are some oils that may be used safely in these cases, but it takes training and experience to use them correctly.) Essential oils are not meant for internal use. Even if diluted, if applied on the ears or nose, burns or increased sensitivity to sunburn may occur. The practitioner should also be very careful around the eyes.

If you are interested in aromatherapy, be aware that often the common name for a plant will include several species. Like herbal medicine, aromatherapy is best practiced when you know the specific botanical (Latin) name of the plant you are dealing with. Properties of two different plants with the same name (such as eucalyptus) can have different properties. In addition, the country of origin, and whether or not a plant is organic, wildcrafted, or ethically farmed makes a difference both in the quality of the oil and the future of the plant (if it is a wild species) and the Earth (in the type of farming used).

If oils are too concentrated when used, they can cause contact dermatitis or respiratory problems in sensitive individuals (Paulsen, 2002). This is especially true for cats. Commonly used carrier oils are sweet almond oil, jojoba oil, and sesame oil. The top 10 essential oils are as follows:

1) Clary sage (*Salvia sclarea*): Aches, pains, insomnia (Seol et al., 2010; Setzer, 2009).
2) Eucalyptus (*Eucalyptus globulus* or *E. radiata*): Respiratory problems such as coughs, colds, and asthma. (But must be used very carefully for asthma because any aromatic oil can also cause asthmatic symptoms in susceptible individuals.) Also can relieve muscle tension (Cermelli et al., 2008; Rakover et al., 2008; Silva et al., 2003).
3) Geranium (*Pelargonium graveolens*): Helps the skin. Can be both relaxing and uplifting (Setzer, 2009).
4) Lavender (*Lavandula angustifolia* and *L. vera*): Skin care, wounds, burns, and relaxation (Cavanagh and Wilkinson, 2002; Louis and Kowalski, 2002; McCaffrey et al., 2009; Setzer, 2009).

5) Lemon (*Citrus limon*): Wounds, infections, and house cleaning and deodorizing (Fisher and Phillips, 2009). Be careful with it around cats.

6) Peppermint (*Mentha piperita*): Muscle aches, respiratory problems, digestive disorders such as indigestion and flatulence. Has some antifungal activity (Duarte et al., 2005; McKay and Blumberg, 2006; Rakover et al., 2008).

7) Roman chamomile (*Anthemis nobilis*): Sleeplessness and anxiety, muscle aches and tension, wounds (Duarte et al., 2005; Rossi et al., 1988).

8) Rosemary (*Rosmarinus officinalis*): Muscle aches, anxiety, the liver, mental stimulation. Good for older animals (Gutiérrez et al., 2010; Rakover et al., 2008).

9) Tea tree (*Melaleuca alternifolia*): A natural antifungal oil, helps with ringworm and yeast infections of the ears (Hammer et al., 2002).

10) Ylang ylang (*Cananga odorata*): Muscle tension and depression, relaxation (Hongratanaworakit and Buchbauer, 2004, 2006).

Veterinarian's Role

Veterinarians who are well-versed in essential oils will use them as part of their practice, especially to calm animals as well as to treat them. Essential oils are in somewhat of a gray area as to who can recommend them. They are easily acquired over the counter, although the quality is variable.

Technician's Role

This is one area in which a technician certified in the use of aromatherapy can contribute to the practice, both in the use of oils to help with anxious patients and in recommending products for home use. Technicians may instruct owners in their correct use and storage at home. Technicians can guide both veterinarians and pet owners to the companies offering the highest quality oils. In addition, technicians may help with the preparation of the products, mixing them with carrier oils to make a much safer product. For most owners, the safest form is the diluted form.

Where to Learn How

Ashi Aromatics Inc.
School for Animal Aromatherapy & Flower Essence Studies
https://www.animalaromatherapy.com/product-category/courses/
https://www.animalaromatherapy.com/membership/animal-aromatherapy-practitioner-certification-course/
individual courses and certification

JennScents Aromatherapy
https://jennscents.com/aromatherapy/aromatherapy-for-animals/guidelines

Dr. Melissa Shelton
https://animaleo.info/
products, information

Christropher Day MRCVS
https://www.natural-animal-health.co.uk/aromatherapy.php

Summary

What can the technician do?

1) The technician can become familiar with aromatherapy and help find the most reliable companies to order them from.
2) The technician can mix and dispense essential oils and help instruct the owner on their use.
3) A technician who is certified in aromatherapy can contribute actively to discussions about appropriate oils to use.
4) A certified or knowledgeable technician can advise pet owners on the correct use of aromatherapy.
5) In most states, people who are trained in aromatherapy can also advise human customers. (Do this as a side business, not in the veterinary hospital.)

Veterinary Orthopedic Manipulation (VOM)

Definition

Veterinary orthopedic manipulation (VOM) is a treatment system that uses specific equipment to treat muscle spasms and restricted range of motion.

History

William Inman, DVM, developed the VOM procedure in his practice between 1982 and 1996. Initially, he used an activator, but as he refined his technique, Dr. Inman developed an electric version of the activator, as well as a Vetrostim for myofascial release. He now includes the use of cold lasers as well. He devotes all his time to training veterinarians, chiropractors, and veterinary technicians and nurses in this technique.

Description

VOM uses some of the language of chiropractic and started by using a chiropractic activator, but practitioners emphasize that it is *not* chiropractic. Chiropractic treats areas that are found through a chiropractic exam. Unlike chiropractic or osteopathy, VOM treats all areas (not just restricted areas), even if the problem is not detected by a veterinary or chiropractic examination. Although VOM may use an activator, it does not use the diagnostic methods of Arlan Fuhr, D.C., who relied on the diagnosis of subluxations by checking leg lengths. Because it treats the whole spine regardless of diagnosis, its use is more like massage and not chiropractic.

Practitioners of VOM believe that human hands are too slow to properly treat fixations, and this is why the VOM system uses specific equipment. The best chiropractors can move a joint in 80 milliseconds, but an animal may react to resist as quickly as 20 milliseconds. The equipment used in VOM acts in 2–5 milliseconds, before an animal can resist.

Veterinarian's Role

A veterinarian can be certified in VOM, or they may be an employer of a VOM-certified technician who can apply VOM as a therapy similar to massage. The veterinarian must be the one to make a diagnosis.

Technician's Role

A certified technician can apply the VOM therapy to an animal under the supervision of a veterinarian. If the technician is in a state that allows animal massage therapists to practice with the referral of a veterinarian, they might be able to add VOM to their massage techniques. They should check with their local licensing board to find out what they are allowed to do.

Where to Learn How

VOM Technology
William L. Inman, DVM, CVCP
3761 E Lookout Drive
Coeur d'Alene, ID 83815
E-mail: drbill@vomtech.com
Phone: (888) 935-4866
https://vomtech.com/non-doctor-or-para-professional-training-and-certification/

Summary

What can the technician do?

1) After the veterinarian has made a diagnosis, a technician that is VOM certified can apply VOM treatment.
2) In some areas, it may be possible for a certified VOM technician to open a VOM treatment practice. Check with local laws to see what would apply to you. There is some discussion about this in the VOM certification course.

Homeopathy

Definition

Homeopathy was developed by Samuel Hahnemann (1755–1843). The practice is based upon the principle of *similia similibus curentur,* or "like cures like." In other words, a substance that causes certain symptoms can cure those same symptoms when given at a lower dose. Homeopaths recommend remedies according to a complex pattern of symptoms, rather than the few that Western medicine considers.

Purpose

Homeopathy is used to treat diseases and chronic problems in animals. Veterinary homeopaths do not reject other methods, such as surgery, where needed. The aim of homeopathy is to treat the whole body, taking into account all symptoms, and to resolve issues that may occur because of past disease.

History

Samuel Hahnemann earned his medical diploma in 1779 and went into medical practice in Mansfeld, Saxony. At that time, bleeding, blistering, and purging were accepted practices, and many accepted medications were poisonous. Hahnemann was disturbed by the side effects of the medicines in use at that time and so gradually gave up his practice in 1784, turning more and more into translating medical texts into German. He also began research into pharmacology.

When translating Materia Medica by a Scottish physician named Cullen, he could not agree with the reasoning behind the statement that Cinchona bark worked on malaria because of its astringent properties on the stomach. Cinchona bark was one of the few medicines of the time to actually work, but other items with even stronger astringent effects on the stomach did nothing for malaria or any other kind of fever. When Hahnemann took Cinchona bark himself, he found that he experienced the symptoms of malaria for a few hours afterward and then recovered. Repeating the experiment, he came to the conclusion that perhaps one could cure a disease by using small doses of remedies that actually cause the disease.

He then tried a number of other herbs and substances from the traditional pharmacopoeia in existence at that time (consisting of plant, animal, and mineral substances) and recorded all his symptoms in great detail (far more detail than most doctors did, then or now). Healthy friends and relatives were enlisted to help in this project. After he had enough information, he reopened his practice in 1796, using these new remedies but in a very dilute form. In 1808, he coined the term *homeopathy*. He published the *Organon* in 1810, a description of his theory of disease and its cure. He tested 67 remedies over a 20-year period.

Hahnemann also recognized the roles that poor hygiene, nursing, diet, bed rest, and isolation of the sick during epidemics can play in disease. During a typhus epidemic in 1812–1813, he treated 180 cases of typhus and lost only two patients (one of whom was very old). In 1831, during a cholera epidemic, Hahnemann treated 154 patients and lost 6 (3.9%). During that same time, orthodox physicians treated 1500 cases, and 821 died (54.7%).

Hahnemann was rather irascible and not afraid to express his contempt for the medicine of the day. This probably contributed to the reluctance of many physicians of his time to follow his lead, not only for homeopathy but also for intelligent nursing care.

Several doctors who had studied homeopathy in Europe brought the practice to the United States, beginning in 1825. Gradually, schools were established, and a homeopathic medical organization was formed. By the mid-1800s, there were several medical colleges that taught homeopathy, including the New England Female Medical College. (This was also the first medical school in the United States to admit women.)

Homeopathy was introduced into the UK by Dr. F.H.F. Quin in the 1930s. Dr. Quin was of aristocratic birth and introduced homeopathy to the British aristocracy, including dukes, counts, lords, minor royals, and baronets. He concentrated on introducing it to medically qualified doctors of these patients and so smoothed the way for its acceptance within the medical establishment. Quin established the British Homeopathic Society in 1843 (which became the Faculty of Homeopathy in 1944), a London Hospital in 1850, and the *British Journal of Homeopathy* (*BJH*) in 1844 (which became the *BHJ* in 1911). The Faculty of Homeopathy is the organization that controls the training and recognition of medical homeopathy in the UK. Quin worked through his influential contacts to obtain an amendment to the 1858 Medical Act, which withheld the original recommendation about the type of medicine approved for use in Great Britain. Because of this, homeopathy was not challenged as a valid medical practice. Also as a result, the practice of lay homeopathy became established in the UK and grew during the 1920s and 1930s, while the number of homeopathic doctors declined.

By the early 1900s, there were 22 homeopathic medical schools and over 100 homeopathic hospitals in the United States. As allopathic medicine gained in favor, these schools and hospitals converted to allopathic medicine or were closed.

In the United States in 1938, the Federal Food, Drug, and Cosmetic Act, passed through Congress by a homeopathic physician who was a senator, recognized as drugs all substances included in the

Homeopathic Pharmacopoeia of the United States. The US FDA requires that homeopathic remedies meet standards for strength, purity, and packaging. Labels on the remedies must include one major medical problem that the remedy is used to treat, a list of ingredients and their potency, and safety instructions. Generally, the FDA lets the company determine whether a remedy is sold over the counter or by prescription only. However, if there is a claim for treatment of a serious disease, the remedy must be sold by prescription. Only remedies for self-limiting diseases such as a headache can be sold without a prescription. The FDA does not require the same safety and efficacy testing of homeopathic items as in conventional medications because they believe the low concentration of active ingredients guarantees their safety.

In the UK in 1978, a group of lay practitioners (or "professional homeopaths") established the Society of Homeopaths, a register, the London College of Homeopathy, a new journal (*The Homeopath*), and a code of ethics. More colleges were established in the 1980s and 1990s. Currently, there are more than 20 colleges in the UK with standardized teaching syllabi and training procedures. The professional homeopaths are separate from the approximately 1,000 medical doctors who also practice homeopathy.

In Europe (especially in England, France, Germany, and Greece) and in India, homeopathy is practiced with conventional medicine. India has over 100 four-year homeopathic medical schools. There are also a large number of practitioners in Argentina, Brazil, Mexico, and South Africa.

In the United States, licensure as a homeopathic physician is available only to medical doctors and doctors of osteopathy in Arizona, Connecticut, and Nevada. Arizona and Nevada also license homeopathic assistants, who are allowed to perform medical services under the supervision of a homeopathic physician. Some states explicitly include homeopathy within the scope of practice of chiropractic, naturopathy, physical therapy, dentistry, nursing, and veterinary medicine.

Description

Many think of homeopathy as the treatment of disease by impossibly dilute amounts of a substance, but there is more to the theory of homeopathy than this. There are a number of tenets upon which homeopathy is founded.

Homeopaths speak of a patient's "vital force." (This echoes the Asian idea of qi or ki.) Disease is something that has a bad effect on this force, and the symptoms are from the reaction of the patient to this attack on the vital force. A homeopathic remedy is the spark that focuses the power of the vital force upon that disease, allowing the body to cure itself. (This is another theme from holistic medicine in general.) The remedy is specific and intended to mimic symptoms as closely as possible in order to direct the body as precisely as possible.

Homeopathy recognizes a "healing crisis," where there may be a brief exacerbation of symptoms just before recovery. The way to determine if this is a healing crisis and not a worsening of the disease is by its duration: the crisis is generally brief, often 24 hours. The symptoms may look worse, but the patient generally feels better. For example, the skin may look horrible, but the patient is not itchy and is eating and sleeping well. Often, it is just one symptom of many that worsens. With acupuncture and chiropractic, a pet may become more sore or lethargic before it shows improvement.

Homeopathy also recognizes a progression of disease, some of which also echo TCM theory: the body tries to prevent disease from spreading through inflammation in an attempt to localize it. The body tries to keep disease on the surface ("superficial" disease in TCM theory). So if a disease is improving, one may see skin lesions where there were none before. If a disease is just being repressed, a skin problem may improve, but one may see something deeper, such as kidney disease.

The body tries to keep disease away from the head and away from the trunk. (So if a skin disease on the face is cleared but the arm breaks out with the same problem, this is actually progress.) And the final effects of a disease can be mental and emotional. (Often if a patient with extreme dermatological problems is also treated with something to decrease anxiety, the skin lesions will improve. The improvement is not just from the pet's decreased scratching because it can be seen in areas difficult for the pet to reach.)

The corollary to this is that if a disease worsens (known as "vicariation"), deeper organs may become involved. If symptoms decrease or disappear, but the pet becomes grouchy or lethargic, the problem may actually be worse, not better. As a chronic disease reverses ("regressive vicariation") and moves from deep in the body to a more superficial location, you can see the previous disease reappearing.

Another facet of homeopathy is the recognition of symptoms of detoxification: if a disease process is being eliminated, one may see some kind of discharge. Discharges include the following:

Abscesses
Skin eruptions
Abnormal urine (dark or strong smelling)
Dark, smelly feces or diarrhea
Vomiting

A central tenet of homeopathy is the idea that "like cures like" (also known as the principle of analogy): a diluted and potentized form of a drug can cure the toxic signs seen when a large amount of the drug is ingested. We can see this in conventional medicine, where the side effects of an overdose of digitalis (usually in the form of digoxin or its derivatives) include heart arrhythmias and other problems related to heart failure. A smaller dose of digoxin may be used to treat congestive heart failure.

Homeopaths believe that conventional medicine is often "antiopathetic," that is, a substance is used to neutralize a problem. If you stop giving the substance, the disease returns or reappears. Homeopathic practitioners are trying to get rid of the problem and consider the disease to be the signs of an underlying problem. Conventional medicine is beginning to recognize this in some diseases, such as chronic fatigue syndrome, the anemia of lead poisoning, and fibromyalgia, and with sensitivities to various substances. Until the substance is removed, the patient will continue to show signs of the disease. Painkillers may help a patient function but do not solve the problem.

Another foundation of homeopathy is the idea that very dilute preparations can be effective, and this effectiveness in part is because of the way that each substance is diluted. One does not just dilute a substance in one step. Dilutions are done serially, mostly in steps of 1 : 10 or 1 : 100, and after each step, the remedy is "succussed" (struck against another object a number of times). Hahnemann used a Bible for this. The whole process of dilution and succussion is referred to as *potentization*. A controversial subject is just how large the volume of diluent can be for the solution to retain its healing effect. Extremely dilute solutions may have no more of the active substance left in the remedy. Homeopaths claim that the properties of the remedy are transmitted to the diluent by shaking and percussing (succussing) the remedy after each dilution. This is hard to substantiate, although there is an interesting paper that suggests the possibility of such a transmission (Witt, 2006).

Most over-the-counter (OTC) remedies are not available in this degree of dilution, but some drugs that are conventionally used are diluted as much as these. For example, a common dilution of digoxin is 0.05 mg/mL. If one started with 5 g/mL of digoxin and diluted it to 0.05 mg/mL, it would be the same dilution as a 5× dilution. OTC homeopathic remedies are often between 1× and 10×. They start with a "mother tincture," which is usually a 1× or 2× potency, prepared in accordance with standards set by the HPUS (Homeopathic Pharmacopeia of the United States). For a homeopathic version of digoxin, the actual leaf of the foxglove plant (*Digitalis* spp.) is used, since the HPUS is based primarily on the original list of plants and minerals in use in Hahnemann's time.

A real-life example of a dilution performed by many veterinarians using interferon is the recommendation to dilute it to a concentration of 3 IU/mL in this way: Mix a 1-cc vial of 3 million IU/mL with 100 cc of sterile water. This gives 30,000 IU/mL. Take 0.1 cc of this mix and add it to 1 liter of sterile saline. The result is now 3 IU/mL, and this is used orally in cats at a dose of 1 cc. This dose is 1/1,000,000 of the original dose, or the same concentration as a 6× or 3 C remedy.

Thus, the lower potencies are within the realms of dilution seen in the conventional medical world. Sometimes patients (including humans) can taste some of these substances, and cats, especially, may object. Remedies are available using lactose tablets at the diluent, or glycerol, or tinctures, and the alcohol content of the tinctures may also be aversive to animals. Leaving the top off the bottle to allow some of the alcohol to evaporate may help with this problem.

Finally, like Chinese and Ayurvedic medicine, homeopathy emphasizes the individual approach. For example, with TCM theory, when one is treating a respiratory condition, one uses different herbs depending on whether it is a heat condition (bloody or yellow thick mucus) or a cold condition (clear mucus) and on what type of disposition the animal might have (fearful, energetic, lethargic, phlegmatic, etc.). Homeopathy has similar concerns, and every case is treated differently, depending on the patient, the history, the signs, and how that patient reacts to a remedy.

For that reason, homeopathy is difficult to study using current scientific methods. You can't just study "diarrhea" because it can be treated by many different remedies depending on all the other factors in a pet's body and life. More than one remedy may be indicated, and one homeopath might choose one while a different homeopath chooses another. Lifestyle and diet often play a big role. Research techniques would usually change only one factor at a time, but this is usually not in the best interests of the patient who often comes to a homeopath very ill, after everything else has failed. In addition, very highly diluted solutions of a substance are difficult to verify.

Remedies should not be given with food because they are less effective this way. The time between a remedy and the time the patient can have food varies from 10 to 60 minutes, depending on the dosing schedule and the problem being treated. Remedies should be stored in an area with relatively constant temperature, away from direct sunlight, and away from strong-smelling solutions. It is best not to touch the pills, but there is some controversy over how much you can touch them without contamination. Some recommend that pills be poured directly into the mouth; poured onto paper and then placed into the mouth; or poured onto a spoon, crushed, and then placed into the mouth. Some recommend they be diluted with distilled water, and then the result dripped into the mouth with an eyedropper. (When using this method, be sure to rinse the eyedropper with distilled water after using it.) Some recommend remedies be kept well away from electromagnetic sources such as microwaves and televisions. Use the recommendations of your own veterinarian when talking to clients.

Some homeopaths believe that homeopathy should never be used with acupuncture because both are forms of energetic medicine. However, many holistic veterinarians treat animals successfully with both methods at the same time.

Veterinarian's Role

Veterinarians can receive training and certification through the Academy of Veterinary Homeopathy (www.theavh.org).

Technician's Role

Technicians are helpful in explaining what homeopathy is to pet owners. They are especially helpful in the correct storage and administration of homeopathic remedies, and in mixing remedies to be dispensed. A technician with training in homeopathy can prepare remedies to dispense to animals. If you have a certification in homeopathy, you might be able to participate more directly or, in some states, practice on your own, especially if homeopathy is not included in the state's veterinary practice act.

Where to Learn How

For technicians

Although there are no certification programs specifically for veterinary technicians or nurses that I have been able to find, the National Center for Homeopathy has a page with links to a number of homeopathy schools and training programs at:
https://homeopathycenter.org/training-practice/

For veterinarians

ANHC Education Programs
https://www.drpitcairn.com/recordings/pc-course/

Summary

What can the technician do?

Technicians can prepare homeopathic prescriptions prescribed by the veterinarian of the practice. Technicians can order supplies in the same way that they would keep a conventional pharmacy stocked for a practice.

Equine Osteopathy

Equine osteopathy is a treatment system that uses high-velocity, low-force thrusts, soft tissue massage, stretching, and rhythmic passive joint movements to treat a horse. It is especially used for pain and lameness and to free up the body to move better. Human osteopathy emphasizes a holistic approach (whole body and the mind–body connection), preventive medicine, nutrition, physical fitness, and the musculoskeletal system.

History

Osteopathy is a form of treatment invented by Andrew Still, MD in 1874. After losing three children to an epidemic of viral meningitis, he began developing his system of treatment. He believed that a problem in one part of the body affects the rest of the body, a belief echoed by many other methods of holistic treatment. He used palpation as a method of diagnosis of internal disorders; referred pain is now recognized as a symptom of a number of internal diseases such as stomach ulcers and kidney disease. In addition, some problems such as tension headaches may be a result of a musculoskeletal problem such as cervical subluxation or trigger points in the neck.

Osteopathy is relatively new to veterinary medicine, although it has been used in human medicine for decades. Human osteopaths go through training similar to that of medical doctors, with the addition of osteopathic manipulation. For humans, osteopaths also emphasize nutrition. Equine osteopathy has been around for only about 20 years. Its use is more widespread in Europe and the UK than it is in the United States. To go through equine osteopathic training, one must already be a veterinarian.

Definition

Osteopathy holds that a body that is in proper balance can heal itself. It also says that if a body is out of balance, the function of the internal organs can be compromised. Osteopathic palpation is also an early warning system that can help a veterinarian detect problems before they show up in a blood test.

Allopathic treatments may be used to treat infections, fractures, or other problems. No osteopathic adjustment will hold if the problem needs medical treatment, but once the problem is fixed, adjustments can improve the function of the body.

Equine osteopathy is based on the normalizing of the body and its functions by following certain osteopathic principles. To correct structural abnormalities, osteopathic therapy uses treatment with the hands or by mechanical means. Methods include massage to relax stiff muscles, stretching to help joint mobility, and manipulation and high-velocity thrust techniques that can restore easy movement to the body. Using these techniques, the osteopath tries to remove strictures and abnormalities and thus reestablish the normal functioning of the body's activities.

Osteopathic medicine holds that true health involves complete physical, mental, and social wellbeing rather than merely the absence of disease. The body is viewed as having a capacity for health that the osteopath can help the individual fulfill by treating the whole patient, considering such factors as nutrition and mental habits in addition to the physical symptoms.

The fundamental principles of osteopathic medicine were formulated in 1874 by the American doctor Andrew Taylor Still. Still organized the first osteopathic medical school at Kirksville, Missouri, in 1892. According to Still, all diseases are caused by obstruction of arteries or nerves because of the pressure of maladjusted bones, especially of the vertebrae of the spinal column. He therefore maintained that most ailments can be prevented or cured by techniques of spinal manipulation.

Osteopaths are generally consulted to treat problems of the musculoskeletal structure such as back pain, and many doctors refer patients to them for such treatments. Osteopathy can also be used to ease pain during pregnancy, for asthma, constipation, and premenstrual syndrome.

The French veterinarian Dominique Giniaux was the first person to translate human osteopathy to horses and is considered the founder of equine osteopathy (Giniaux, 1996). Osteopaths such as Pascal Evrard and Janek Vluggen have furthered this study.

Description

Equine osteopathy is the application of human osteopathic theory, modified to fit the equine physical structure, to horses. In the same way that a human osteopath manipulates the body to maintain its natural equilibrium, an equine osteopath ensures the horse's optimal health without the use of surgery or medication.

A holistic approach to health means that every part of the body is seen to affect the rest. As all the organs and systems of the body are interconnected, we cannot treat one part without influencing and changing the whole. This may mean that the cause of a problem may be far from where the symptoms are found.

Veterinarian's Role

Veterinarians can receive training at the Vluggen Institute. Currently, only horses are covered in the courses.

Technician's Role

The Vluggen Institute also trains osteopaths (DO), licensed physical and massage therapists, and licensed practitioners. According to their website, a licensed veterinary technician or nurse may also be able to take the course if he or she has enough background education.

It can be difficult to find an equine osteopath, and there are no small animal osteopaths. However, many of the principles of human osteopathic medicine are shared by holistic veterinarians (preventive health and nutrition, for example). A technician can help clients who are really interested in this modality, by knowing where to search on the Web.

Where to Learn How

Vluggen Institute for Equine Osteopathy and Education
Austin, TX 78745 and
Puth, Netherlands
https://www.vluggeninstitute.com

The Vluggen Institute certifies students in equine osteopathy (EDO) following instructions in 10–12 intensive modules. These modules are taught at various times throughout the year and can be attended in the US or Europe. Courses must be attended consecutively as each module builds on the knowledge of the prior.

Courses are open to veterinarians, physical therapists, doctors of osteopathy, and massage therapists. They are willing to train veterinary technicians who have enough equine experience.

Summary

What can the technician do?

With basic knowledge about osteopathy, technicians who work in an equine practice can assist any veterinarian who has had training in osteopathy, and can help answer client questions about osteopathy and how it is different than chiropractic.

A technician might be able to be certified in equine osteopathy, with enough background in equine care. This is on an individual basis.

A technician who is certified in equine osteopathy could work in an equine practice under direct supervision of a veterinarian. They might be able to work independently, depending upon the local laws.

Do not attempt any type of osteopathic adjustment without training. Book learning alone is not enough.

Acupuncture/Acupressure

Definition

Acupuncture is one method of treatment covered by TCM and is the most commonly used Chinese medicine method among veterinarians using TCVM therapy. The word *acupuncture* comes from the roots *acus*, for needle and *punct*, to puncture. Technically, acupuncture means puncturing the skin with an acupuncture needle in specific acupuncture points. However, it has come to mean stimulating these points by many means, such as very small electrical currents, pressure, or injections of vitamin B12 or Bc complex as well as with acupuncture needles. Points are chosen depending on the disease condition and what the practitioner is trying to do.

Purpose

In the United States, acupuncture is widely used for pain relief in both humans and animals. It is also used to a lesser extent for many other functions, such as to stimulate the gastrointestinal tract (for megacolon), stimulate hormone production (to aid in conception), relieve muscle spasms, induce labor, calm an animal, decrease or abolish paralysis, etc. Acupressure is also used, to a lesser extent, for the same reasons.

History

Acupuncture has been practiced in China for over 2000 years, originally for agriculturally important species such as cattle, pigs, and horses. The first acupuncture points used were those that were related to the way the animals were used as well as for common problems. For horses, points for lameness and for colic were very important. For cattle, points to increase milk production and to help diseases of the udder were emphasized. After veterinarians in the United States and Europe began using acupuncture for pets, human charts and points were adapted for them, reflecting the fact that they were being treated as companions, rather than for food and transportation.

From China, acupuncture spread to other parts of Asia, most notably Japan and Korea. It may also have been practiced elsewhere in the world. Ötsi, the Stone-Age mummy found in the Alps, had 61 tattoos mostly over acupuncture points (Samadelli et al., 2015). They may have been placed to help Ötsi perform acupressure on himself or as part of acupuncture treatments.

The French learned about acupuncture during their involvement with Vietnam. In the United States, veterinarians became interested after President Nixon's visit to China. There, major surgery performed with no anesthesia other than the deep analgesia produced by electroacupuncture machines was filmed. Initially, there was some suspicion that some of the effect was from the stoicism or belief system of the Chinese, but it was later shown that it worked on animals as well.

Initial interest in the United States was to use acupuncture for pain relief, which was verified by research showing the release of endorphins, enkephalins, and serotonin in the central nervous system. Research also showed that acupuncture results could be blocked by administering a narcotic antagonist. Later research indicated that hormone levels could be manipulated by acupuncture, and that smooth muscle contractions could be stimulated by acupuncture.

Initially, the North American Veterinary Acupuncture Society was founded by a group of interested veterinarians based mostly in California. This evolved into the International Veterinary Acupuncture Society, which has spun off local associations such as the American Association for Veterinary Acupuncture and similar associations in other countries.

Description

Acupuncture points are generally very rich in nerve endings. Western research has shown that stimulation of these points results in the release of endorphins and serotonin, the body's natural painkillers. Certain points can also stimulate changes in hormone levels. Up to 75% of these points also have less electrical resistance compared to the rest of the skin.

Not all acupuncture points can be detected in this way, but enough can be detected that beginning veterinary acupuncturists may use a "point finder" (an instrument measuring current flow in millivolts and microamps) to help locate the points until the practitioner can find them without help. The voltage at an acupuncture point at the ends of meridians is consistently about 50 mV (millivolts). To use such a measurement as a diagnosis, it takes practice to be consistent because the result can be different depending on the amount of pressure on the probe, how wet or dry the skin is, and how thick the skin is. Some researchers have not found consistency for some points. There is a device that consistently shows lower resistance for acupuncture points than for normal skin, but it consists of an array of probes so it is best for research, not treatment.

In TCM theory, disease comes from a blockage of the normal flow of the basic energy of the body, or *Qi* (pronounced "chee"). Acupuncture regulates the flow of Qi and can help unblock restrictions to it.

Almost all acupuncture consists of stimulating specific points on the body. Stimulation may be done by insertion of acupuncture needles; injection of substances (such as vitamin B_{12}, lidocaine, or even corticosteroids) at acupuncture points (aquapuncture); stimulating the points electrically (electroacupuncture); applying heat to the points with moxa (moxibustion); applying specific types of laser light to the points (cold laser treatment); or by applying pressure to the points (acupressure).

The needles used for acupuncture are much smaller than regular hypodermic needles (Figure 10.1). The smallest needle commonly used by conventional small animal veterinarians for injections is 25 gauge. (The largest is usually 18 gauge.) Acupuncture needles are usually 35–37 gauge in size. Usually, a ½-inch or 1-inch needle is used in small animals.

Moxibustion is performed with mugwort (*Artemisia vulgaris*), which has been dried and formed into rolls that resemble cigars. The roll is lit and the hot ember on the end is used to heat the needles, points, or areas.

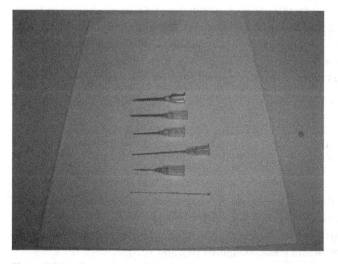

Figure 10.1 Comparison of the size of hypodermic needles (beginning with 16 gauge on the top) to an acupuncture needle (on the bottom).

Acupressure can be performed by owners to help prolong the effects of acupuncture or to treat minor problems between acupuncture sessions. A veterinary technician who is familiar with acupuncture points can help clients locate these points and, if the veterinarian agrees, demonstrate the proper technique. Acupressure can be used around the face, where some animals might object.

Acupuncture is excellent for relieving pain. In addition, it can help with other chronic diseases such as asthma and chronic renal disease. It will often boost the effect of Western medicine, and the two work well together.

Some conditions, for instance lameness in young dogs from activities such as herding, agility trials, flyball trials, etc., can be helped with just a few treatments. Some chronic conditions, because of permanent damage, may need treatment for life. Usually, a patient is seen initially once or twice a week, then sessions become farther apart as the patient improves. A few need only three or four treatments, but the majority require long-term therapy, sometimes weekly, sometimes monthly, or even farther apart.

Medical Acupuncture

There is a subset of acupuncture known as medical acupuncture, a system that is based strictly on Western research. This type of acupuncture does not treat as wide a variety of conditions as TCM does because Western research is primarily concerned with pain relief. Veterinary medical acupuncture proponents claim that TCM theory was developed during the Chinese Cultural Revolution of the 1950s, ignoring all previous Chinese texts (Robinson, 2010). This view is not necessarily shared by those in the human medical acupuncture field (Beyens, 1998).

Medical acupuncture ignores TCM theory and emphasizes the relationship of the nervous system to various effects in the body when stimulating the various points. Choice of acupuncture points is based on modern research rather than on TCM theory. However, the majority of modern research is on pain, so other disease problems tend to be neglected (White et al., 2009).

Veterinarian's Role

In most states, acupuncture can be performed only by a veterinarian with extra training or by an licensed acupuncturist under the direct supervision of a veterinarian. Acupuncture is considered by the AVMA to be a part of the practice of veterinary medicine. Acupuncturists for humans are governed by separate licensing boards, must complete a degree in TCM, and take a licensing exam. Medical acupuncture courses are available only to veterinarians or people with human medical degrees.

Technician's Role

The RVT can play a crucial part in educating the public about acupuncture. Common questions that clients ask include the following.

"How do you keep the animals still?"
This is not a problem for most animals. The needles are very small, so most barely feel them. Some animals don't react at all. Others will flinch slightly if a needle is inserted in a spot that is especially sensitive. Once they learn they feel better, most animals immediately relax when they see they are going to have an acupuncture session (Figures 10.2 and 10.3).

"How do you know it works?"
Pets treated with acupuncture often fall asleep in the exam room once the needles are placed. We often see rapid improvement in cases that did not respond to conventional therapy for months.

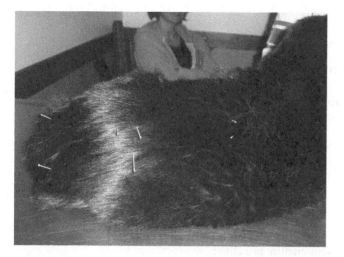

Figure 10.2 Needles placed in the back of a cat.

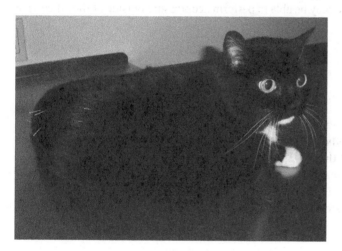

Figure 10.3 The cat stays on the table without restraint.

"How does the doctor know where to put the needles?"

The doctor has had special education in addition to his or her regular veterinary training, in order to know the correct points to use.

"Why does your doctor do it differently from the other acupuncturists?"

There are many ways to treat a problem, just as there are many antibiotics to choose from. Different doctors use different points and different ways of stimulating them. As long as the treatment works, it is the correct treatment.

"How many treatments does it take?"

The number of treatments varies with the problem and with the patient. Sometimes you will see great improvement with a single treatment. At other times, it may take a number of treatments to finally see results. In addition, some drugs such as corticosteroids may partially interfere with the process, which means it can take longer for a good result.

Where to Learn How

Veterinarians become certified in veterinary acupuncture through the following:

AAVA (American Academy of Veterinary Acupuncture)
Chi University
IVAS (International Veterinary Acupuncture Society)

For technicians

A technician cannot perform acupuncture, but they can learn and perform acupressure. (See Chapter 6.)

Summary

What can the technician do?

1) The technician can help explain acupuncture to a client.
2) The technician can set up rooms and equipment for acupuncture and electroacupuncture.
3) The technician can become certified in acupressure and perform it in a veterinary practice. If their laws permit, the technician may be able to perform acupressure outside of the office. (For more, see Chapter 6.)

Chinese Herbal Medicine

The three biggest concerns heard about using Chinese herbs are the safety of the herbs, which companies to order from, and whether to get started without a deep knowledge of Chinese medicine. The first two are related, and the FDA has found repeated problems with imported Chinese herbal formulas. To order safely, one must order from a company that does regular, reliable testing and that has people you can talk to. Formulas based on ancient remedies or formulated by experienced herbalists are the best and safest to use. Formulas from Taiwan or Hong Kong are the most likely to be contaminated.

History in the United States

In 1974, four cases of agranulocytosis were linked to the use of specific imported Chinese herbal formulas. These resulted in one death and three extensive hospitalizations. FDA analysis of these formulas revealed phenylbutazone and aminopyrine. This led to analyses of other Chinese herbal medicines that revealed methyl testosterone, prednisolone, diazepam, chlorzoxazone (a muscle relaxant), and acetaminophen. The cases were reported in the *Journal of the American Medical Association* (Ries and Sahud, 1975).

The FDA issued an import alert on December 30, 1975, banning the importation of the product and seven other Chinese patent medicines, all of which were suspected of containing undisclosed prescription drugs. Five of the banned products were manufactured by the Nan Lien Pharmaceutical Co., Ltd., of Hong Kong. However, the herbal formulas continued to resurface in the United States.

In 1980, another death, along with several illnesses, was linked to chuifong toukuwan, which was found to contain indomethacin, hydrochlorothiazide, chlordiazepoxide, lead, and cadmium.

This is a relatively new formula for arthritis and is not listed in ancient Chinese formularies. The packages listed only the herbs, but the pills contained the adulterants.

Much publicity followed, with articles in the *New York Times* and the *L.A. Times*. It is believed that all the adulterated pills came from Hong Kong and Taiwan rather than mainland China. The government of the People's Republic of China was cooperative throughout the investigation.

In May 1988, the states of California, Oregon, and New York responded by publishing and distributing a list of 40 Chinese herbal formulas that contained controlled substances, unapproved ingredients, potential hazards, or that were mislabeled. Trade groups of Chinese merchants in California voluntarily cooperated with officials on this issue. Additionally, Dr. Dharmananda of the American Botanical Council issued a bulletin (2004) to over 400 practitioners of acupuncture and Oriental medicine, alerting them to the presence of the drugs in these products.

Medical writer Leigh Fenly (1989) noted that over $11 million worth of chuifong was confiscated by health officials in Hong Kong in 1983. Company officials were reportedly given suspended jail sentences and fined $10,000. K.Y. Li, chief pharmacist for Hong Kong's Medical and Health Department, is quoted in the article as having had his agents raid the Nan Lien premises on November 29, 1989. Agents reportedly seized "enough of the product to fill two cargo containers." The pills allegedly contained mefenamic acid, an anti-inflammatory, and the factory also had supplies of Feldene, another anti-inflammatory drug.

The presence of prescription drugs in chuifong and related products has been confirmed by the U.S. FDA, the DEA, the state of Washington, Canadian Health officials, the Texas Department of Health, and the Herb Research Foundation through a series of independent laboratory tests using a variety of analytical techniques.

One way the producer of chuifong was able to evade detection was to manufacture it as both brown pills and black pills. The brown pills had no drugs, but the black ones did. They were marketed in the United States under a number of different names, but the one that got the most publicity was Miracle Herb. Unfortunately, in the trial of a Texas distributor, it was portrayed as an attack by the FDA on Chinese medicine. In this case, it was not.

In January 2001, the American Association of Oriental Medicine (AAOM), an organization representing the professional Oriental medicine community, held an emergency meeting to create a representative coalition to work with the FDA to develop acceptable guidelines for the safe production and use of Chinese herbal medicines, working in a way somewhat similar to the National Animal Supplement Council (NASC). They created the Chinese Herbal Medicine Coalition (CHMC) with the mission of promoting and ensuring the safe, effective, and responsible use of Chinese herbs in the US. The CHMC represents Chinese herbal manufacturers, distributors, and practitioners who work to promote education and certification standards for the practice of CHM and to develop informational material and recommendations for the safe and effective use of these products. Manufacturers promote good manufacturing standards that include thorough testing to ensure proper identification of raw products, cleanliness, freedom from contamination, and other standards that apply to the manufacturing process. The updated book *Chinese Herbal Patent Medicine* (Fratkin, 2001) is an excellent reference for more detailed information on Chinese patent medicines, including tainted ones. The website https://www.aaaomonline.org/45055.asp also gives more details.

There were still problems in China. On May 29, 2007, *The Washington Post* reported that the ex-head of the Chinese FDA was sentenced to death for taking "huge bribes" to approve faulty medicine in general, including a batch of antibiotics that killed 6 patients and sickened 80 (Cody, 2007).

The moral of the story is to deal with companies whose representatives you can talk to and who follow good manufacturing practices (GMPs). The companies to trust have certificates of analysis for their products, they comply with the Chinese GMPs, and have been certified by the Australian Therapeutic Goods Administration (TGA).

Herb Companies

The following companies are based in the United States or Canada and have herbalists (often the founder) ready and willing to talk to you. The omission of a company does not mean it is not a good company. It merely means they do not deal with veterinarians as often.

Health Concerns

This company imports raw herbs from China (wildcrafted or organically grown when possible). They do not use herbs that are endangered, sprayed, or fumigated. The herbs are evaluated by trained herbalists for quality on the basis of smell, taste, and appearance. Samples are sent to independent labs to screen for pesticides, sulfites, and bacterial contamination, using capillary electrophoresis, high-pressure liquid chromatography (HPLC), gas chromatography, and thin-layer chromatography (TLC), among other methods.

Once the herbs have passed inspection, they are processed according to tradition to maximize potency and eliminate undesired effects (a problem when improperly chosen or prepared, such as in kava.) A sample of each batch of the final product is sent to an outside lab to ensure the accuracy, purity, and potency of the finished formula. The founder is an Oriental medical doctor (OMD) available for consultation. Health Concerns also adds nutraceuticals or Western herbs when it will improve a product.

Jing Tang Herbals

The herbs from this company come from China. Most are grown by farmers, but some are wildcrafted. Every batch of herbs is tested before, during, and after processing. TLC, HPLC, and gas chromatography/mass spectrometry (GC/MS) are used to test them for active constituents, insuring potency. All these raw materials and herbal products comply with the new stringent Chinese GMPs and have also been certified by the Australian Therapeutic Goods Administration. Tests for moisture content, dissolution, heavy metals (lead, arsenic, mercury, cadmium), and microbial content (including bacteria and fungi) are performed on every batch of finished product. Following extensive in-house testing, heavy metal testing is conducted again at third-party labs to confirm results. More sophisticated analyses, such as aristolochic acid testing and chloramphenicol testing, are conducted at outside certified labs. When the products arrive in the US, they are subject to an additional review by the FDA. Certificates of analysis for herbal quality are provided by independent laboratories including ADPEN Laboratories Inc. and Mayway Corp. labs.

Dr. Huisheng Xie is the founder of Jing Tang Herbals and the author of 12 textbooks about Chinese medicine, including Xie's Chinese Veterinary Herbology (see bibliography at the end of this chapter). He is a third-generation Chinese herbalist and a veterinarian. He has created a certification course in Chinese herbal medicine for veterinarians, as well as numerous courses about Chinese medicine for veterinarians and veterinary technicians. He is Professor Emeritus at the Veterinary Medical Center of the University of Florida, founder of the Chi University, and a regular lecturer for the AHVMA, IVAS, and AAVA.

Golden Flower Chinese Herbs

This company is located in Albuquerque, New Mexico. Like the others, they submit incoming herbs to intense testing to be sure they are the correct herbs and are free from contaminants. Dr. Signe Beebe is their veterinary advisor. She has also coauthored the book *Clinical Handbook of Chinese Veterinary Herbal Medicine* (2006).

Kan Herbs

Herbs sold by Kan Herbs are imported from China and tested for pesticides, contaminants, excess sulfur, etc. They are processed in a plant in Northern California, where they are first assembled into specific Chinese herbal formulas. Then they are processed into liquid extracts and tablets and tested again for potency.

Dr. Steve Marsden is the formulator for their pet line of Chinese herbs.

Mayway

Founded in 1969 in Chinatown, San Francisco, Mayway is run by second-generation owners.

Each of the internationally GMP-certified factories in which their products are produced in China has an in-house lab where extensive quality control analysis is performed. All raw materials are identified and basic tests are performed before use. Chemical analyses, including TLC and HPLC, are also used to confirm identification, ensure potency, and test for active constituents when necessary.

Tests for moisture content, dissolution, heavy metals (lead, arsenic, mercury, cadmium), and microbial content are performed on every batch of finished product. Plum Flower's (a Mayway brand) restrictions on heavy metal and microbial contaminants are stringent and in line with international requirements. Following extensive in-house testing, heavy metal testing is conducted again at third-party labs to confirm results and to ensure that the standards of purity and safety are met. More sophisticated analyses, such as aristolochic acid testing and chloramphenicol testing, are conducted at outside certified labs. When the products arrive in the US, they are subject to an additional review by the FDA. Mayway has cooperated with the FDA ever since the first identified problems in 1974.

Natural Path

Dr. Steve Marsden founded Natural Path and formulates its compounds. According to Marsden, their source of herbs is Herbasin, a German–Chinese venture, which is the only FDA-certified organic Chinese herb company in the world. It meets German standards as well, making it the only worldwide GMP-certified Chinese herb manufacturing company.

Organic certification is only possible because Herbasin grows its own herbs. The dried raw herbs are checked to confirm identification, then assayed for heavy metal content, and confirmed to be free of lead, arsenicals, mercury, etc.

Upon manufacture, extracts are analyzed to confirm that appropriate chemical constituents are present. The extracts then undergo accelerated decomposition over a simulated 3-month period to calculate expiration dates. Expiration dates are 1 year less than the time period for which the herbs are shown to be potent.

The formulas are then cultured to ensure bacterial counts are negligible.

Dr. Marsden, DVM, OMD, Ph.D., ND, is a frequent speaker at AHVMA meetings and is available for consultation.

Natural PetRx (Formerly Darcy Naturals)

Herbs used by Natural PetRx are certified by labs and are organic or wild-crafted where possible. Products are powders or in vegetarian capsules, with no fillers. The founder is an OMD available for consultation. Natural PetRx also adds nutraceuticals and a wide range of other herbs to their formulas.

Useful Formulas

The following is a list of the top 10 useful formulas from Health Concerns. The Americanized name, listed first, is the product from Health Concerns. The traditional Chinese name is in parentheses. These compounds can be ordered by the traditional Chinese name from most of the companies listed above.

1) Mobility 2 (Shu Jing Huo Xue Tang) for arthritis with inflammation
2) Skin Balance (Health Concerns original formula) (atopy)+/−Xanthium Relieve Surface (Bi Yan Pian) (allergic rhinitis/conjunctivitis) used with or without Si Wu Xiao Feng Yin No. 3 (Darcy Herbs, for severe itch)
3) Astra C (modified Jade Screen Formula) for upper respiratory problems
4) SPZM (Shao Yao Gan Cao Tang) for severe muscle spasm
5) Ease 2 (Chai Hu Gui Zhi Tang, or Bupleurum and cinnamon) for muscle spasms/Ease Plus (Chai Hu Mu Li Long Gu Tang or Bupleurum and Dragon Bone) to calm, and the combination is used for seizures
6) Calm Spirit (Modified Ding Xin Wan) for anxiety/Shen Gem (Gui Pi Tang) can also be used for anxiety
7) Astra 8 (Si Jun Zi Tang)/Enhance (Quan Yin formula designed by Misha Cohen OMC, L. Ac.) immune modulator, cancer
8) Essence Chamber (Combination Western/Chinese formula) for prostate problems
9) Rehmannia 8 (Shen Qi Wan)/Backbone (Bu Shen Huo Xue) for lower back pain, and urinary and fecal incontinence
10) Clear Air for asthma (Ding Chuan Tang) for asthma

Other companies have many of these formulas, usually listed under the Chinese (Pin Yin) name.

Bi Yan Pian: Mayway
Jade Screen Formula: Golden Flowers: Jade Screen and Xanthium. Jade Screen Formula: Mayway (Jade Screen teapills)
Chai Hu Gui Zhi Tang: Golden Flowers
Chai Hu Mu Li Long Gu Tang: Golden Flowers. Natural Path has Chai Hu Jia Long Gu Mu Li Tang
Ding Chuan Tang: Mayway (Mayway also has the original Xiao Zing Long Wan, also known as minor blue dragon, formerly carried by Health Concerns, but not at present—2023)
Gui Pi Tang: Golden Flowers and Natural Path.
Gui Pi Tang teapills: Mayway.
Shao Yao Gan Cao Tang: Golden Flowers.
Shao Yao Gan Cao Tang: Mayway (Peony and Licorice teapills)
Jin Gui Shen Qi Wan: Mayway (Golden Book teapills)
Shu Jing Huo Xue Tang: Golden Flowers
Si Jun Zi Tang: Golden Flowers

Other formulas to consider are as follows:

Ba Zheng San (cystitis)
Aquilaria 22 (diarrhea, internal parasites)
Artestatin (giardia), with Aquilaria 22
Astra Essence or Zuo Gui Wan (stress, chronic fatigue, chemotherapy)
Channel Flow or Huo Luo Xiao Ling Dan (pain relief)
Clear Phlegm or Wen Dang Tan (chronic bronchitis)
Ecliptix (hepatitis)
Enhance (immunomodulant—demodectic mange)
Flavonex (canine cognitive dysfunction)
Gastrodia Relieve Wind or Tian Ma Gou Teng Yin (hypertension and vestibular syndrome)
Isatis Cooling or Chien Chi Tai Wan/Quiet Digestion or Shen Chu Gu Ya (irritable bowel syndrome)
Marrow Plus (bone marrow suppression, including from chemotherapy)
Nasal Tabs 2 (chronic sinusitis)
Phellostatin (*Malassezia* or other yeast conditions)
Power Mushrooms (cancer)

Veterinarian's Role

Veterinarians make a Chinese diagnosis and prescribe herbs according to the Chinese diagnosis. They may also use acupuncture.

Technician's Role

Currently, there is no certification for technicians. Chinese herbs are considered drugs by the FDA. A technician's role is basically the same as the role played in the way they treat prescription drugs: filling them according to their veterinarian's diagnosis and prescription, and explaining their use to pet owners.

Where to Learn How

Veterinarians can become certified by taking courses given by Chi University, IVAS, and by CIVT. At this time, technicians cannot become certified, although they can take a course that introduces them to TCVM therapy. Such a course is offered by Chi University and by CIVT.

Summary

What can the technician do?

The technician can offer support by helping to explain the use of herbs prescribed by a veterinarian certified in Chinese herbal medicine.
The technician can fill Chinese herbal prescriptions in the same way that they fill conventional prescriptions.

Ayurvedic Medicine

Definition

Just as Chinese herbal medicine is best used with a knowledge of traditional Chinese medical theory, Ayurvedic herbs are best used with an understanding of Ayurvedic medicine. In India, Ayurvedic practitioners must first complete a Western medical degree and then undergo an additional 8 years of training in Ayurvedic medicine.

Purpose

Ayurvedic medicine combines the use of herbs, diet, massage, exercise, detoxification, and meditation. It aims to not only treat disease but also to maintain individual health and well-being. Like other holistic modalities, its emphasis is on preventive care, balance, and helping the body to heal itself. Like Chinese medicine, one can still use certain aspects of the system, including Ayurvedic herbs, to help patients without having to know the entire system.

History

Ancient texts, up to 6000 years old, describe the use of Ayurvedic herbs in the treatment of animals. Horses and elephants were very important in ancient times, and famous veterinarians were named who specialized in their treatment. One such specialist, Shalihotra, compiled an Indian Materia Medica in Sanskrit around 2500 BC (*The Shalihotra*), considered to be the first book written to describe specific techniques in veterinary medicine, including herbal medicine for working animals. The first Indian veterinary hospital was built in 300 BC by King Ashoka, predating the European one by 1400 years. Ayurvedic medicine also contributed to TCM, and there are a number of similarities between the two.

Description

The main points in Ayurvedic medicine that correspond to similar principles in TCM theory are the following:

Purusha (energy) and Prakruti (matter) are complementary forces similar to Yin and Yang.
Disease is a result of imbalance.
Prana is the life force (like Qi).
Certain types of energy travel through Srotas, similar to TCM meridians.
Ayurvedic medicine also uses tongue and pulse diagnosis, similar to TCM.
Ayurvedic herbs are usually used in combinations, comprising specific herbal formulas.

Disease can also come from an imbalance of the three doshas (Vata, Pitta, and Kapha), and there are a number of constitutions based on these three, similar to the five-element theory of TCM.

Vata qualities include dryness, lightness, coldness, clearness, and motion. A Vata constitution is anxious, fearful, light, and ectomorphic. Vata tends toward instability, restlessness, and avoidance of confrontation.

Pitta qualities include hotness, sharpness, liquidity, fleshiness, pungency, and sourness. A Pitta constitution is aggressive, hotheaded, and mesomorphic.

Kapha qualities include heaviness, coolness, softness, viscosity, sliminess, sturdiness, plumpness, and wisdom. Kapha constitutions may be lethargic and phlegmatic, a stable personality, or an endomorph.

A living being must have all three of the doshas to be alive. However, they usually show one or two that are dominant. A balance of all three traits is rare. Some herbal formulas are designed to address imbalances in the doshas.

This description is a very small part of Ayurvedic medicine. However, one does not need a complete understanding to be able to use Ayurvedic herbs.

A number of Ayurvedic herbs have entered the consciousness of those interested in herbal medicine. Some, such as aloe vera, have been used by Western herbalists for years. Others, such as *Azadirachta indica* (Neem), are newer, but as their properties are explored by Western herbalists and researchers they have been embraced by the herbal community.

Where to Learn More

Ayush Herbs Inc. carries formulas for animals created by a holistic veterinarian whose family is from India and is a good source of information for anyone who wants to use them in their practice. Their blog has some articles specifically for pets, with references.

Ayush Herbs
2239 152nd Ave. NE
Redmond, WA98052
https://ruved.com/pages/ayushpet
https://ruved.com/blogs/rooted-in-health

Book recommended by a veterinarian who uses Ayurveda in her practice:
The Way of Ayurvedic Herbs: A Contemporary Introduction and Useful Manual for the World's Oldest Healing System, by Karta Purkh Singh Khalsa and Michael Tierra (see bibliography).

Certification in Ayurvedic medicine is available through The Ayurvedic Institute. They offer three levels: Ayurvedic Health Counselor, Ayurvedic Practitioner, and Ayurvedic Doctor. (Although the third level is "Doctor," in most states, you would not be able to call yourself a doctor.) They can be taken mostly online, but all three require an in-person portion. This certification is for Ayurvedic medicine used for humans and they emphasize practice in Ayurveda. The first-level course offers enough depth for a basic understanding of Ayurveda. The second level includes herbology and manual therapy. The third level is at the clinical level, including some studies in India. This is much more in-depth than needed in a veterinary practice.

The Ayurvedic Institute
62 Orange Street
Asheville, NC 28801
https://www.ayurveda.com/education-ayurvedic-studies-programs/

Veterinarian's Role

In a veterinary practice, the veterinarian is the only one who can diagnose or prescribe, so they would be the person responsible for Ayurvedic diagnosis and prescriptions as well.

Technician's Role

If a technician is interested and knowledgeable in Ayurvedic herbs, he or she can be a great resource for both the veterinarian and for clients. If a veterinarian uses Ayurvedic herbs, then the technician should learn as much as possible about them to help explain their use to clients.

Where to Learn How

The National Institute of Ayurvedic Medicine, in association with The Institute of Indian Medicine in Poona, India, offers a correspondence course. There currently are no courses specifically for veterinarians or veterinary technicians in the United States.

National Institute of Ayurvedic Medicine
https://niam.com/corp-web/index.htm.

Summary

What can the technician do?

1) A technician can learn Ayurvedic principles and help explain them to clients
2) A technician cannot diagnose or prescribe, even if it is only when using Ayurvedic medicine

Chiropractic

Definition

Chiropractic is the manipulation of the spine (especially) and other joints (sometimes) to relieve pain. Chiropractic uses the term *subluxations* to describe areas of fixation in the joints or backbone, including slight changes in position of the articulating bones, with accompanying muscle spasms or imbalance and pain. Abnormal blood flow in vertebral arteries has also been verified in these situations. These areas are treated to release spasms and allow them to move normally again.

Purpose

The purpose of chiropractic in veterinary medicine is to relieve pain. Chiropractic points out that fixation in joints or spasms in muscles will affect nerves and nerves influence the body and body processes. We rely on other means to treat other diseases. Nevertheless, with a decrease in stress from the pain, clients may see an improvement in hair coat or decreased susceptibility to disease. This can also happen with other natural means of pain relief.

History

D.D. Palmer founded chiropractic in 1895. He was not the first to perform manipulative therapy, however. As early as 2700 BC, Kong-Fou gave the first written description of a manipulative therapy, and many ancient civilizations, in both the Old World and New World, practiced manipulative therapies (Leach, 1986).

Palmer's son, B.J. Palmer, continued the tradition. He contributed to chiropractic research by using every instrument known at the time to measure the difference between normal systems and those with subluxations.

In 1951, L.A. Hadley, a physician and radiologist, verified the existence of subluxations and also described the histological appearance of nerve roots compressed by a subluxation (Hadley, 1951).

In 1953, J.R. Verner was instrumental in getting chiropractors to recognize the role of bacteria in diseases. (Verner et al., 1953).

In 1989, Sharon Willoughby, DVM, DC, formed the American Veterinary Chiropractic Association (AVCA). Dr. Willoughby became interested in chiropractic when she saw the improvement in one of her animal patients after it received chiropractic care. She attended a human chiropractic school and received her doctor of chiropractic degree in order to be able to administer chiropractic treatments to her patients.

The AVCA currently oversees the certification process for animal chiropractic, for both veterinarians and chiropractors. It approves courses in animal chiropractic.

Description

Veterinary chiropractic starts with a general health exam (which may also include blood tests if the pet has not had a full exam recently), a neurologic exam, stance and gait analysis, and motion and static palpation. Prior X-rays are reviewed. If there is any chance of fractures (for example, after being hit by a car), X-rays should be taken. After a thorough exam, the areas of fixation are identified and chiropractic treatment is started. The extent and duration of treatment depend upon an animal's intended use. Equine and canine athletes, because of their activity, are more likely to require regular treatment after each competition. Geriatric patients are most likely to require multiple sessions for long-term problems.

Chiropractic finds areas of fixation or limited to no range of motion in the back and joints. These areas can be freed up by a thrust that moves the joint just past its normal range of motion. This stimulates joint movement receptors and allows the joint to move more freely. The bones of the spine and joints are maintained in a specific alignment.

The nerves that surround each joint and vertebral articulation are in constant communication with the central nervous system, brain, and all organs.

When even a subtle change in the alignment occurs, it is called a subluxation. Subluxations affect the nervous system, local muscles, joints, and even distant organs, glands, and body functions. They can also affect circulation in the vertebral artery.

Any time an animal shows difficulty in moving, such as problems getting up or down from a sitting or lying position, problems jumping, problems going up or down stairs, or lameness, it can be helped by chiropractic. It can help athletes who compete in agility events such as herding, flyball, etc. If a behavior problem is related to pain or discomfort, chiropractic can help that as well.

The initial visit often lasts for 30–45 minutes, with each follow-up visit lasting approximately 15 minutes. The longer a problem has been present, the longer it takes the body to heal; thus, more visits may be required for a period of weeks to months. Older pets heal more slowly, and visits are timed to allow optimal healing to occur between each adjustment. Gradual onset of a problem may indicate more extensive nerve cell damage and prolong the healing process.

Manipulation may be performed by using the hands or by using an instrument such as an activator. Chiropractic may also include advice about rehabilitation exercises and prevention of further problems. A chiropractic adjustment is defined as a short-lever, high-velocity controlled thrust by hand or instrument that is directed at specific articulations to correct vertebral subluxations.

Veterinarian's Role

Chiropractic is performed by either a veterinarian certified in chiropractic or by a chiropractor. If the veterinarian has training, then treatment is done by the vet in the hospital. Otherwise, the veterinarian may employ a chiropractor on the premises or may refer the patient to another practice with a chiropractor or veterinarian who has proper training. In that case, the referring veterinarian may not know a lot about chiropractic except that it can help, or he may be able to explain it to the animal owner.

Technician's Role

A technician can be very helpful here. If treatment is to be done at the hospital, the technician can answer questions about a veterinarian's training, how a pet will respond, how many treatments are required, how it is done, etc. The technician can also suggest other holistic treatments the owner might want to consider (such as nutritional supplements, acupuncture, massage therapy, or swim therapy). If the technician is trained in physical therapy, he or she can help design an entire physical therapy program.

Where to Learn How

These courses are only open to veterinarians and chiropractors, not veterinary technicians. However, Healing Oasis in Wisconsin also offers massage and rehabilitation classes for technicians.

United States:
Healing Oasis Wellness Center
Sturtevant, WI
https://www.thehealingoasis.com/

Options for Animals
Wellsville, KS
www.animalchiro.com

Training may be done outside the United States, but certification is given only by the AVCA. After completion of the course, a veterinarian or chiropractor must pass a written exam and a clinical competency exam and complete a 40-hour internship with a veterinarian certified in animal chiropractic.

Summary

What can the technician do?
1) Like other veterinarian-only training, the courses are not open to technicians. However, when working in a practice with a veterinarian who uses chiropractic, knowledge of the basic principles will help a technician answer questions that owners may have.

Applied Kinesiology

Definition

Applied kinesiology (AK) is a method of testing muscle strength in reaction to various stimuli. The stimulus can be something held in the testee's hand or from a touch at specific places on the body. It may also be performed by having the testee think of a specific item and then testing whether the muscle is strengthened or weakened. This is done for various purposes, using various forms, and there are now over 80 procedures using the term *kinesiology* that have sprung from this form.

History

AK started in 1964 when Dr. George J. Goodheart, a chiropractor, was searching for ways to strengthen weak muscles. He found factors that could strengthen or weaken muscles immediately. Dr. Goodheart chose to call this *applied kinesiology* in order to differentiate it from *kinesiology*, which means the study of movement and muscle function.

Description

AK is also known as "muscle testing." It has a number of offshoots, including contact reflex analysis (CRA) and Nambudripad's allergy elimination technique (NAET®).

AK was originally designed to be performed on the patients themselves, but in veterinary medicine, we use the patient's owner or another person as a surrogate for that patient. The owner either holds the patient in his or her lap or has other contact with the patient in order to perform the test.

The tester uses the same muscle or muscle group to perform the test. Most often, the arm is extended, either to the front of the body (see Figure 10.4) or to the side (see Figure 10.5), and the tester applies downward pressure to test the strength of the muscle.

By applying the same pressure and using different stimuli, muscle strength and weakness is evaluated. The results are interpreted variously, depending on the circumstances. For example, it may be used to locate a problem in the body, make a diagnosis, or choose a food, herb, drug, or other treatment.

Even if AK is not used regularly in your practice, the knowledge of how to apply its use to help the owner choose a pet food, for example, will bring in owners who will use your practice for medical problems also. It will also encourage them to tell you about things they are trying and people they are seeing who might be helpful or might interfere with what you are doing.

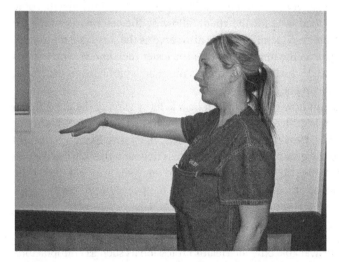

Figure 10.4 Arm extended to the front, ready for testing. For muscle testing, pressure is applied to the top of the wrist.

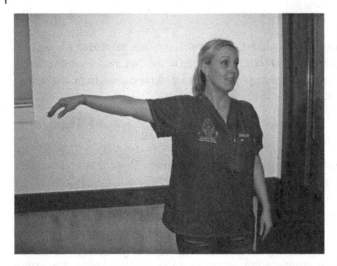

Figure 10.5 Arm extended to the side, ready for testing. For muscle testing, pressure is applied to the top of the wrist.

Veterinarian's Role

Veterinarians who use AK regularly generally use it for diagnosis and/or treatment. They get their training from various places and usually complete their education by reading further, attending lectures, and experimenting for themselves. The International College of Applied Kinesiology (ICAK) has a training program and a certification program available.

Technician's Role

Some clients may want to test every food and/or every possible treatment for their animals. Some holistic veterinarians may do this as a general rule, but many do not. A good technician with some basic knowledge of AK can perform food tests for the client, allowing the veterinarian time for other methods of diagnosis and treatment. A technician may also serve as the surrogate for testing. Using the same person as the surrogate all the time means that the tester then knows which items will consistently test better or worse and which areas or organs may show problems in the testee. This can be compensated for before testing begins.

Although there is much written about how the testing can be faked (by varying the pressure on the arm when pressing downward), it is difficult to find any neutral research for AK. Whether or not you believe in the usefulness of AK, if you have never experienced it, try this: Extend your right arm straight out until it is parallel to the ground. Have a friend press down on the wrist while you resist the pressure as strongly as possible. Now hold some sugar in your left arm and repeat the process, with your friend using the same amount of pressure. What happened? And why?

Where to Learn How

Training and certification at ICAK are available only for Health Professionals such as chiropractors, MDs, and osteopaths, as well as dentists. The training is very rigorous and certification involves submitting case studies as well as an exam. ICAK has chosen this route because they want AK practitioners to know anatomy, physiology, and various diseases before they start.

References

American Botanical Council. 2004. Review of adulteration of Chinese patent medicines with synthetic drugs. *Herbal Gram* 61:22–23.

Beebe S., et al. 2006. *Clinical Handbook of Chinese Veterinary Herbal Medicine*. Placitas, NM: Herbal Medicine Press.

Beyens F. 1998. Reinterpretations of traditional concepts in acupuncture. In: Filshie J. and White A. eds., *Medical Acupuncture, A Western Scientific Approach*, chapter 20. Edinburgh: Churchill Livingstone.

Cavanagh H.M. and Wilkinson J.M. 2002. Biological activities of lavender essential oil. *Phytother Res* 16(4):301–308.

Cermelli C., et al. 2008. Effect of eucalyptus essential oil on respiratory bacteria and viruses. *Curr Microbiol* 56(1):89–92.

Cody E. 2007. Ex-head of China FDA sentenced to death; ruling comes after alarm over tainted exports. *The Washington Post*, May 30, D-1.

Duarte M.C., et al. 2005. Anti-*Candida* activity of Brazilian medicinal plants. *J Ethnopharmacol* 97(2):305–311.

Fenly L. 1989. Vast supply of Oriental remedies are seized here. *The San Diego Union*, Dec 17, D-3.

Fisher K. and Phillips C. 2009. *In vitro* inhibition of vancomycin-susceptible and vancomycin-resistant *Enterococcus faecium* and *E. faecalis* in the presence of citrus essential oils. *Br J Biomed Sci* 66(4):180–185.

Fowler, M and Xie, H. 2020. *Integrative and Traditional Chinese Veterinary Medicine Food Therapy Small Animal and Equine*. Chi University Press.

Fratkin J. 2001. *Chinese Herbal Patent Medicines: The Clinical Desk Reference*. Boulder, CO: Shya Publications.

Giniaux D. 1996. *What the Horses Have Told Me: An Essay on Equine Osteopathy*. Franktown, VA: Xenophon Press.

Gutiérrez R., et al. 2010. Oxidative stress modulation by *Rosmarinus officinalis* in CCl_4-induced liver cirrhosis. *Phytother Res* 24(4):595–601.

Hadley L.A. 1951. Intervertebral joint subluxation, boney impingement and foramen encroachment with nerve root change. *Am J Roentgenol Rad Ther* 65:377–402.

Hammer K., et al. 2002. *In vitro* activity of *Melaleuca alternifolia* (tea tree) oil against dermatophytes and other filamentous fungi. *J Antimicrob Chemother* 50(2):195–199.

Hongratanaworakit T. and Buchbauer G. 2004. Evaluation of the harmonizing effect of ylang-ylang oil on humans after inhalation. *Planta Med* 70(7):632–636.

Hongratanaworakit T. and Buchbauer G. 2006. Relaxing effect of ylang ylang oil on humans after transdermal absorption. *Phytother Res* 20(9):758–763.

Leach R. 1986. *The Chiropractic Theories*. Baltimore, MD: Williams & Wilkins, p. 24.

Louis M. and Kowalski S.D. 2002. Use of aromatherapy with hospice patients to decrease pain, anxiety, and depression and to promote an increased sense of wellbeing. *Am J Hosp Palliat Care* 19(6):381–386.

McCaffrey R., et al. 2009. The effects of lavender and rosemary essential oils on test-taking anxiety among graduate nursing students. *Holist Nurs Pract* 23(2):88–93.

McKay D.L. and Blumberg J.B. 2006. A review of the bioactivity and potential health benefits of peppermint tea (*Mentha piperita L.*). *Phytother Res* 20(8):619–633.

Paulsen E. 2002. Contact sensitization from compositae-containing herbal remedies and cosmetics. *Contact Dermatitis* 47(4):189–198.

Rakover Y., et al. 2008. The treatment of respiratory ailments with essential oils of some aromatic medicinal plants. *Harefuah* 147(10):783–788, 838.

Ries C.A. and Sahud M.A. 1975. Agranulocytosis caused by Chinese herbal medicines: Dangers of medications containing aminopyrine and phenylbutazone. *JAMA* 231(4):352–355.

Robinson N. 2010. Medical Acupuncture for Veterinarians Brochure. Accessed online 5/22/2010 at https://scienceofacupuncture.com/Fort Collins: Colorado State University.

Rossi T., et al. 1988. Sedative, anti-inflammatory, and anti-diuretic effects induced in rats by essential oils of varieties of *Anthemis nobilis*: a comparative study. *Pharmacol Res Commun* 20(Suppl 5):71–74.

Samadelli M, et al. 2015. Complete mapping of the tattoos of the 5300-year-old Tyrolean Iceman. 16(5):753–758.

Seol G.H., et al. 2010. Antidepressant-like effect of *Salvia sclarea* is explained by modulation of dopamine activities in rats. *J Ethnopharmacol* 130(1):187–190.

Setzer W.N. 2009. Essential oils and anxiolytic aromatherapy. *Nat Prod Commun* 4(9):1305–1316.

Silva J., et al. 2003. Analgesic and anti-inflammatory effects of essential oils of Eucalyptus. *J Ethnopharmacol* 89(2–3):277–283.

Valentine R. and Valentine R. 1998. Veterinary NAET: The veterinary application of NAET; A breakthrough approach to allergy resolution. *J Amer Holistic Vet Med Assoc.* 14(1):30–32.

Verner J.R., et al. 1953. *Rational Bacteriology*. New York: Wolf.

White A., et al. 2009. Western medical acupuncture: a definition. *Acupunct Med* 27(1):33–35.

Witt C.M. 2006. The role of trace elements in homeopathic preparations and the influence of container material, storage duration, and potentisation. *Forsch Komplementmed* 13(1):15–21.

Bibliography

Acupuncture

Filshe J. and White A. 1998. *Medical Acupuncture*. Edinburgh: Churchill Livingstone.

Schoen A., ed. 2000. *Veterinary Acupuncture: Ancient Art to Modern Medicine* 2nd Edition. St. Louis, MO: Mosby.

Chinese Herbs

Gaeddart A. 2010. *Health Concerns Clinical Handbook*. Oakland, CA: Health Concerns.

Xie H. 2004. *Chinese Veterinary Herbal Handbook*. Reddick, FL: Chi Institute of Chinese Medicine.

Xie H. 2010. Xie's *Chinese Veterinary Herbology*. Wiley-Blackwell.

Western Herbs

Blumenthal M., et al. 1998. *The Complete German Commission E Monographs: Therapeutic Guide to Herbal Medicines*. Austin, TX: American Botanical Council.

Goldstein R., ed. 2008. *Integrating Complementary Medicine into Veterinary Practice*. Ames, IA: Wiley-Blackwell.

Thomson Healthcare Staff. 2007. *PDR for Herbal Medicine*, 4th edition Nottingham, UK: Thomson Reuters.

Wynn S. and Fougere B. 2007. *Veterinary Herbal Medicine*. St. Louis, MO: Mosby.

Ayurvedic Medicine

Pole S. 2006. *Ayurvedic Medicine: The Principles of Traditional Practice*. Edinburgh: Churchill Livingstone.

Khalsa K.P.S. and Tierra M. 2008. *The Way of Ayurvedic Herbs: A Contemporary Introduction and Useful Manual for the World's Oldest Healing System*. Lotus Press.

Lad V. 2001. *Textbook of Ayurveda, Volume One: Fundamental Principles*. Albuquerque, NM: Ayurvedic Press.

Lad V.L. 2007. *Textbook of Ayurveda, Volume Two: A Complete Guide to Clinical Assessment*. Albuquerque, NM: The Ayurvedic Press.

Williamson E. 2002. *Major Herbs of Ayurveda*. Edinburgh: Churchill Livingstone.

Chiropractic

Kamen D. 1998. *The Well Adjusted Horse: Equine Chiropractic Methods You Can Do*. Brookline, MA: Brookline Books.

Snader M.L., et al. 1993. *Healing Your Horse: Alternative Therapies*. Stuttgart: MacMillan.

Verhoef M.J., et al. 1997. The chiropractic outcome study: Pain, functional ability and satisfaction with care. *J Manipulative Physiol Ther* 20(4):235–240.

Homeopathy

Day C. 1990. *The Homoeopathic Treatment of Small Animals, Principles and Practice*. Essex: Danile Co.

Hamilton D. 1999. *Homeopathic Care for Cats and Dogs: Small Doses for Small Animals*. Berkeley, CA: North Atlantic Books.

McLeod G. 2004. *A Veterinary Materia Medica and Clinical Repertory*. London: Random House UK.

McLeod G. 2005. *Dogs: Homeopathic Remedies*. London: Random House UK.

McLeod G. 2005. *Cats: Homeopathic Remedies*. London: Random House UK.

McLeod G. 2006. *The Treatment of Horses by Homeopathy*. London: Ebury Press.

Pitcairn R. and Pitcairn S.H. 2005. *Dr. Pitcairn's New Complete Guide to Natural Health for Dogs and Cats*. Emmaus, PA: Rodale Books.

Aromatherapy

Bell K.L. 2002. *Holistic Aromatherapy for Animals*. Forres, Scotland: Findhorn Press.

Gattefossé R.M. 1993. *Gattefossé's Aromatherapy*. Saffron Walden, UK: The C.W. Daniel Company Limited.

Manniche L. 1999. *Sacred Luxuries: Fragrance, Aromatherapy & Cosmetics in Ancient Egypt*. Ithaca, NY: Cornell University Press.

Tisserand R. and Balacs T. 1995. *Essential Oil Safety: A Guide for Health Care Professionals*. Edinburgh: Churchill Livingstone.

Tisserand R.B. 1997. *The Art of Aromatherapy*. Rochester, VT: Healing Arts Press.

Physiological Therapy

Nilsson N., et al. 1997. The effect of spinal manipulation in the treatment of cervicogenic headache. *J Manipulative Physiol Ther* 20:326–330.

Webliography

Western Herbs

Natural Pet Rx
http://www.naturalpetrx.com/index.php?main_page=page&id=43&chapter=10
Besides being a source of Western herbs, this website has links to videos, slide shows, webinars, and
   articles about Western herbal medicine

Herbalist and Alchemist
https://www.herbalist-alchemist.com/need-to-know/educational-resources/
Founded by David Winston, who has contributed to quality Western herbal medicine for over 40 years.
   Besides herbal products for animals, the resources page (above) lists associations and other
   resources for Western herbal medicine, as well as links to his own courses

Thorne Research
https://thornevet.com/thornevet-blog/
Has a veterinary line, designed by veterinarians with an interest in nutritional supplements for
   individual disease processes. The blog describes some individual products and problems.

Veterinary Botanical Medical Association
https://www.vbma.org/herbalist-certification.html
Veterinary organization for all who are interested in herbal medicine for animals. Some information is
   in the public sector, but much of the most in-depth information is available to members only.
   Certification for vet techs and pet owners is available at the link above. Veterinary technicians
   interested in becoming a member must have extensive experience with herbs.

Veterinary Information Network
https://www.vin.com
Great source of information for veterinarians. They also have a discussion group for alternative
   veterinary medicine: see the VIN Alternative Medicine board (available to veterinarians only).

Vetriscience
http://www.vetriscience.com
Makes a number of nutritional supplements for animals.

Ayurvedic Herbs

Ayush Pets
https://ruved.com/pages/ayushpet
AyushPets are ayurvedic herbs formulated for pets
https://ruved.com/blogs/rooted-in-health
Their blog has a number of articles about their products and ayurvedic medicine for animals.

Chiropractic

Chiropractic training is not available for veterinary technicians or nurses.

VOM

Veterinary Orthopedic Manipulation
https://www.vomtech.com/

Offers education in the VOM technique to veterinarians and to veterinary technicians and nurses

Equine Osteopathy

The Vluggen Institute
https://www.vluggeninstitute.com/education-non-vet

Offers training for all animal therapists and all equal and comparable certified education holders in the US and Germany

Meridian Institute
https://www.meridianinstitute.com/manual-therapy/
Collections of early manuals on various types of manual therapy, especially osteopathy

Osteopathic Educational Society
https://www.osteohome.com/
Site with an explanation of human osteopathy.

Homeopathy

Alternative Medicine Foundation
https://www.amfoundation.org/homeopathinfo.htm
This is currently an archival source only, no longer being updated since 2010. But it still has a lot of links to homeopathic information

Boiron
https://www.boironusa.com/education/online-training/
Boiron is a manufacturer of homeopathic remedies. Their website has webinars about various aspects of homeopathy

Homeopathic Pharmacopoeia of the United States
https://www.hpus.com/
legal standards of strength, quality, purity, and packaging as well as identification and quality standards of homeopathic starting materials and tinctures

Homeopathy Family Medicine
https://homeopathic.com/a-condensed-history-of-homeopathy/
Besides this history, has articles and videos and links to books about homeopathy

U.S. Food and Drug Administration
https://www.fda.gov/drugs/information-drug-class/homeopathic-products

Web site for the FDA, which regulates both food (including supplements) and drugs, for both humans and animals. This webpage includes a link to download their "final guidance" (as of December 2022) for Homeopathic Drug Products

Aromatherapy

Aromaweb
www.aromaweb.com
Website with lots of information about aromatherapy.

The National Association for Holistic Aromatherapy
https://www.naha.org
Organization for practitioners of aromatherapy. Good article on safety at https://www.naha.org/safety.htm.

Applied Kinesiology

International College on Applied Kinesiology
https://www.icak.com/
Website for licensed health practitioners training and certification in Applied Kinesiology

11

Other Commonly Employed Modalities

Nambudripad's Allergy Elimination Technique

Definition

NAET® (Nambudripad's allergy elimination technique) is a method that combines diagnosis and treatment of what the practitioners call "allergies" to substances and environmental problems. By *allergies*, they are referring to hypersensitivity and altered reactions (usually overreactions) to the various items. These are termed *allergies* in NAET, although they include reactions that are not always recognized as allergic reactions in Western medicine. For example, psychological or emotional overreaction to certain stimuli may be called "allergies." In addition, there may be items tested for (such as emotions) that Western medicine may not recognize as allergy provoking.

NAET uses a combination of applied kinesiology and acupressure to test and treat these allergies.

Purpose

The reason for using NAET is to eliminate hypersensitivity to the various allergens as defined by NAET. It may be used to help patients with dermatological problems or to help them better deal with chronic disease.

History

The technique was developed for humans in 1985 by Dr. Devi Nambudripad, L.Ac., D.C., Ph.D.; further modified for animals by Rahmie Valentine L.Ac., O.M.D.; and used for animals since 1994 (Valentine and Valentine, 1998).

Description

NAET borrows from traditional Chinese medical theory to explain what occurs with an allergy: qi (energy) flows through meridians, and allergic responses can cause a blockage of this flow of qi. Acupuncture or acupressure, administered while the patient or surrogate is in contact with the offending substance, can clear the blockage and restore normal qi flow. When this happens, the body's reaction becomes normal again.

Muscle response testing (applied kinesiology) is used to determine which items cause a hypersensitivity reaction. In humans, the actual patient is tested, whereas in animals, a human surrogate

Complementary Medicine for Veterinary Technicians and Nurses, Second Edition. Nancy Scanlan.
© 2024 John Wiley & Sons, Inc. Published 2024 by John Wiley & Sons, Inc.

(usually the owner) is used. The surrogate places one hand on the patient, and their free arm is used for muscle testing. There are usually numerous items identified as allergies. Not all are treated at the same time, just the most critical.

Acupressure is used to treat (or "clear") these reactions while the surrogate (touching the patient) holds a sample of the allergen. For humans, 10 of the most common allergens are usually cleared first. Animals are usually in an acute state (such as severe reaction to pollen allergies), and the acute state is addressed first. After this is done, the patient is tested again through applied kinesiology to see whether their response has changed. If so, other items will be cleared. For maximum effect, the patient should avoid the allergens for 25 hours after this procedure. Nutritional supplements are also often recommended to help with the problem.

On subsequent visits, previous allergies are retested first. If they remain cleared, the practitioner progresses to new items. If not, they must be cleared again. Sometimes results are seen immediately. At other times, all identified allergens must be cleared before a reduction in symptoms is seen. For humans, about two-thirds have responded within 15–25 visits.

A session can last from 30 minutes to 1 hour.

Veterinarian's Role

NAET certification course is available to everyone interested in NAET is a procedure for both diagnosis and treatment of a problem (two of the three veterinarian-only functions of diagnosis, treatment, and surgery). Thus, in states that consider NAET a veterinary diagnostic technique, this may be a procedure that only a veterinarian can legally perform.

Technician's Role

Depending on state law, technicians may be able to perform NAET. Technicians can be used as a surrogate for the testing procedure. They also can help explain the whole process.

Where to Learn How

Certification in NAET is available at https://www.naet.com/training/become-a-naet-practitioner/.
There is no specific training for veterinary technicians.

Bach Flower Remedies

Definition

Bach flower remedies were developed to address seven groups of mental reactions to diseases. They have been found to be useful in human clinical settings (Oliva, 2009; Thaler et al., 2009).

(Note: If you try a little Rescue Remedy—a mixture of five of Bach's remedies—on anxious animals in your practice, you will often be pleasantly surprised. Even if the effect is on the owners, with the pet reacting to their reaction, it is still a useful way to calm an animal without side effects.)

Purpose

Dr. Edmund Bach, developer of the remedies, was a medical doctor who believed that the way a person reacted mentally to a disease determined the way that the disease would progress and that by treating the mental state, one could best treat the disease. Currently, the remedies are more often used to treat the states (such as fear or anxiety) themselves or as an adjunct to other methods of healing, rather than as the primary remedy itself.

History

Dr. Edward Bach (1886–1936) was a house surgeon at the University College Hospital in London and also had a general medical practice. He was a bacteriologist and a pathologist, worked on vaccines, and developed a set of homeopathic nosodes (vaccines) to prevent or treat diseases. He was dissatisfied with treating only the disease and wanted to help the people themselves feel better. He felt that different personality types responded differently to the same disease and that their feelings were a primary part of the whole disease. (We see this today with anxiety induced by severe allergic dermatitis or aggression associated with pain.) He was inspired by homeopathy but wanted to work with gentler remedies rather than those that caused disease symptoms when used in high doses.

In 1930, he left practice and began his search for these substances. He relied upon his own intuition to enumerate the emotional states and to find remedies for each of them. In spring and summer, he would search in nature to find and prepare remedies, and in fall and winter, he would treat those who came to him for help. Most Bach remedies are derived from flowers.

He found that disease symptoms often decreased and people were able to heal better when they were treated according to their personalities and feelings. He believed that their moods not only guided him to the proper treatment but also that a mood could warn of impending disease; thus by treating a mood he could also fend off a disease. According to one of his publications, "It is not the disease that is of importance, it is the patient. . . ." This is a basic tenet of holistic medicine in general.

Description

Two methods are used to make the remedies themselves. Remedies made from delicate flowers are prepared by floating the blooms in pure water for 3 hours in direct sunlight. Woody plants, and flowers that bloom when the sun is weaker, are boiled in pure water for half an hour. After this initial phase, 40% brandy is mixed half-and-half with the suffused water. This creates the mother tincture. Two drops of the mother tincture are diluted in 30 mL of brandy for a stock solution. The stock solution is further diluted to create the Bach remedies.

These remedies are treated differently from homeopathic remedies: they may be put into hot drinks for owners. A drop may be placed on the forehead and/or paws of the pet, or it may be given directly to the pet.

Bach identified seven main mental states. Each has a number of subdivisions, not all of which are problematic, and he created 38 remedies in all to account for each individual mental state. Even for those mental states considered healthy, Bach believed that the use of a corresponding remedy could still be helpful as part of the treatment for whatever disease they might be suffering. The most popular Bach remedy is Rescue Remedy, a combination of five of his remedies. It is used for general worry and anxiety and is the most commonly used item for pets. It is very gentle and takes the edge off the emotion, without dizziness, ataxia, or sleepiness. Because it is so gentle, immediate effects can be seen for an animal with moderate anxiety in a veterinary office, but it should not be relied upon to control fear biting or other extreme anxiety. Like other modalities, it can be used as part of a program in multicat households to help situations such as aggression or territorial marking. It can also help some pets with carsickness.

The seven primary mental states identified by Bach are as follows:

- Fear
- Uncertainty
- Insufficient interest in present circumstances
- Loneliness
- Oversensitivity to influences and ideas
- Despondency or despair
- Over-care for the welfare of others

Fear

Bach divided fear into five types:

- *Terror or panic*, with the feeling that there is no hope. (Rock rose, *Helianthemum vulgare*, is the main remedy, but Bach said you may need to use others with this state.)
- *Ordinary everyday fears* (of accidents, illness, the dark, being alone, burglars, animals, other people, etc.), whether there is a reason to fear or not (mimulus, *Mimulus luteus*).
- *Vague fear that something dreadful is going to happen*, but not being able to say what it is. Real to the patient, but not to the observer (aspen, *Populus tremula*).
- *Fear of stress*, that the mind is being overworked and that you can't stand the mental strain. Includes the impulse to do something bad that you would normally not do (cherry plum, *Prunus cerasifera*).
- *Fear for others*, especially those near and dear to us (red chestnut blossom, *Aesculus hippocastanum*).

Uncertainty

The following may remind you of many pet owners who come to your practice. Their pets may pick up on their owner's problems and echo them in some way. The characteristics of this category and the remedy used to treat them are as follows:

- Those who have no confidence in themselves to make their own decisions and who are constantly looking to others for advice. (Besides your clients, a lot of toy poodles act this way.) (Cerato, *Ceratostigma willmottianum*)
- Those who have an inability to decide between two things. (Scleranthus, *Scleranthus annuus*)
- Those who are easily discouraged, even if things are progressing well. (Gentian, *Gentiana amarella*)
- Those who are unable to believe that any more can be done. Even if something is tried, they will assure others that it isn't going to work. (Gorse, *Ulex europaeus*)
- Those who have the feeling that they don't have enough mental or physical strength to carry on or that something—mind or body—needs to be strengthened before anything will work. (Hornbeam, *Carpinus betulus*)
- Those who have no great calling to any one thing but who want to do something great, to live life to the fullest. This can cause dissatisfaction in their life. (Wild oat, *Bromus asper*)

Insufficient Interest in Present Circumstances

The characteristics of this category and the remedy used to treat them are as follows:

- Those who are not happy in present circumstances, and have no great interest in life. They may look forward to death, believing they will be better off or meet someone who has gone before them. (This complicates the healing process and weakens their life force.) (Clematis, *Clematis vitalba*)

- Those who are living in the past, when things were better for them, believing they will never be as good again. (This can be a problem for abandoned pets or pets whose owners have died, especially parrots.) (Honeysuckle, *Lonicera caprifolium*)
- Those who are just gliding resignedly through life without any effort to find joy or happiness. (Wild Rose, *Rosa canina*)
- Those who have suffered so much mentally or physically that they have given up (another issue for abandoned pets). (Olive, *Olea europaea*)
- Those who have an obsession and who can't prevent unpleasant thoughts from entering their minds repeatedly. This interferes with being able to think about anything else. (White chestnut, *Aesculus hippocastanum*)
- Those who have clinical depression, a feeling of gloom and despair, like a dark cloud is hiding any sign of light. (Mustard, *Sinapis arvensis*)
- Those who can't learn easily from past experience and keep doing the same things wrong, repeatedly. (Chestnut bud, *Aesculus hippocastanum*)

Loneliness

The characteristics of this category and the remedy used to treat them are as follows:

- Those who are quiet, aloof, independent, self-reliant types who prefer to be alone in health or illness. Their peace and calmness is a blessing to those around them. (Water violet, *Hottonia palustris*)
- Those who always want everything to happen or be done faster and think that they should get better more quickly. Also used for excruciating pain. (Another personality you may see among pet owners.) (Impatiens, *Impatiens roylei*)
- Those who always need to be with others, discussing themselves and their own problems with the nearest person, friend, or stranger. They are very unhappy if they have to be alone for very long (another abandoned pet issue). (Heather, *Calluna vulgaris*)

Oversensitivity to Influences and Ideas

The characteristics of this category and the remedy used to treat them are as follows:

- Those who are cheerful and humorous who love peace and are distressed by fighting. They may agree just to keep the peace, but inside tend to be anxious or tormented. Humans may turn to alcohol or drugs to help this. Pets may do something silly or bring the owners a favorite toy when owners are arguing. (Agrimony, *Agrimonia eupatoria*)
- Those who want to serve others so much that they neglect themselves. (Centaury, *Erythraea centaurium*)
- Those who occasionally are swayed from their own ideals and ambitions by others who influence them by the force of their convictions. This remedy helps them keep to their own path. (May help dogs who were obedient but are led into mischief by a new puppy.) (Walnut, *Juglans regia*)
- Those who feel jealousy, envy, revenge, suspicion when there is no need for such feelings. (This is a good remedy if a pet resents a new pet in the household.) (Holly, *Ilex aquifolium*)

Despondency or Despair

The characteristics of this category and the remedy used to treat them are as follows:

- Those who think they are never as good as those around them and who expect failure. (Larch, *Larix europa*)

- Those who always blame themselves no matter what happens. They think they always could have done better. (Pine, *Pinus sylvestris*)
- Those who are depressed because they feel that whatever they are doing is too hard for any person to be able to achieve. (Elm, *Umus campestris*)
- Those who feel like they have endured all they can and that life is unbearable and there is nothing but destruction left. (Another abandoned pet issue, and also for pets whose owners have died.) (Sweet chestnut, *Castanea vulgaris*)
- Those who find that sudden misfortune brings great unhappiness. (Star of Bethlehem, *Ornithogalum umbellatum*)
- Those who are unable to accept misfortune without complaint or resentment. (Willow, *Salix vitellina*)
- Those who are fighting strongly to get well, even though their case may seem hopeless. (Oak, *Quercus pedunculata*)
- Those who feel there is something dirty in their body that they must get rid of. (Crab apple, *Pyrus malus*)

Over-Care for the Welfare of Others

The characteristics of this category and the remedy used to treat them are as follows:

- Those who are always worried about their owners and family. They are worried when the family is away from them. (Guard dog breeds may have this problem.) (Chicory, *Cichorium intybus*)
- Those who have fixed principles and ideas that rarely change, and that they believe others should share, to the point of wanting to convert everyone else to their own ways and ideas. (Like a lot of cats!) (Vervain, *Verbena officinalis*)
- Those who are capable, certain of their own ability, confident of their success. They also believe others would benefit from doing things the way they do. They are of great value in an emergency. (Grapevine, *Vitis vinifera*)
- Those who see the good and beauty in all that surrounds them, and within all people. They understand that there are different ways each person and all things work to their own final perfection. (Beech, *Fagus sylvatica*)
- Those who are ascetics that deny themselves some pleasures in life because it might interfere with their work. They will do anything to keep themselves well, strong, and active, and hope to set examples for others. They tend to expect too much of themselves. (Rock water)

Veterinarian's Role

Most holistic veterinarians know about Rescue Remedy, the five-flower combination for general problems with fear and anxiety. They often recommend it and may also use it in their practice to help anxious patients. Some have studied more or taken a course about the other remedies as well. Practitioners recognize that the remedies are best used in conjunction with other methods of treatment, but they can be very useful for the mental/emotional part of the treatment.

Technician's Role

A technician who recognizes when a pet might need a little help for its anxiety can be responsible for administering Rescue Remedy and making the rest of the experience better for the pet and for the veterinarian. A technician who is well-versed in Bach flower remedies can be helpful to both veterinarians and clients, when the situation warrants it.

Where to Learn How

You can earn a certificate of completion with a short course designed to give you familiarity with the remedies and their use at Directly From Nature. Their website also has a page specifically about animals. This is not the same as the BFRP (Bach Foundation Registered Practitioner) or the BFAP (Bach Foundation Animal Practitioner) certifications recognized by the Bach Centre. To become a BFAP you must complete the BFRP course first and then be approved by the center.

The Directly From Nature course is available at
https://www.directlyfromnature.com/Online_Bach_Flower_Education_s/2123.htm

They also have information about pets and 27 of the remedies useful them at
https://www.directlyfromnature.com/Bach_Pet_Indication_s/1943.htm

A book that is often recommended which discusses their use in animals is:
Bach Flower Remedies for Animals by Helen Graham and Gregory Vlamis (see bibliography)

Glandular Therapy

Definition

"Glandulars" are various tissues, usually in a dried or processed form, that are used to help an animal heal. They include organs and other tissues as well as glands found in the body. Glandular materials have tissue-specific activity and contain physiologically active substances capable of exerting significant biologic and therapeutic effects. Popular hormones such as insulin and thyroxine are commonly derived from animal glands (usually hogs or cattle). Bionutritional therapy uses whole glandulars (containing cells, cell extracts, and antibodies).

Purpose

One purpose for using tissue is the principle that everything you need to grow or heal in a tissue is in the tissue itself. For example, extra taurine can be given to help heal heart tissue, or one can give actual heart itself to supply the extra taurine (and other elements the heart has that are not found in muscle meat or vegetarian protein).

History

The use of animal tissues for healing purposes is mentioned throughout written history.

Description

Besides dried tissue, tissue extracts may be used. One company uses extracts of nuclei of the tissues. Tissues often originate from pigs and are named in Latin for their origin. For example, *cor suis* means pig heart. With the presence of various diseases such as mad cow disease and the problem of contamination with *Salmonella* spp. and *Escherichia coli* from meats processed in both the United States and China, one must be careful of the origin (both species and country) of the glandulars and the way they are processed.

Veterinarian's Role

It is the veterinarian who generally recommends or uses glandulars. The veterinarian is also the primary person who will be discussing their use with pet owners.

Technician's Role

The role of the technician again lies in explanations of the use of glandulars and in helping a client evaluate the companies that sell them.

Standard Process is a reputable company that uses glandulars in their products as well as whole foods. They have a specific line for products for animals, as well as their human line.

Standard Process
1200 W. Royal Lee Drive
Palmyra, WI 53156
https://www.standardprocess.com

Magnetic Therapy

Definition

Magnets are used on acupuncture points in various items made to be secured on the body (including collars and harnesses) and in pet beds.

Purpose

Magnets are most often used to help pain, especially pain from arthritis.

History

- 4th century: Magnets were used for painful hands and feet by a French physician (Martel).
- 6th century: Magnets were used for joint pain by Tralles and for spasms and foot pain by Abbas.
- 16th century: Magnets were used for inflammation by Paracelsus.
- 17th century: William Gilbert wrote *De Magnete*, a book on magnetism and used magnets to stop bleeding.
- 18th century: French Royal Society of Medicine stated that magnets were antispasmodic and helped pain.
- 19th century: Magnets were used by Drs. Magiorani and Charcot.
- 1925: A book about magneto therapy was written by French physician Durville.
- 1976: The First International Conference on Magnetism was held in Boston.
- 1983: Rare earth neodymium magnets were developed (more powerful than previous magnets and can hold their magnetism with almost no decline in strength for at least 10 years).
- 1991: The Eighth International Conference on Magnetism was held in Munster, Germany.
- Today: Magnetic therapy is approved in over 45 countries.

Description

Stationary magnet therapy is more controversial than pulsed magnetic field therapy. There are a number of studies showing no effect and a number of others showing good effect. One problem lies in the fact that the magnets used are of variable strength and are used in a number of ways (beds, bracelets, on acupuncture points, etc.) Comparison of different studies generally shows that those finding no effect are, as a group, using magnets that are of lower strength than those used in studies that found beneficial effect.

Magnets may be glued on to acupuncture points using surgical glue, after the area is shaved. This is the most specific method of treating with magnets. Or magnets may be placed at regular intervals in beds, collars, and harnesses.

Veterinarian's Role

When using magnets on acupuncture points, the veterinarian must have knowledge of where those points are located. Otherwise, there is no special knowledge necessary for the use of magnets.

Ozone Therapy

Definition

Ozone therapy is the application of ozone from an ozone generator (requiring input from a tank of oxygen) for medical purposes.

Purpose

Ozone therapy is used to kill pathogens and to treat chronic diseases. It may also have a part to play in decreasing the harmful side effects of chemotherapy.

History

Ozone was discovered in 1840 by Joseph Lloyd Martin. In 1856, it was used to disinfect operating rooms and sterilize surgical instruments. Later in the century, it was also used to disinfect drinking water throughout Europe. An article in 1892 in the British journal, *The Lancet,* described the administration of ozone to treat tuberculosis. During World War I, it was used for infected wounds, including severe osteomyelitis in the femur and tibia (Stoker, 1916). (This was a big problem before antibiotics: Teddy Roosevelt died of complications from osteomyelitis affecting his leg after years of repeated surgeries.) It was also studied in Great Britain for the treatment of wounds in World War II (Quain, 1940). The European Cooperation of Medical Ozone Societies was founded in 1972. They publish guidelines on medical indications and contraindications of ozone. They also host training seminars (www.ozone-association.com). In the United States, ozone therapy can be used for humans in Alaska, Arizona, Colorado, Georgia, Minnesota, New York, New Jersey, North Carolina, Ohio, Oklahoma, Oregon, South Carolina, and Washington without fear of prosecution. The FDA recently approved its use in the food-processing industry as a disinfectant. Publications on the medical uses of ozone therapy are primarily published in peer-reviewed medical journals in non-English-speaking countries. They are available through Medline, but this lack of availability contributes to the idea that there is no research supporting the use of ozone therapy.

Description

Ozone is harmful when breathed and does damage to the lungs (Folinsbee, 1981). For this reason, many believe it must be equally harmful to other tissues. However, medical ozone therapy involves the use of ozone in small, precisely controlled concentrations, and it is administered through other parts of the body. The administration of ozone therapy to humans is condemned in the US, with the exception of the states listed above, and thus it is not widely practiced in human medicine.

A controversial use of ozone therapy is in the ozonation of blood. Since ozone has pathological effects on the lungs, especially seen in bad smog, one would think it would also oxidize the blood and other tissues if used in the blood. However, autohemotherapy, practiced in Europe for over 50 years (Haferkamp, 1950), has been investigated for harmful effects multiple times, with none being found. Autotherapy in humans involves withdrawing up to 200 mL of blood, mixing it with a little anticoagulant and therapeutic concentrations of ozone, and then reinfusing it into the patient. Veterinarians use this same method.

Research was published in 2000 by three biochemists from the Scripps Research Institute in California, which showed no effect on red blood cell integrity or on red blood cell enzymes (Zimran et al., 2000). A Canadian study showed no adverse effects after 12 weeks of treatment (Garber et al., 1991). This has been confirmed by Italian (Bocci et al., 1993; Travagli et al., 2006); Israeli (Margalit et al., 2001); Japanese (Shinriki et al., 1998) and Polish (Tylicki et al., 2004a,b; Biedunkiewicz et al., 2004, 2006) studies. Human blood tolerates ozone in concentrations up to at least 42 mcg/mL, whereas pathogens are adversely affected by the same concentrations (Carpendale and Freeberg, 1991). There is evidence that human neutrophils may naturally create ozone as part of their function as immune cells (Babior et al., 2003; Wentworth et al., 2002), although others argue that the biomarkers used could also be evident with some other reactions (Kettle and Winterbourn, 2005).

It must be stressed that ozone must never be administered directly in the vein because there is a chance of a fatal air embolism occurring. Ozone generators designed to "purify" the air can also generate lung damage because one of the elements of smog is created in your house. Nitrous oxide may be generated by an ozone generator, and if it is not dispersed, may cause problems.

Ozone therapy is also administered through rectal insufflation (Carpendale et al., 1993; Guerra et al., 1998) and by ozonating oils for topical use (Menéndez et al., 2002). Olive oil is commonly used for this purpose, and aloe vera juice may also be ozonated. These treatments are used topically for psoriasis and dry skin. Ozonated oils may help burns, decubital ulcers, fistulas, infections, and gangrene.

Ozone therapy has been used successfully for necrotizing fasciitis (Di Paolo et al., 2002). It has been investigated as a good sterilizing method (Murphy, 2006) and as a nontoxic way to sterilize drinking water (Suchkov, 1964; Wang et al., 2006; Wolfe et al., 1989). Another study found some improvement when used to treat herniated lumbar discs (Muto et al., 2004).

The American Cancer Society recommends against ozone therapy for cancer patients. However, a French study reported that ozone enhanced the treatment of tumors that were resistant to chemotherapy. Hypoxia of tumors is known to adversely affect treatment with radiation and chemotherapy (Dunn, 1997; Gray et al., 1953), and ozone therapy has been shown to improve oxygenation in hypoxic tumors (Bocci et al., 2005; Clavo et al., 2004a). A 2004 study in a Spanish cancer research institute involved 19 patients with incurable head and neck tumors. All received radiation therapy and tegafur. Twelve patients received additional chemotherapy during radiation, and seven patients whose disease was much more advanced received ozone therapy during radiation. The ozone group survived an additional 8 months, whereas the chemotherapy group survived an additional 6 months, suggesting that ozone therapy might be a good adjunct to radiation therapy, especially if applied earlier in the disease (Clavo et al., 2004b). Other studies have shown that ozone therapy may help decrease the side effects of radiation and chemotherapy (Borrego et al., 2004; Clavo et al., 2004a, 2005; González et al., 2004; Gretchkanev et al., 2002; Kontorschikova et al., 2001;

Potanin et al., 2000). Blood ozonation has also helped in the treatment of hepatitis C (Kontorschikova et al., 1996; Nedogoda et al., 1998).

For veterinarians, the use of ozone therapy shows promise in the treatment of chronic disease and, perhaps, for the treatment of cancer.

Veterinarian's Role

Medical-grade ozonators require a tank of oxygen in order to generate a high enough level of ozone. Oxygen is a prescription item and, thus, is available to veterinarians only.

Technician's Role

The technician's role is confined to helping restrain animals and to discussing the pros and cons of ozone therapy.

Hyperbaric Oxygen Therapy

Definition

Hyperbaric oxygen therapy (HBOT) is the administration of 100% oxygen at pressures above 1 atm. It is used to increase the oxygen saturation of tissues. For humans, hyperbaric therapy is used to rescue those with "the bends," or decompression sickness. It can help with medical problems that result in decreased oxygenation of tissues.

Purpose

In veterinary medicine, HBOT is especially useful for infections or injuries with insufficient circulation. In addition, it also enhances the effects of chemotherapy and radiation therapy.

History

Hyperbaric oxygen has been used clinically since the mid-1800s, especially for respiratory disease and to raise the oxygen content of the blood of patients anesthetized with nitrous oxide. In 1896, compressed air was pumped into the tunnel being constructed under the Hudson River. Workers coming up from the tunnel were affected with decompression sickness (and about one-fourth of them died). The bent postures they assumed in response to their pain coined the term *the bends* for this problem. Moir, an engineer, built a hyperbaric chamber for the workers and successfully treated the workers with recompression and then slow decompression; the death toll dropped dramatically (Moir, 1896).

Since the 1930s, hyperbaric treatment has been used for decompression sickness in deep-sea divers. However, because oxygen is so explosive; initially, only air was used. Because hyperbaric oxygen forces nitrogen out of tissues, making treatment much faster, as soon as a way was found to safely incorporate it, hyperbaric oxygen therapy became the treatment of choice for the divers.

In the 1950s, the Dutch were the first to use hyperbaric oxygen for other medical purposes (heart surgery). To do so, they pressurized the entire surgical suite. Later, HBOT was found to be of use for anaerobic infections, especially gas gangrene, and for carbon monoxide poisoning.

In 1967, the Undersea and Hyperbaric Medical Society (UHMS) was founded to foster the exchange of data on the physiology and medicine of commercial and military diving, and HBOT is now recognized by the American Board of Medical Specialties as a subspecialty of both emergency medicine and preventive medicine.

Description

For veterinarians, hyperbaric oxygen can be used to help anaerobic infections, slow-healing wounds, carbon monoxide poisoning, and severe lung disease. It has been shown to help decrease the side effects of chemotherapy and radiation therapy.

For humans, it is used for the following:

- Carbon monoxide poisoning
- Decompression sickness
- Arterial gas embolism
- Radiation-induced tissue injury
- Brain injury
- Stroke
- Spinal cord injury
- Clostridial myonecrosis
- Necrotizing fasciitis
- Refractory osteomyelitis
- Acute traumatic ischemic injury
- Compromised skin grafts and flaps
- Anemia due to exceptional blood loss
- Thermal burns
- Nonhealing wounds

It also enhances the effects of chemotherapy and radiation.

Veterinarian's Role

Individual hyperbaric chambers are expensive, and oxygen is usually a prescription item. Thus, generally, this technology is limited to veterinarians.

Technician's Role

Technicians are helpful in monitoring a patient inside a chamber and in informing clients about the usefulness of HBOT.

Prolotherapy

Definition

Prolotherapy is a method of stimulating the body to heal itself by creating scar tissue to stabilize joints. It is done by injecting a solution, usually concentrated dextrose into tissue surrounding a joint. This produces scar tissue and can stabilize unstable joints (such as luxating patellas).

Purpose

In veterinary medicine, prolotherapy currently is primarily used for back and joint pain.

History

In the late 1800s, injections of irritant solutions were used to build up scar tissue in order to repair hernias. In the early 1900s, the technique was used for temporomandibular joint (TMJ) disease. In the 1940s, Dr. George S. Hackett developed the technique further to help lax joints in general. Initially, he used a fatty acid mixture to induce inflammation.

Dr. Gustav A. Hemwall, one of Hackett's students, started treating patients with prolotherapy in the 1950s. He continued until the 1990s and documented almost 10,000 cases.

Today, prolotherapy is recognized as a special procedure by the American Association of Orthopaedic Medicine.

Description

Prolotherapy is also known as nonsurgical ligament reconstruction. It is used for chronic musculoskeletal pain. The "prolo" in prolotherapy comes from *proliferation* and is so-named because the method causes the proliferation of connective tissue around a joint. Normally, ligaments and tendons have limited blood supply, so healing tends to be limited. In hip dysplasia, these structures are often lax to begin with.

Currently, a mixture of 50% dextrose with lidocaine and other substances, such as B_{12}, is used to induce inflammation and stimulate fibroblasts to proliferate. Fibroblasts are present in tendons, ligaments, fascia, and cartilage. Although dextrose in low concentrations is well tolerated by tissues, high concentrations are not and cause inflammation. With inflammation, scar tissue builds up, helping stabilize an area. Most pets tolerate the procedure well, but some may need sedation.

Treatments are repeated at intervals varying from once a week to once a month. Because there is inflammation, some pain is common, varying from mild to severe enough to need analgesics. Narcotics such as tramadol can be helpful, but anything that also has an anti-inflammatory action (aspirin, deracoxib, carprofen, white willow bark, etc.) will interfere with the inflammation necessary to stimulate maximum repair of ligaments and tendons. Exercise is encouraged but not enough to break down the joint. (Owners are often so encouraged by initial improvement they make things worse by over-exercising the pet. Young, active dogs also may have this problem.) Between four and eight treatments are usually necessary and eventually, they often need to be repeated.

There are six mechanisms for this strengthening to occur:

- Mechanical trauma from the needle causes cellular damage, which stimulates inflammation.
- Compression of tissue by the injected solution stimulates intracellular growth factors.
- Inflammatory products induce cytokines and multiple growth factors, stimulating collagen growth.
- Inflammatory products also cause chemoneuromodulation of nociceptors and modulate nerve transmissions.
- Change in intraosseous pressure leads to the reduction of pain. (Dextrose plus lidocaine seems to have a longer effect than lidocaine alone.)

The joint is stabilized temporarily because of the inflammatory response each time the substance is injected. This allows ligament and tendon repair without reinjury from excessive movement.

Prolotherapy is used for the following conditions:

- Cruciate ligament laxity or partial rupture
- Hip dysplasia
- Patellar luxations
- Other stifle injuries
- Intervertebral disc disease
- Shoulder, elbow, carpal, sacroiliac instability
- Wobblers syndrome
- Carpal and tarsal luxations
- TMJ luxation

Prolotherapy is contraindicated if there is any of the following:

- Allergy to the injected solutions
- Dislocated joint that has not been reduced
- Septic arthritis or hemarthrosis
- Acute bursitis or tendonitis
- Recent onset of a progressive neurological deficit
- Spinal or articular neoplasia
- Severe exacerbation of pain

Veterinarian's Role

Prolotherapy involves injections and a thorough knowledge of animal anatomy, so it is reserved for veterinarians alone.

Technician's Role

The technician is helpful in restraining the animal and in explaining the procedure, as well as for follow-up care to the owner.

Where to Learn How

Many veterinarians find a human prolotherapist and study with him or her before venturing out on their own. Others find a veterinarian who is experienced in the procedure and study with him or her.

Homotoxicology

Homotoxicology remedies are no longer available in the United States or Canada. They are still available in the UK.

Definition

Homotoxicology uses remedies that are similar to those used by homeopathy and shares some of the same theories of disease. However, homotoxicology uses combined low-potency dilutions and places a bigger emphasis on detoxification. In addition, homotoxicology relies upon a Western diagnosis rather than the homeopathic method of case-taking (which enumerates multiple and unusual symptoms overlooked by Western methods of diagnosis) in order to decide which formulas should be used.

Purpose

Homotoxicology is used to treat diseases, either alone or in combination with Western medicine (depending on the disease).

History

Homotoxicology was begun by a German physician, Hans-Heinrich Reckeweg, M.D., who developed various combinations of low-potency homeopathic remedies in order to treat the diseases that he diagnosed allopathically. He chose the remedies according to the symptom patterns he saw in each disease. In 1936, he founded the company Heel GmbH to manufacture and market his products. More recently, a few other companies have started making similar products.

Description

Dr. Reckeweg believed that disease is the body's reaction to toxic substances, which he called *homotoxins*, that are stored in the intercellular spaces (or matrix) of the body. (The existence of toxic substances stored in the body's fat as well as intercellular space and connective tissue was not proven until decades later; see the chapter on detoxification.)

According to Dr. Reckeweg, the type and severity of an illness are determined by the amount of toxins in the matrix and how long they have been there as well as how effectively the body is able to detoxify and get rid of the toxins. (Again, the role of phase I and phase II enzymes in the liver, which are responsible for much of the detoxification process, as well as the variability of those actions among individuals, was verified decades later.)

Local action of the toxins can cause inflammation, distortion, and destruction of nearby cells. These substances also disrupt the movement of nutrients from capillaries to cells and waste products from cells back into the circulation. Helping the body to remove the homotoxins restores the body's biochemical balance, enabling healing.

Reckeweg developed a six-phase chart (Figure 11.1) showing the diseases each body system develops as the disease process travels deeper into the body (from top to bottom in the chart) or increases toxicity in a body system (from left to right in the chart). It is a way for a practitioner with conventional medical training to see where a conventional diagnosis corresponds to the internalization of a disease, whether the disease is progressing or regressing, and helps in the choice of remedies. Disease progresses from left to right, through the phases of excretion, inflammation/reaction, deposition, impregnation, degeneration, and dedifferentiation/neoplasia, and from top to bottom, starting with tissues originating from the ectodermal layer of the embryo (starting with the skin), through entodermal, mesenchymal, and mesodermal tissues, and ending with emotional problems. (The emotional stage was added by Reckeweg later in the development of his theory and echoes homeopathic theory.) With healing, you see a progression of signs going in the opposite direction.

In addition, the chart divides the depth of disease along the "biological divide." Milder diseases (to the left of the divide) have the potential for complete cure, whereas severe diseases (to the right

Recovery and Self Healing ⟵⟵⟵   ⟶⟶⟶ **Chronic Disease**

Embryonic Tissue	Excretion Phase	Inflammation Phase	Deposition Phase		Impregnation Phase	Degeneration Phase	Dedifferentiation Phase
Ectodermal 1. Epidermal	Sebum, cerumen	Pyoderma, erythema	Keratosis, pigmentation		Chronic pigmentation	Dermatosis	Basal cell neophasia, squamous cell tumor
2. Orodermal	Saliva	Stomatitis	Nasal polyps		Chronic stomatitis	Chronic atrophic rhinitis	Oral and nasal neoplasia
3. Neurodermal	Neuro-homones	Feline herpes dermatitis	Neuralgia, neuroma		Viral infection	Paresis, nerve atrophy	Neuroma
4. Sympathico-dermal	Neuro-hormones	Feline herpes dermatitis	Neuroalgia, neuroma		Viral infection	Paresis, nerve atrophy	Neuroma
Entodermal 1. Mucodermal	GI secretion	Pharygitis, enterocolitis	Constipation		Asthma, duodenal ulcers	Chronic bronchial disease, COPD	Cancer of stomach, small & lg intestines
2. Organodermal	Pancreatic secretions	Hepatitis, pneumonia	Gall stones		Chronic hepatitis, viral diseases	Liver cirrhosis, hyperthyroidism	Cancer—liver, lung, gall bladder, pancreas
Mesenchymal 1. Interstitiodermal	Hyaluronic acid, GAGs	Abscess, deep pyoderma	Edema, adiposis		Influenza virus infection	Cachexia	Various fibrosarcomas
2. Osteodermal	WBC production	Osteomyelitis	Exostoses		Osteomalacia	Spondylitis deformans	Osteosarcoma
3. Hemodermal	RBC, lymph production	Embolism, sepsis	Thrombus		Endocardiosis	Anemia	Leukemia, hemangiosarcoma
4. Lymphodermal	Antibodies, lymph	Tonsilitis	Swollen lymph nodes		Lymphatism	Lymphogranulo-matosis	Lymphosarcoma
5. Cavodermal	Synovial fluid	Polyarthritis	Dropsy		Hydrocephalus	Coxarthrosis	Chondrosarcoma, synoviosarcoma
Mesodermal 1. Nephrodermal	Urine	Nephritis, cystitis	Nephroliths, BPH		Hydronephrosis, albuminuria	Polycystic kidney disease	Renal carcinoma
2. Serodermal	Serous secretions	Pericarditis, peritonitis	Ascites		Preliminary tumor phase	Tuberculosis of the serosa	Serous membrane neoplasia
4. Germinodermal	Ovary, sperm	Prostatitis	Ovarian cysts		Preliminary tumor phase	Sterility	Ovaries, testes, and uterine neoplasia
5. Musculodermal	Lactate	Myositis	Myogelosis		Myositis	Musc. dystrophy	Myosarcoma

(The vertical label between the two halves of the table reads "Biological Divide.")

Figure 11.1 Reckeweg's six-phase table. *Source:* Reprinted with permission from Goldstein et al. (2008).

of the divide) involve irreversible cell damage. These diseases can be helped, but there will always be some residual problems.

One can follow improvement of a disease by matching symptoms with those on the chart. As a patient improves, signs or symptoms of diseases that they had previously in their lives may appear. This process is called regressive vicariation. The process will follow the chart from right to left and from bottom to top. The chart also indicates that if damage is deep-seated enough, permanent cell damage is possible. In this case, the patient can be helped to a certain extent but cannot be completely cured.

Homotoxicological treatment is chosen according to two considerations: diagnosis of the disease and the homotoxic formula specific to the disease. Other formulas designed to help detoxify the body (by increasing drainage of toxins from the matrix, activating metabolic detoxification pathways, improving the function of specific organs, strengthening the immune system, etc.) are used as well. In addition, if possible, there should be a reduction of any external toxic substances (such as artificial colors in foods, toxic chemicals in cleaning products, etc.).

There are a number of types of cancer in animals that develop after prolonged inflammation (for instance, squamous cell carcinoma on the ears of white cats, lymphoma of the intestinal system of cats after prolonged inflammatory bowel disease, and squamous cell carcinoma in a lick granuloma that had been present for years). Research has verified cellular damage from build-up of toxic products in the body, especially in the case of fibromyalgia, diseases linked to Agent Orange, and chronic fatigue disease.

There have been a number of clinical studies verifying the action of some of the homotoxicological formulas. For example, the formula "Zeel" has been shown to have the same painkilling effect after 6 weeks of use as two Cox-2 inhibitors (Celebrex and Vioxx) without the potential for gastrointestinal inflammation or liver or kidney damage (Heinz et al., 2003). Traumeel, in a double-blind study, was shown to significantly decrease the incidence of stomatitis in children receiving chemotherapy during bone marrow transplant procedures (Oberbaum et al., 2001). Unfortunately, most of the research on homotoxicology is in German and thus unavailable to most of the English-speaking population. This adds to the myth that there is no research that supports holistic medicine in general and homotoxicology in particular.

There are a number of ways to use homotoxicology, but one way for the beginner to get started is to find the disease problem on the six-phase chart. Use one phase remedy (depending on which phase the disease is in) and one symptom remedy. Another method is to use one remedy related to the symptoms, one remedy related to the organ involved, one related to which of the six phases it lies in, and one related to detoxification. Remedies are given twice a day and work best when given on an empty stomach, not near mealtime. (See the chart in Appendix 12 for amounts.) Doses may be given for a few days or weeks or for life, depending upon the problem being treated. (This is different from homeopathy, and you may need to explain this to clients.)

Veterinarian's Role

Homotoxicological preparations are available only to licensed veterinarians, medical doctors, and other medical practitioners. Use of homotoxicology preparations involves diagnosis and prescribing; thus, it is limited to veterinarians. Access to homotoxicology preparations is extremely limited in the US and Canada, but they are much easier to access throughout the rest of the world.

Technician's Role

The technician can help the veterinarian by providing explanations to the pet owner: what homotoxicology is, how it works, how to store the remedies, and how to administer them. As is so often the case, this is an area in which people are often confused. Clients may think they understand and then call back to ask for more information on how to give remedies, if it is harmful that the puppy ate a whole bottle of them (no), and how to store the remedy (out of direct sun, in a cool place, or the refrigerator, depending on how it is prepared). The homotoxicology theory of disease progression is useful to know to explain the idea of progression of disease from external to internal, which echoes the same ideas in Traditional Chinese Medicine. The idea of detoxification is a central part of Homotoxicology treatment.

Where to Learn How

There is no certifying body for veterinary homotoxicology. A course in homotoxicology is available online at https://www.schoolofhealth.com/naturopathy/homotoxicology/, through The School of Health, in the UK. It is oriented toward humans, not animals, but is very helpful in understanding the homotoxicology approach to health.

A PDF version of the Heel Practitioner's Handbook is available at:
https://www.healingedge.net/pdf/heel_practitioners_handbook.pdf

The Biological Medicine Institute is a source of information about homotoxicology and related practices:

The Biological Medicine Institute
305 North Lyndon Lane,
Louisville, KY 40222
https://www.biologicalmedicineinstitute.com/
https://www.biologicalmedicineinstitute.com/homotoxicology
https://www.naturaltherapypages.com.au/article/what-is-homotoxicology

Summary

What can the technician do?

1) Familiarize yourself with any of these modalities that your practice uses so that you may answer commonly asked questions.
2) Serve as a surrogate for applied kinesiology. You may be asked to help restrain pets, watch pets, or operate equipment for items such as pulsed magnetic therapy or hyperbaric oxygen.
3) Rotate stock, order appropriate quantities, and let the veterinarian know if there is anything new that the distributor has to offer.

References

Babior B.M., et al. 2003. Investigating antibody-catalyzed ozone generation by human neutrophils. *Proc Natl Acad Sci USA* 100(6):3031–3034.

Biedunkiewicz B., et al. 2004. Natural killer cell activity unaffected by ozonated autohemotherapy in patients with end-stage renal disease on maintenance renal replacement therapy. *Int J Artif Organs* 27(9):766–771.

Biedunkiewicz B., et al. 2006. Blood coagulation unaffected by ozonated autohemotherapy in patients on maintenance hemodialysis. *Arch Med Res* 37(8): 1034–1037.

Birnesser, Heinz & Klein, Peter & Weiser, Michael. (2003). A Modern Homeopathic Medication Works as well as COX 2 Inhibitors. *Der Allg* 25.

Bocci V., et al. 1993. Studies on the biological effects of ozone: 5. Evaluation of immunological parameters and tolerability in normal volunteers receiving ambulatory autohaemotherapy. *Biotherapy* 7(2):83–90.

Bocci V., et al. 2005. Restoration of normoxia by ozone therapy may control neoplastic growth: a review and a working hypothesis. *J Altern Complement Med* 11(2):257–265.

Borrego A., et al. 2004. Protection by ozone preconditioning is mediated by the antioxidant system in cisplatin-induced nephrotoxicity in rats. *Mediators Inflamm* 13(1):13–19.

Carpendale M.T., et al. 1993. Does ozone alleviate AIDS diarrhea? *J Clin Gastroenterol* 17(2):142–145.

Carpendale M.T. and Freeberg J.K. 1991. Ozone inactivates HIV at noncytotoxic concentrations. *Antiviral Res* 16(3):281–292.

Clavo B., et al. 2004a. Ozone therapy for tumor oxygenation: a pilot study. *Evid Based Complement Alternat Med* 1(1):93–98.

Clavo B., et al. 2004b. Adjuvant ozonetherapy in advanced head and neck tumors: a comparative study. *Evid Based Complement Alternat Med* 1(3):321–325.

Clavo B., et al. 2005. Intravesical ozone therapy for progressive radiation-induced hematuria. *J Altern Complement Med* 11(3):539–541.

Di Paolo N., et al. 2002. Necrotizing fasciitis successfully treated with extracorporeal blood oxygenation and ozonization (EBOO). *Int J Artif Organs* 25(12):1194–1198.

Dunn T. 1997. Oxygen and cancer. *N C Med J* 58(2):140–143.

Folinsbee L.J. 1981. Effects of ozone exposure on lung function in man: a review. *Rev Environ Health* 3(3):211–240.

Garber G.E., et al. 1991. The use of ozone-treated blood in the therapy of HIV infection and immune disease: a pilot study of safety and efficacy. *AIDS* 5(8):981–984.

Goldstein R. et al., 2008. *Integrating Complementary Medicine into Veterinary Practice*. Hoboken, NJ: Wiley-Blackwell.

González R., et al. 2004. Reversion by ozone treatment of acute nephrotoxicity induced by cisplatin in rats. *Mediators Inflamm* 13(5–6):307–312.

Gray L.H., et al. 1953. The concentration of oxygen dissolved in tissues at the time of irradiation as a factor in radiotherapy. *Br J Radiol* 26(312):638–648.

Gretchkanev G.O., et al. 2002. Role of ozone therapy in prevention and treatment of complications of drug therapy for ovarian cancer. *Akusherstvo Ginekologiya* 4:57–58.

Guerra V.X., et al. 1998. The nurse's work in the application of ozone therapy in retinitis pigmentosa. *Rev Cubana Enferm* 14(2):99–102.

Haferkamp H. 1950. Effect of autohemotherapy on the blood and blood picture. *Hippokrates* 21(15–16):475–478.

Heinz B. et al. 2003. A modern homeopathic medication works as well as COX2 inhibitors. *Der Allgemeinarzt* 25(4):261–264.

Kettle A.J. and Winterbourn C.C. 2005. Do neutrophils produce ozone? An appraisal of current evidence *Biofactors* 24(1–4):41–45. Access at https://iospress.metapress.com/openurl.asp?genre= article&issn=0951-6433&volume=24&issue=1&spage=41.

Kontorschikova K.N., et al. 1996. Effect of ozone on the liver state in experimental chronic hepatitis. (In Russian). *Biull Eksp Biol Med* 122(8):238–240.

Kontorschikova K.N., et al. 2001. Ozonetherapy in a complex treatment of breast cancer. In: *Proceedings of the 15th Ozone World Congress*, 11–15th Sept 2001, Medical Therapy Conference (IOA 2001, Ed.). Ealing, London, UK: Speedprint Macmedia Ltd.

Margalit M., et al. 2001. Effect of ozone on neutrophil function *in vitro*. *Clin Lab Haematol* 23(4):243–247. Access online at https://www.blackwell-synergy.com/openurl?genre=article&sid= nlm:pubmed&issn=0141-9854&date=2001&volume=23&issue=4&spage=243.

Menéndez S., et al. 2002. Efficacy of ozonized sunflower oil in the treatment of *tinea pedis*. *Mycoses* 45(8):329–332.

Moir E.W. 1896. Tunnelling by compressed air. *J Soc Arts* 44:567.

Murphy L. 2006. Ozone—the latest advance in sterilization of medical devices. *Can Oper Room Nurs J* 24(2):28, 30–32, 37–38.

Muto M., et al. 2004. Treatment of herniated lumbar disc by intradiscal and intraforaminal oxygen-ozone (O_2–O_3) injection. *J Neuroradiol* 31(3):183–189.

Nedogoda V.V., et al. 1998. Liver: influence of ozonotherapy on antioxidant protective system of patients with chronic hepatitis. *Scand J Gastroenterol* 33(Suppl. 227: P23):29.

Oberbaum Y., et al. 2001. Randomized, controlled clinical trial of the homeopathic medication traumel S in the treatment of chemotherapy-induced stomatitis in children undergoing stem cell transplantation. *Cancer* 92(3):684–690.

Oliva S.M. 2009. Emotional support and Bach flower therapy. *Rev Enferm* 32(10):16–19.

Potanin V.P., et al. 2000. Ozonotherapy in the early postoperative period in the surgical treatment of the lung cancer. *Kazanskij Medicinskij Zurnal* 4:263–265.

Quain J.R. 1940. Ozone treatment of wounds. *Lancet I* 1(6)1028–1029.

Shinriki N., et al. 1998. Susceptibilities of plasma antioxidants and erythrocyte constituents to low levels of ozone. *Haematologia (Budap)* 29(3):229–239.

Stoker G. 1916. The surgical uses of ozone. *Lancet II* 188(4860): 712. Accessed online 9/16/2010 at https://www.musa-group.com/premotes/stoker1916.pdf.

Suchkov B.P. 1964. Study of the ozonization of drinking water containing pathogenic bacteria and viruses. *Gig Sanit* 29:22–29.

Thaler K., et al. 2009. Bach flower remedies for psychological problems and pain: a systematic review. *BMC Complement Altern Med* 26(9):16.

Travagli V., et al. 2006. A realistic evaluation of the action of ozone on whole human blood. *Int J Biol Macromol* 39(4–5):317–320.

Tylicki L., et al. 2004a. No effects of ozonated autohemotherapy on inflammation response in hemodialyzed patients. *Mediators Inflamm* 13(5–6):377–380.

Tylicki L., et al. 2004b. Platelet function unaffected by ozonated autohaemotherapy in chronically haemodialysed patients. *Blood Coagul Fibrinolysis* 15(7):619–622. Access online at https://meta.wkhealth.com/pt/pt-core/template-journal/lwwgateway/media/landingpage.htm?issn=0957-5235&volume=15&issue=7&spage=619.

Valentine R. and Valentine R. 1998. Veterinary NAET: The veterinary application of NAET; A breakthrough approach to allergy resolution. *J Amer Holistic Vet Med Assoc* 14(1): 30–32.

Wang X.C., et al. 2006. Safety of treated water for re-use purposes—comparison of filtration and disinfection processes. *Water Sci Technol* 53(9):213–220.

Wentworth P., et al. 2002. Evidence for antibody-catalyzed ozone formation in bacterial killing and inflammation. *Science* 298(5601):2195–2199.

Wolfe R.L., et al. 1989. Disinfection of model indicator organisms in a drinking water pilot plant by using PEROXONE. *Appl Environ Microbiol* 55(9):2230–2241. Access online at https://aem.asm.org/cgi/pmidlookup?view=long&pmid=2679383.

Zimran A., et al. 2000. Effect of ozone on red blood cell enzymes and intermediates. *Acta Haematol* 102(3):148–151. Access online at https://content.karger.com/produktedb/produkte.asp?typ=fulltext&file=aha02148.

Bibliography

Veterinary NAET

Nambudripad's Allergy Elimination Techniques
www.naet.com
Web site of Dr. Devi Nambudripad, originator of NAET. NAET studies are available at https://www.naet.com/about/studies

Homotoxicology

Bellavite P. 1995. *The Emerging Science of Homeopathy: Complexity, Biodynamics and Nanopharmacology.* Berkeley, CA: North Atlantic Books.

Goldstein R., et al. 2007. *Integrating Complementary Medicine into Veterinary Practice.* Ames, IA: Wiley.

Heel, Inc. 2000. Biotherapeutic Index: Ordanatio Antihomotoxica et Materia Medica 5th edition. Germany: Konkordia Druck GmbH, Bühl. Accessed online 10/21/2002 at http://homotoxicology.net/Documents/biotherapy.pdf

Heel, Inc. Veterinary Materia Medica. Access the online interactive version at https://data.urenus.com/ heel-vet-index/ and the online pdf book at http://www.homotoxicology.net/Documents/vetguidefinal.pdf

Smit A., et al. 2010. *Introduction to Bioregulatory Medicine.* New York: Thieme.

Van Brandt B. 2004. *Inflammation Means Healing,* 3rd edition Evansville, MN: Inspiration Publishing.

Bach Flower Remedies

Bach E. and Wheeler E.J. 1998. *The Bach Flower Remedies.* Essex, UK: CW Daniel.

Graham H and Vlamis G 1999. *Bach Flower Remedies for Animals.* Findhorn Press

Magnet Therapy

Harlow T., et al. 2004. Randomised controlled trial of magnetic bracelets for relieving pain in osteoarthritis of the hip and knee. *BMJ* 329:1450–1454.

Pelka R.B., et al. 2001. Impulse magnetic-field therapy for migraine and other headaches: a double-blind, placebo-controlled study. *Adv Ther* 18(3):101–109.

Philpott W.H. and Kalita D.K. 2002. Magnet therapy. In: Anderson J., et al. eds. *Alternative Medicine the Definitive Guide,* p. 23. Berkeley, CA: Celestial Arts.

Ozone Therapy

Lara P.C., et al. 2009. Severe hypoxia induces chemo-resistance in clinical cervical tumors through MVP over-expression. *Radiat Oncol* 4:29.

Hyperbaric Oxygen Therapy

Boerema I., et al. 1956. High atmospheric pressure as an aid to cardiac surgery. *Archivum Chirurgicum Neerlandicum* 8:193.

Brummelkamp W.H., et al. 1961. Treatment of anaerobic infections (*clostridial myositis*) by drenching tissues with oxygen under high atmospheric pressure. *Surgery* 49:299.

Fontaine J.A. 1879. Emploi chirurgical de l'air comprime. *Union Med* 28:445.

Grim P.S., et al. 1990. Hyperbaric oxygen therapy. *JAMA* 263(16):2216–2220.

Jacobson J.H., et al. 1965. The historical perspective of hyperbaric therapy. *Ann N Y Acad Sci* 117:651.

Kawasoe Y., et al. Hyperbaric oxygen as a chemotherapy adjuvant in the treatment of osteosarcoma. *Oncol Rep* 22(5):1045–1050.

Morrison D.S. and Kirby R.D. 2006. Hyperbaric medicine: a brief history. Access online 10/23/2023 at https://sabahyperbaricmedicine.wordpress.com/2006/10/19/brief-history-of-hyperberic-medicine/

National Academy of Sciences and National Research Council. 1966. Fundamentals of Hyperbaric Medicine. Publication #1298.

Sheridan R.L. and Shank E.S. 1999. Hyperbaric oxygen treatment: a brief overview of a controversial topic. *J Trauma* 47:426–435.

Simpson I. 1857. *Compressed Air as a Therapeutic Agent in the Treatment of Consumption, Asthma, Chronic Bronchitis and Other Diseases.* Edinburgh: Sutherland & Knox.

Smith G. and Sharp G.R. 1962. Treatment of coal gas poisoning with oxygen at two atmospheres pressure. *Lancet* 1:816.

Tibble P.M. and Edelsberg J.S. 1996. Hyperbaric-oxygen therapy. *N Engl J Med* 334:1642–1648.

Prolotherapy

DeHaan R.L. 2004. My experience with prolotherapy. *Animals: An Alternative Answer to Anterior Cruciate Ligament and Hip Dysplasia Degeneration*. From the AHVMA 2004 Conference Proceedings: *Journal of Prolotherapy*. 1:54–58. Access online at https://www.getprolo.com/.

Webliography

Homotoxicology

Heel, Inc.
www.heel-vet.com
Homotoxicology for animals, with education for veterinarians
https://www.heel.com/
The company that was started by Reckeweg.

Applied Kinesiology

International College of Applied Kinesiology
https://www.icak.com/
Information about applied kinesiology and practitioners of it.

Bach Flower Remedies

The Bach Centre
https://www.bachcentre.com/
The original Bach Centre, run from Dr. Bach's home.

The Original Bach Flower Remedies
https://www.bachflower.com/
Source of Bach flower remedies, made according to the original methods of Dr. Bach.

Hyperbaric Therapy

Undersea and Hyperbaric Medical Society
https://www.uhms.org/
Interesting information about hyperbaric chambers.

Sechrist Veterinary Health
https://sivethealth.com/product-details/
Hyperbaric chambers for animals and information about hyperbaric oxygen therapy for pets

Prolotherapy

GetProlo.com
https://www.getprolo.com/
Web site to find prolotherapists for humans.

Prolotherapy.com
www.prolotherapy.com
Information on prolotherapy for humans.

The Medical Acupuncture web page
https://med-vetacupuncture.org/english/articles/prolovet.html
Primarily a site about veterinary acupuncture, web page has information about prolotherapy.

12

Other Less Commonly Used Modalities

Immuno-Augmentive Therapy

Definition

Immuno-augmentive therapy (IAT) is a type of cancer therapy. It measures and uses blocking and unblocking proteins, complement, and antibodies to help a body's immune system destroy cancer cells.

Purpose

IAT is designed to help prolong and improve the lives of cancer patients. The IAT website specifically states that it does not promise to cure cancer, just to prolong survival time, and IAT is used in conjunction with other methods such as nutrition.

History

IAT therapy was developed in the early 1970s by Lawrence Burton, PhD, based on his research with fruit flies and mice. He developed a mixture of blood proteins that he believed would slow or stop the growth of cancer cells. He first offered his treatment to human cancer patients in 1973 in Great Neck, New York. In 1974, he submitted a new drug application to the US FDA to begin human trials, but he later withdrew it.

In 1977, Dr. Burton closed his New York clinic and opened the Immunology Researching Centre in the Bahamas (which was later closed). In the late 1980s, he opened additional clinics in West Germany and Mexico. He died in 1993, but his clinic still operates (although since 2003, it has used a different name: IAT Clinic).

Dr. Burton never came to an agreement with the Office of Technology Assessment on research methods and refused to disclose his methods of isolating the specific blood products used in his treatment. In 1980, MetPath (now Quest Diagnostics, a biomedical lab) terminated their contract with Dr. Burton because they had too many false positives and false negatives when trying to develop a test based on his methods. In 1985, the clinic was closed by Bahamian health authorities because some compounds may have been contaminated with hepatitis B virus and HIV. It reopened 1 year later.

Complementary Medicine for Veterinary Technicians and Nurses, Second Edition. Nancy Scanlan.
© 2024 John Wiley & Sons, Inc. Published 2024 by John Wiley & Sons, Inc.

Two studies by Burton were published. His mesothelioma study did show some promise. Burton's case presentations were incomplete and poorly presented, prompting skeptics to say that IAT has no promise (Cassileth et al., 1987; Clement et al., 1988). The practice moved to new, upgraded facilities in 2017 with the help of a $250,000 grant from a grateful patient. Dr. Eric Brown, MD, who had worked with Burton and Clement previously, is the current medical director. The practice has been renamed to Quantum Immunotherapy and more information can be found at https://quantumimmunotherapy.net/.

Description

IAT is based on measurement of complement, unblocking and blocking proteins, and anti-tumor antibodies, which are said to be unbalanced in cancer patients. Injections of certain amounts of these substances are based on measurement of the amounts in the patient's blood. (This is not the same as the use of cancer vaccines and cytokines by conventional veterinary oncologists.)

Some veterinarians in the US use IAT. You can find them on the American Holistic Veterinary Medical Association's website. Click on Find a Member and put IAT in the search box.

Ironically, current (2023) research in human medicine has abundant studies on multiple aspects of the immune system and how to harness it in the fight against cancer. They are not based on Burton's studies, however.

Color Therapy

Definition

Color therapy is used for humans more often than for animals. Color is used to affect mood, personality traits, and the body's ability to fight disease. Along with colors of surroundings, color therapy may involve colored lights, gemstones, candles/lamps, crystal and glass prisms, and colored fabrics.

Purpose

Colors are used to influence mood and to influence certain disease states through the *chakras*. For humans, this has been applied more to advertising and home decorating than to therapy, although there are those who use it for therapy as well. It has been used to help design radiology suites to be less foreboding. For animals, the question is whether it influences them directly or if the effect is more on the owners, with the animals picking up on the owners' moods. Birds, monkeys, and apes see colors. Other animals do not see colors as intensely as we do, although there has been some research suggesting they do have some color vision.

History

Color healing has roots in ancient Egypt. Just as in modern times, the color red was associated with both vitality and danger by ancient Egyptians. They also associated black with night, death, and magic; green was the color of life. White was the symbol of purity, as it is today. Red was masculine, and white was considered to be feminine.

Ayurvedic medicine associates a specific color with each major chakra. With this system, a specific color helps with problems associated with each chakra.

Research by Dr. Max Luscher during the early 1900s, showed how color can affect behavior through emotional responses. He found that color preferences can also reveal personality traits. His test is used by some businesses as part of the hiring process.

SAD (seasonal affective disorder), where people become depressed or lethargic during the winter, has been linked to a lack of exposure to full-spectrum sunlight. When treated by exposing those affected to time under a full-spectrum light, their energy and optimism can be restored. This is cited by some as a type of color therapy, but it is more correctly termed phototherapy.

Angela Wright is a major force in color psychology. She began her studies in the 1970s, studying psychoanalytical psychology at Queen Mary's Hospital in Roehampton, England, before traveling to Carmel, California, to study the dynamics of color. She found links between patterns of color and patterns of human behavior and developed her hypothesis of four color palettes and the four corresponding personality types. In 1998, she was invited to become a Fellow of the Royal Society of Arts and is recognized worldwide as an expert on the unconscious effects of color. Her theories have been tested throughout the industry.

Another type of color therapy attributes specific traits to specific colors. This is less well-researched but does have some support.

Description

Proponents of color therapy note that warm colors (red, yellow, magenta) are generally viewed as more stimulating, and cool colors (violet, blue, green, and gray) are more calming. Red light increases blood pressure, and blue light decreases blood pressure.

The psychological properties of colors are said to be as follows:

- Red: physical strength, warmth, energy, action, optimism
- Blue: intelligence, serenity, idealism, rationalism, coolness, reflection, aloofness
- Yellow: emotion, friendliness, creativity, confidence, fear, depression
- Green: balance, harmony, restoration, healing, sympathy, peace, environmental awareness
- Violet: spirituality, vision, authenticity, truth, introversion (helps with contemplation and meditation)
- Brown: warmth, earthiness, supportive, reliability, obstinance, conscientiousness, deprivation, frivolity, immaturity, heaviness, unsophistication
- Orange: food, warmth, security, passion
- Gray: cold, neutral
- Cyan (turquoise): calm, refreshing, enhancing self-confidence
- Pink: feminine, love, physical tranquility, physical weakness
- Black: sophistication, glamour, security, coldness, menace, heaviness
- White: sterility, purity, cleanliness, simplicity, sophistication, coldness, elitism

The Colour Affects System

Angela Wright's research became the basis of her Colour Affects System. She found that colors have different effects on people depending on the color palette and the person's personality. There are four groups (palettes) of colors. Colors within each group are more harmonious than colors outside each group. (In the 1990s, mathematical correlations between wavelengths within each group were found, which were different for each group. There was no similar correlation between each group.) There are also four personality types with respect to color. Each personality type reacts best to a corresponding color group. The personality types have been characterized as Spring,

Summer, Fall, and Winter or Morninglight, Dreamlight, Firelight, and Starlight. This is not the same system used in the fashion industry to classify consumers based on hair color and complexion (also named after the four seasons).

Her theories have been tested multiple times in humans by various industries. One study in 2003–2004, sponsored by Oki Printing Solutions and administered by the Colour and Imaging Institute at the University of Derby, tested the connection between specific adjectives and her color palettes and tested her theories on color harmony. (http://www.colour-affects.co.uk/research) Subjects were tested in Great Britain, France, Germany, Spain, and Sweden, and native Chinese residing in the UK were also included. Subjects were asked to match colors with adjectives describing emotional states. Wright used these answers to determine which personality type each person had and how they would mentally interpret a color. There was a high correlation between her theory and the answers of all the subjects, suggesting that this is a universal human trait, not just a European one.*

Colors do affect moods and emotions of people, but the same colors tend to affect various people in different ways. For animals, the application of color therapy lies in exposing an animal (and maybe its owner) to specific colors in order to get specific responses. Another application is in the design of the waiting room, exam rooms, website, and business cards to reflect the philosophy of the holistic veterinary practice itself.

Siemens, a company specializing in electronics and electrical engineering, has designed colored lighting systems for magnetic resonance imaging (MRI) and computed tomography (CT) rooms in Denmark and Germany after consulting with Ms. Wright. The result is less movement artifact for MRIs, fewer patients who need sedation, and more relaxed patients.

For chakras, the colors of the rainbow are each associated with a specific chakra (see Table 12.1), starting with the first one at the base of the spine (Figure 12.1). To treat a problem or chakra, surround the pet with that color—on the bed, on favorite furniture, or with a rug where the pet likes to lie. For hyperthyroidism, put the appropriate color in the area of the throat.

Table 12.1 The chakras.

Chakra	Color	Effects
First	Red	Stimulates immune system, helps with detox, anti-tumor, antiviral
Second	Orange	Appetite stimulant, lung problems
Third	Yellow	GI system, diabetes, kidneys
Fourth	Green	Bronchodilator, infections
Fifth	Blue	Burns, fevers, infections
Sixth	Indigo	Hyperthyroidism
Seventh	Violet	Spleen, white blood count

---

* For a copy of the full report, you can telephone Colour Affects at +44 (0)20 7233 9904 or email them at info@colour-affects.co.uk

Figure 12.1 Locations of the seven chakras.

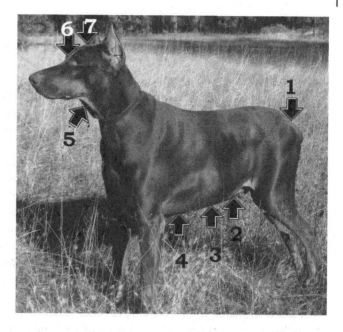

Veterinarian's Role

It is the veterinarian who decides whether color therapy is used to help a pet or to set the whole mood for the practice itself. It does take some study to use color for healing purposes, but there are no specialized classes for use in pets.

Technician's Role

Technicians can help in a number of ways: If they are cognizant of the Chinese five-element theory, they can supply a different color towel for a pet to lie on, depending on the patient's Chinese personality. If technicians are conversant in Angela Wright's theory, they can have some input into color schemes of the exam rooms. And if they have some knowledge of healing colors, they can help with appropriate lighting or other healing methods for treatment of a pet.

Royal Rife's Microscope and Beam Ray Machine

Royal Rife was an American inventor who became famous for two of his many inventions: a microscope and his therapy device that he believed could treat cancer and many other diseases. Discussions of him and his inventions get bogged down in speculations about conspiracies against him, whether he was a genius or crazy, how his partners ruined him and his company, how quacks claim to have replicated his equipment, and whether his inventions did something wonderful or nothing at all. If you read original writings by doctors and researchers of the time, you can find some facts that would probably be worth pursuing by people who can integrate optical, medical, and electronic knowledge.

The Microscope

Rife became interested in microscopes when working for Carl Zeiss, a manufacturer of camera lenses and microscopes. He moved from New York to Heidelberg, Germany and continued working there for a while before returning to the United States at the outbreak of World War I.

Microscopes are limited in resolution, depending upon the wavelength of the light passing through them. The shorter the wavelength, the smaller the size of the organism that can be clearly seen. In addition, the lenses must be made carefully and be of uniform consistency of clarity, for optimum viewing.

Ultraviolet light and X-rays are two wavelengths that are shorter than visible light. However, they are invisible to the naked eye. Rife microscopes use two beams of ultraviolet light, a patented high-intensity light source, a variable monochromatic beam, and Risley prisms (to polarize the light beams) to visualize live bacteria and viruses at a magnification larger than standard microscopes. The reason for monochromatic light is that different parts and organelles of a cell fluoresce differently depending on the wavelengths of light. So observing the same cell with different wavelengths makes different organelles and cell processes appear more prominently. Electron microscopes can magnify even more, but in order for them to work well, the subject must be stationary (dead) and fixed either chemically, by freezing, by dehydration, or stained using heavy metals. Rife invented a stain based on alfalfa hay and mercury to better visualize the flagella, but the bacteria and viruses themselves were not stained. The advantage of a Rife microscope is that you can see life processes inside living cells and movements of bacterial flagella, things not easily visualized with standard microscopes. (Photomicrographs can be viewed online at the bottom of the page https://rife.org/microscopes.)

Only five of these microscopes were made, the third of which (his Universal Microscope) was the most complex. (Rife claimed it could magnify items up to 60,000 times their normal size.) The microscopes were extremely expensive because of the requirements. Besides the prism and ultraviolet light source, the focusing mechanism was extremely precise: seven turns of the dial moved the lenses 1 micron. Lenses had to be spaced differently because of the extra-long length of the body tube. Rife discussed the production of his microscope with Bausch and Lomb, but their conclusion was that the expense would be too great for doctors, and there was not enough of a demand, even for research, for it to be commercially viable. Microscope number 5 is in the London Science Museum. It is not on exhibit to the public and can be seen only by special appointment. It is not in working order and may not even be assembled correctly. The only other known existing microscope sold at Bonhams Auction House in November 2009 for 14,400 pounds. This microscope was possibly number 2, although Professor John Hubbard, professor of pathology at the State University of New York at Buffalo in 1978 (who has been interested in Rife technology since the mid-1940s), stated that it had been cannibalized for later microscopes, along with number 1. Rife number 4 may still be in existence in the United States.

The Spencer Lens Company tested the microscope in the 1930s and did not find its performance any better than that of others with similar apertures. Professor Hubbard believed that people who had problems with the Rife microscope did not know how to select and prepare specimens with adequate care and did not operate it properly. The few people from Bausch and Lomb who looked at it (and pronounced it no better than other microscopes) were not well-versed in microscope theory, and so their opinions were considered invalid by some (including the curator of the London museum). Hubbard stated that he thought the instrument combined fluorescence, polarization, and interference microscopy. He had seen photomicrographs taken from the Universal and estimated that features shown were about 10 nanometers in size, whereas for regular light microscopes, the resolution is only down to about 200 nm. There are three papers from this general time period, with descriptions by scientists who saw the fine details described by Rife (Rosenow 1932a,b; Seidel and Winter 1944).

When the Wellcome Museum in London (original receiver of the scope) obtained Rife's microscope number 5, they dismantled it and found it impossible to obtain any image. Borrowing some parts from a Reichart microscope, they obtained a very poor image, about 30% larger than expected. This did not match any photomicrographs published. (However, the original microscope used quartz, not glass lenses because glass does not pass ultraviolet light.) There was no discussion of using monochromatic light of varying wavelengths to see different organisms. The curator found using the scope to be impossibly tedious, with extremely small adjustments for each of its parts. He believed this was because Rife liked to tinker. A better explanation would be that perhaps it allowed for all the adjustments needed for each specimen because Rife found that a different color of the monochromatic light was needed for each organism, and different colors could also pick out different organelles. Part of the problem is that nobody really talked to Rife about proper adjustment of the microscope, and current investigators have often not read original papers describing some of the important items to consider.

Mr. John Crane, Rife's former partner and the person who took some of Rife's equipment from his lab after his death, was not a good caretaker for the items. When Professor Ronald Cowden, emeritus professor of biophysics at East Tennessee State University, inspected the microscope Crane had taken, he found a main part missing, with no explanation of what it might have been used for. This illustrates some of the problems trying to reconstruct the Rife microscope (Rife's Notes, 1993).

More recently, two different websites were started to collect and make available all the information about Rife's life and discoveries that they could find. The founder of one website (Stanley x) and his partner built a microscope that duplicated the more outstanding abilities of Rife's microscopes: to see living organisms under higher magnification than is normally possible with conventional light microscopes. A picture of a functioning chloroplast can be seen on YouTube at https://www.youtube.com/watch?v=qToOzzB579Y.

Rife's Beam Ray Machine

With his observations from the microscope and with experiments on filtering bacteria, Rife believed he had proven that bacteria could change into viruses and that viruses caused cancer. If you read the part of the 1944 report of the Smithsonian titled "The New Microscopes" (at https://static1.squarespace.com/static/6120fd6cda3b62095f7499c9/t/615dda1b997cb074cceb78f0/1633540647875/Smithsonian+Report+The+New+Microscopes+1945.pdf) you can see that they did not really understand things like organelles. Rife and the Smithsonian talked about cells inside the cells. In addition, the first bacteria he studied were the bacteria causing typhus. This is a rickettsial bacteria. Rickettsia are known to be pleiomorphic, readily changing their size and shape depending on their environment. It is likely that the bacterial transformation he was seeing included the smallest rickettsial form rather than a virus.

Rife did see something in cancer cells that was not in normal cells. He thought it was a virus. It is more likely to be either an abnormal organelle (we know many cancer cells have abnormal mitochondria) or other common abnormality.

He found that the abnormality could be destroyed by auditory waves, using a different wavelength for each bacterium. Auditory waves don't penetrate far into tissues, so he used radio waves as carrier waves for the audio frequencies. (This is currently against FCC regulations because the radio waves are strong enough to interfere with local broadcasts.) He also found that certain frequencies helped with pain and, perhaps, some other diseases. There is a description of improvement of cataracts after a series of his treatments. The tube of a beam ray machine works similarly to an X-ray tube, focusing the waves in a directed beam toward the patient. Rife found that the frequencies destroyed cancer cells without harming normal cells. Recent research has found that pulsed low-frequency electromagnetic fields, in vitro, destroy tumor cells but not normal cells (IEEE, 1997; Mainguy et al., 1997).

There are some early case studies published recounting cures for cancer and tuberculosis using his machine. Rife established the Beam Ray Company to develop and promote his equipment, which was copied by others. In an attempt to preserve his hold on the process, he did not publish the frequencies needed for each type of disease. Rife ran into problems with the American Medical Association, the American Cancer Society, and with his business partners. Others made equipment that they called Rife machines, but that were not the same as Rife's original equipment. There is an argument among Rife's proponents on how to make the equipment, whether or not the color of the beam matters, what the various frequencies are, whether you need tubes in the machine, what gas should be in the main tube, how far away should the patient be, and on ad infinitum. It is hard to believe that any current equipment is the same as Rife's original beam ray or that it is being used in the way that Rife had determined. Reports of cancer cured by a Rife machine seem to be from someone who knows someone who heard of. ... There are, however, anecdotal reports of cancer pain helped by Rife machines.

CANCER PAIN CONTROLLED BY TREATMENT WITH A RIFE MACHINE

One of my patients with sternal osteosarcoma (bone cancer in the sternum), with pain uncontrolled by any combination of analgesics or holistic medicine, got instant relief from a Rife machine. (I have no idea which version or where they got it.) The pain relief lasted until the dog was euthanized 8 months later after the cancer had spread to his lungs. I have talked to other veterinarians who have seen the same effect. This would be well worth investigating.

Why Are Rife's Ideas Worthwhile?

The idea that we can see live microorganisms at a size and clarity large enough to directly watch their interactions with each other, with body cells (especially leukocytes), and with various drugs (and herbs, for that matter) is something worth pursuing. We might get a new insight into the body's defense mechanisms. We may never completely figure out the Rife microscope, but several people have been able to combine a number of his ideas into new microscopes with similar properties.

As for the Rife machine, no side effects on normal tissues were recorded, and none was seen when turning the frequencies on blood cells and watching them under the Rife microscope. How does this relate to other electromagnetic phenomena, such as pulsed magnetic therapy, for example? Can it affect wound healing? It is worth looking into the profound analgesic effect to see if another electronic instrument can be designed for pain relief, especially for the pain of cancer. If the observation about cataracts is confirmed, this is another possible area for examination.

When there is evidence for profound beneficial effect, what is the harm in pursuing this?

Electro-Acupuncture and Other Equipment

In the early 1950s, a German physician, Reinhold Voll, developed a way to find acupuncture points electrically. He found that acupuncture points have a lower electrical resistance than surrounding tissues. He then began searching for the correlation between different disease states and changes in resistance to various acupuncture points. Ultimately, he measured the resistance of skin at acupuncture points at the ends of meridians (on fingers and toes); 50 mV is considered normal, and charges above and below this indicate abnormalities. Abnormalities are treated either by applying an electrical charge to the same point (Voll's method) or by recommending various herbs, homeopathic remedies, or nutraceuticals for the problem. The goal is to return the resting voltage to 50 mV.

Animal Communicators

There are people who have a deep bond with animals and who believe they can communicate with animals, even at a distance. The quality of their communication varies, but there are some who are truly talented. The best of them will ask little to no information from you before they begin to tell you about your pet. Sometimes they can give *you* insight into a pet's strange behavior.

Sometimes they can give *your pet* insight into your strange (to the pet) behavior. Some of these communicators can help find a lost pet by describing what the pet is seeing. One communicator led an owner to their lost cat hiding under the neighbor's house in this way.

HELP FROM AN ANIMAL COMMUNICATOR

One of my patients suddenly began tossing his food dish around, scattering his meal all over the floor. Then he would clean it up off the floor. The first thing a communicator told the owner (without being told of the behavior) was, "He hates his new dish. He likes his old dog dish and wants it back." The owner dug the old dish out of the trash, exchanged it for the new one, and the behavior stopped.

Some can help owners communicate with their own pets, but it is rare for them to be able to transfer the full extent of their talent to others.

There can be a danger if owners rely too much on a communicator and distrust their veterinarian. A good communicator will encourage pet owners to see a veterinarian if it seems important for their pet. Because a communicator relies upon input from the animal's mind, they may not realize that certain things may be wrong. Owners may seek a second or third opinion because a communicator told them their pet did not have cancer (or some other equally serious disease), and they trusted him or her more than a veterinarian. The best way to avoid this problem is to be aware of the communicators in your area and their reputations. Work with the those who work willingly with you. Advise owners to ask others for recommendations also.

Summary

What can the technician do?

Most of these items are modalities that will be practiced by veterinarians. They are less common than other techniques discussed in this book, and the technician can be a big help by explaining the basics of the treatment to the owner (who may be reluctant to ask too many questions). The exceptions are color therapy and animal communication. A technician who knows color therapy can help with general colors for the clinic as well as exam rooms, and a technician who understands how colors relate to chakras can add benefits there. Some veterinarians choose a color of a towel for their patient to lie on related to which of the five Chinese elements the animal is most like, or the color according to color therapy that could help their anxiety or boost their immune system. Some animal communicators hold classes, and if you have a talent for it, you may be able to help clients or your veterinarian with some additional insight into the emotional state of an animal.

References

Cassileth B.R., et al. 1987. Report of a survey of patients receiving immuno-augmentative therapy. Unpublished study cited in published U.S. Congressional Office of Technology Assessment Report 1990. Archived at Princeton University. Immunoaugmentative Therapy Chapter. 1990.

Clement R.J., et al. 1988. Peritoneal mesothelioma. *Quantum Medicine: A J Comp Thera* 1:68–73.

IEEE. 1997. Effect of pulsed electric fields on biological cells: experiments and applications. *IEEE Trans Plasma Sci* 25:2. Access online at: https://ieeexplore.ieee.org/abstract/document/602501.

Mainguy J., et al. 1997. Evolution of neoplastic cells in tissue culture under the influence of electromagnetic fields. (In German.) *Erfahrungsheilkunde* 46: 398–404.

Rife's Notes. 1993. Synopsis from The Science Museum. C.N. Browne, curator. Access online 7/21/2023 at: https://users.navi.net/~rsc/scisyn.htm.

Rosenow E.C. 1932a. Observations on filter-passing forms of *Eberthella typhi* (*Bacillus typhosus*) and of the streptococcus from poliomyelitis. *Proc Staff Meet Mayo Clin* 7:28.

Rosenow E.C. 1932b. Observations with the Rife microscope of filter-passing forms of microorganisms. *Science* 76:192–199.

Seidel, R.E. and Winter M.E. 1944. The new microscopes. *J Franklin Inst* 237:2.

Bibliography

Color Therapy

Fischer S. 2009. *Color Palette for the Radiology Suite*. Siemens customer magazine. Access online 7/21/2023 at https://www.medical.siemens.com/siemens/en_GB/rg_marcom_FBAs/images/News/2009_10_lightsound/Medical_Solutions_September09_Colors_Radiology.pdf.

Wright A. 1998. *The Beginner's Guide to Colour Psychology* London: Colour Affects Ltd.

Rife

Haley D. 2000. *Politics in Healing*. Washington, D.C.: Potomac Valley Press.

Kenall A.I. and Rife R.R. 1931. Observations *on Bacillus typhosus* in its filterable state: a preliminary communication. *Cal West Med* 35:6.

Lynes B. 1987. *The Cancer Cure that Worked*. Minneapolis, MN: CompCare Publications.

Silver N. 2001. *The Handbook of Rife Frequency Healing*. Stone Ridge, NY: Center for Frequency Education.

IAT

American Cancer Society. 1991. Questionable methods of cancer management. Immuno-augmentative therapy (IAT). *CA Cancer J Clin* 41:357–364.

Coulter I., et al. 2003. Best-Case Series for the Use of Immuno-Augmentation Therapy and Naltrexone for the Treatment of Cancer. Evidence Report/Technology Assessment No. 78. Prepared by Southern California-RAND Evidence-based Practice Center under Contract No 290-97-0001. AHRQ Publication No. 03-E030. Rockville, MD: Agency for Healthcare Research and Quality.

Pfeifer B.L. and Jonas W.B. 2003. Clinical evaluation of immunoaugmentative therapy (IAT): an unconventional cancer treatment. *Integr Cancer Ther* 2(2):112–119.

U.S. Congress, Office of Technology Assessment. 1990. *Unconventional Cancer Treatments*. Washington, DC: US Government Printing Office; Publication OTA-H-405.

Webliography

Color Therapy

Colour Affects
www.colour-affects.co.uk
The Colour Affects System and how it can help people.

Color Matters
https://colormatters.thinkific.com/courses/color-psychology-for-logos-and-branding
Psychological properties of colors and how they affect us.

Color Quiz.com
www.colorquiz.com
Quiz based on work by Dr. Max Luscher. Links color with emotions.

Rife

Web site about Royal Rife
www.rife.org
Archive of articles, photos, letters, etc. about Royal Rife. Information about a Rife-like microscope made by Stanley Truman in the US
https://www.youtube.com/watch?v=qToOzzB579Y&t=113s
YouTube video of a chloroplast made with Stanley Truman's microscope

https://rife.de/index.html
Compilation of current (as of 2023) information about Rife and his inventions with links to similar information and to companies who have made Rife-like microscopes

https://www.grayfieldoptical.com/
Company which has created microscopes with characteristics of Rife's microscopes, but which use white light, not UV light. (Lots of illustrations comparing standard and other experimental microscopes with their microscopes)

https://www.psychotronics.org/aiovg_videos/2007-stanley-truman-and-erik-rowley-the-pursuit-of-the-rife-microscope-paradox/
Video of talk by Stanley Truman's partner Erik Rowley about the Rife microscope and developing their own

EAV

Oliveira, A. 2016. Electroacupuncture according to Voll: historical background and literature review. *J Acupunct Orient Med* 3: 5–10, 40.

Appendix 1

Glossary

Acupuncture: An ancient Chinese practice, thousands of years old, consisting of inserting needles into specific spots on the body to create specific physiologic results.

Aflatoxin: Toxins produced by species of *Aspergillus*, a fungus.

Albumin: A protein produced by the liver and responsible for liquid remaining in blood vessels. If albumin level is too low, edema occurs.

Allopathic: Referring to conventional veterinary medicine as taught at veterinary schools.

Animal communicators: People who have the ability to communicate with animals, usually in pictures rather than words.

Applied kinesiology: Using the strength or weakness of a muscle (often by pressing down on an outstretched arm) to determine if a substance is good or bad for a patient. Comes in various forms.

Aromatherapy: Use of essential oils from plants, usually diluted in carrier oils, to treat mental and physical problems.

Ayurvedic herbal medicine: Uses herbs from India and may also incorporate Indian theory of disease.

Bach flower remedies: Homeopathically prepared essences of a specific number of flowers, each of which is used for a specific type of mental state (such as fear).

Chinese herbal medicine: Chinese herbs are used in formulas that are designed using specific guidelines (for master herbs, helper herbs, etc.), and usually used according to a TCM diagnosis.

Chiropractic: A treatment system based on finding fixations in joints and treating them with fast acceleration, short-lever manipulations.

Cold laser therapy: Use of a "cold" laser of specific wavelength (usually in the red end of the spectrum) to reduce injury and speed healing.

Color therapy: Use of colors to affect mood and the immune system of animals.

Complementary veterinary medicine: Nontraditional treatments, such as acupuncture or herbal medicine, that may be used in conjunction with allopathic (conventional) medicine.

Detox: *See* Detoxification.

Detoxification: Elimination of various harmful substances (toxins) from the body. It usually involves diet change (sometimes fasting) and various nutraceuticals.

Electro-acupuncture (EAV): Biotron and other electronic diagnostic and treatment equipment measure electric resistance of the skin in various parts of the body (especially, but not always, at various acupuncture points) to determine health problems. Electroacupuncture can also be used to treat specific acupuncture points.

Complementary Medicine for Veterinary Technicians and Nurses, Second Edition. Nancy Scanlan.
© 2024 John Wiley & Sons, Inc. Published 2024 by John Wiley & Sons, Inc.

Essential oils: Oils that have been distilled from plants, using steam distillation.

Glandular therapy: Use of small amounts of tissue or tissue extracts (such as liver, thymus, thyroid, etc.) orally to help heal that tissue or boost its function.

Goitrogenic: Literally, causing a goiter, or enlarged thyroid. Goitrogenic substances interfere with thyroid activity and may cause hypothyroidism (decreased thyroid activity—more common in dogs) or hyperthyroidism (increased thyroid activity—more common in cats).

Herbal medicine: Use of herbs for specific pharmaceutical effects.

Holistic veterinary medicine: Nontraditional veterinary medicine, such as acupuncture and herbal medicine, emphasizing the idea that the whole animal is being treated, not just the part suffering from the disease. May include mind–body influences when considering a treatment.

Homeopathy: A system of medication based on the following principles: (1) a substance that causes specific signs when used in a high dose can be used to treat those same signs when used in low doses; (2) the more dilute the substance, the stronger its action; and (3) previous diseases may have been repressed rather than cured.

Homotoxicology: A system that emphasizes detoxification as part of the treatment process. It uses combinations of homeopathic remedies for detoxification as well as for treatment of specific disorders.

Hospice care and grief therapy: Care is for animals with a terminal illness, emphasizing comfort and no heroic efforts to keep them alive. Part of hospice care is grief therapy—mostly for the owner, but sometimes for the animal.

Hyperbaric therapy: The use of a 100% oxygen atmosphere with pressure more than 1 atm to treat various diseases.

Immuno-augmentive therapy (IAT): Helps boost certain components in the blood to fight cancer. This is currently unavailable to veterinarians.

Inflammatory bowel disease (IBD): An autoimmune disease causing chronic inflammation of the intestinal tract. Signs can include vomiting, diarrhea, or both.

Magnetic therapy: Use of magnets placed on the body or in a bed to help pain. Magnets may also be taped to specific acupuncture points to prolong treatment at those points.

Massage therapy: Often part of a physical therapy program, massage techniques include shiatsu (Japanese massage), Tui-Na (Chinese massage), and trigger point therapy (myofascial release). These may be used alone or as part of a general massage program or rehabilitation program.

Mutagenic: Causing mutations in cells. Often leads to cancer.

Nambrudipad's Allergy Elimination Technique (NAET): Uses applied kinesiology and other methods to determine allergies and a form of acupressure to desensitize patients to those allergens.

Nutraceuticals: Substances such as vitamins, minerals, and amino acids that are used for specific disease problems.

Nutrition: Holistic nutrition is based upon the use of fresh, whole foods with no artificial flavors, colors, preservatives, or derivatives such as corn gluten meal.

Osteopathy: Looks for problems in both muscles and joints that impact the patient. By helping restore function to a local area, the rest of the body can be helped.

Ozone therapy: Generated from oxygen by an ozone generator, ozone is usually administered rectally, although sometimes a patient's blood is withdrawn, mixed with ozone, and the combination reinjected into the patient. It is used for pain and some degenerative diseases.

Physical therapy: Formerly referring to both humans and animals. Now referring strictly to humans for therapy used to rehabilitate people who have received injuries and to help strengthen people who are disabled by age or disease. It consists of a number of different methods, including, but not limited to massage, acupuncture, chiropractic, water therapy, and balancing and strengthening exercises.

Pulsing magnetic field therapy (PEMFT): Use of a machine that creates pulsed magnetic waves to alleviate pain, speed healing, decrease edema, decrease inflammation, and decrease anxiety. (See also targeted pulsing magnetic field therapy, or tPEMFT.)

Rehabilitation: Therapy used to rehabilitate animals that have received injuries and to help strengthen animals that are disabled by age or disease. It consists of a number of different methods, including, but not limited to massage, acupuncture, chiropractic, water therapy, and balancing and strengthening exercises.

Reiki: A Japanese technique to reduce stress and promote healing. It emphasizes application of "life force energy" through the hands placed on or above the animal.

Rife machine: A machine based on Royal Rife's work that emits various electromagnetic frequencies used to treat disease.

Targeted pulsing magnetic field therapy (tPEMFT): Use of a machine that creates pulsed magnetic waves to alleviate pain, speed healing, decrease edema, decrease inflammation, and decrease anxiety. The waves are modified to narrow their action so that they have an effect primarily on one or a few related actions, rather than a broad effect.

Traditional Chinese medicine (TCM): A system of Chinese medicine thousands of years old that is based on the concept of yin and yang and organ functions that go beyond the Western understanding of how they work. It includes acupuncture and Chinese herbs as the main methods of treatment used by veterinarians.

Traditional Chinese Veterinary Medicine (TCVM): TCM with special application to animals and veterinary practice.

Trigger point therapy (myofascial release): Locates trigger points (areas of tight and tender fibers) in muscles and releases them in a variety of ways.

TTouch: Tellington TTouch is based on circular motions made by the fingers and hands in a form of gentle massage applied all over the body. It also includes specific exercises. Its purpose is not to physically massage muscles but to reconnect an animal with its body. It helps healing and behavior problems.

Veterinary-Client-Patient Relationship (VCPR): The establishment of a professional relationship between the veterinarian, a client, and their pet(s). It must include a physical, hands-on exam of the patient. This is required before veterinary procedures can occur and, in most states, must be renewed each year.

Veterinary orthopedic manipulation (VOM): A type of manipulation using instruments similar to those used by some chiropractors (but not making adjustments by hand).

Western herbal medicine: Based on a combination of European herbs and those found in the Americas, Western herbal medicine may use single herbs or combinations to treat various diseases.

Appendix 2

Alphabetical List of Holistic Veterinary Modalities

Acupuncture: An ancient Chinese practice, thousands of years old, consisting of inserting needles into specific spots on the body to create specific physiologic results. Many of these points can be found with a point finder (which is actually just an ohmmeter that measures current flow in millivolts and microamperes), and others have common anatomical features (such as penetration of fascia by nerves and blood vessels). Most commonly used for pain, acupuncture can also help many other problems. It is the most commonly used aspect of TCM theory in the United States.

Animal communicators: People who have the ability to communicate with animals, usually in pictures rather than words.

Applied kinesiology: Comes in various forms, using the strength or weakness of a muscle (often by pressing down on an outstretched arm) to determine if a substance is good or bad for a patient. It may also be used to determine whether a treatment has helped a patient.

Aromatherapy: Use of essential oils from plants, usually diluted in carrier oils, to treat mental and physical problems. Oils are distilled from plant materials and hence are very strong. The dilute oils may be applied to the patient (carefully!) or to the environment.

Ayurvedic herbal medicine: Uses herbs from India and may also incorporate Indian theory of disease.

Bach flower remedies: Homeopathically prepared essences of a specific number of flowers, each of which is used for a specific type of mental state (such as fear). Rescue Remedy is a commonly used combination of five of the remedies and is used for anxiety.

Chinese herbal medicine: Chinese herbs are used in formulas that are designed using specific guidelines (for master herbs, helper herbs, etc.) and usually are used according to a TCM diagnosis.

Chiropractic: A treatment system based on finding fixations in joints (limitation of joint movement) and treating them with fast acceleration, short-lever manipulations. Chiropractic emphasizes the effect of these fixations and their relief on the nervous system and, from there, on the entire body. Especially used for pain and lameness.

Cold laser therapy: Use of a "cold" laser of specific wavelength (usually in the red end of the spectrum) to reduce injury and speed healing. (A hot laser is a cutting laser used in surgery.)

Color therapy: Use of colors to affect mood and the immune system of animals. Used more often in people than in animals. (Can be useful in setting the mood of a room for clients.)

Detoxification: A process to eliminate various harmful substances (toxins) from the body. These toxins may be leftover drugs or chemicals or just leftover natural substances that the

Complementary Medicine for Veterinary Technicians and Nurses, Second Edition. Nancy Scanlan.
© 2024 John Wiley & Sons, Inc. Published 2024 by John Wiley & Sons, Inc.

body has not yet dealt with. It usually involves diet change (sometimes fasting) and various nutraceuticals to help the process. Detoxification is recognized by a number of different holistic specialties, and the Institute of Functional Medicine has created a large body of research on this topic for humans.

Electro-acupuncture (EAV), Biotron, and other electronic diagnostic and treatment equipment: Often used by holistic veterinarians. This equipment often measures electric resistance of the skin in various parts of the body (especially, but not always, at various acupuncture points). Treatment may be performed by these machines or be based on the readings from these machines.

Glandular therapy: Use of small amounts of tissue or tissue extracts (such as liver, thymus, thyroid, etc.) administered orally to help heal that tissue or boost its function.

Herbal medicine: There are two main groups of herbal supplements used most commonly by holistic veterinarians: Chinese herbs and Western herbs. Unless you or your veterinarian are very familiar with Chinese medicine, Chinese herbs should always be used in a balanced formula, not as individual items. They are best used if someone in the practice has a basic knowledge of Chinese medical theory. However, there are some formulas that are general enough to be used by a beginner. Western herbs are used more like conventional drugs: either alone or in combination, for various disease problems. Herbs are beginning to become a common part of conventional practice.

Some other herbal systems, such as Ayurvedic and South American, are also beginning to be used. Ayurvedic herbs depend upon another ancient medical theory from India, whereas South American herbs are used more like Western herbs.

The chapters on herbal medicine discuss some herbs commonly used in practice and how they are used.

Homeopathy: A system of medication based on several principles: (1) a substance that causes specific signs when used in a high dose can be used to treat those same signs when used in low doses; (2) the more dilute the substance, the stronger its action; (3) previous diseases may have been repressed rather than cured, so when the disease process is reversed, there may be temporary recurrence of these previous conditions as the patient improves. A very complete history of the patient is taken, and remedies are selected by how well they fit this disease pattern. Usually, single remedies are used.

Homotoxicology: A system that emphasizes detoxification as part of the treatment process. It uses combinations of homeopathic remedies for detoxification as well as treatment of specific disorders. Homotoxicology also shares some other philosophy with homeopathy, including the idea that a more dilute substance has a stronger effect and the concept of regressive vicariation. Usually, combinations of remedies are used, and the dilution is often less than that used in classical homeopathy.

Hospice care and grief therapy: We all would like our pets to die peacefully in their sleep. In addition, there are owners who want to help their pets transition peacefully. Hospice care helps an animal stay comfortable and pain-free during this transition. The intent is to relieve pain and suffering without extensive treatment to prolong the life of a dying animal. Part of hospice care is also the support of the owners and helping them through the grieving process. Pets may grieve also, and there is information that can help them, too.

Human–animal bond: Many pet owners have a strong bond with their pets that the human medical world often does not recognize. Therapy dogs and service dogs have been ambassadors for this idea, and there are ways the technician can become involved with them or even help support their use.

Hyperbaric therapy: The use of a 100% oxygen atmosphere with pressure of more than 1 atm to treat various diseases. (Hyperbaric chambers first were used for deep sea divers suffering from the bends.)

Immuno–augmentive therapy (IAT): A therapy that helps boost certain components in the blood to fight cancer. This is currently unavailable to veterinarians, although it is still practiced in the Bahamas for humans and you can still see references to it on the Internet.

Magnetic therapy: Use of magnets placed on the body or in a bed to help pain. Magnets may also be taped to specific acupuncture points to prolong treatment at those points.

Massage therapy: Massage therapy comes in many forms and can be used to help animals when done properly. Not all human massage therapists know how to properly massage an animal, so it is important to learn the technique from someone who is successful with animals. Massage therapy techniques include shiatsu (Japanese massage), Tui-Na (Chinese massage), and trigger point therapy, among others. These may be used alone or as part of a general massage program. In addition, massage therapy is often a part of a program of physical therapy.

Nambudripad's allergy elimination technique (NAET®): Uses applied kinesiology and other methods to determine allergies and uses a form of acupressure to desensitize patients to those allergens. "Allergens" are any item that can cause hypersensitivity reactions and thus can include things we normally do not associate with allergens, such as emotional responses.

Nutraceuticals: Nutraceuticals are substances such as vitamins, minerals, and amino acids that are used for specific disease problems. Nutritional supplements are ingested products, not food, that add to the health of an animal. Vitamins, minerals, antioxidants, amino acids, and fatty acids are examples of nutritional supplements.

Nutrition: Holistic nutrition is based upon the use of fresh, whole foods with no artificial flavors, colors, preservatives, or derivatives such as corn gluten meal. In addition, it attempts to recreate the ancestral diet of an animal.

Osteopathy: Osteopathy looks for problems in both muscles and joints that impact the patient. These problems impinge upon both the nervous system and the circulatory system. By helping restore function to a local area, the rest of the body can be helped because of action on the nervous and circulatory system.

Ozone therapy: Ozone is generated from oxygen by an ozone generator. It is usually administered rectally, although sometimes a patient's blood is withdrawn, mixed with ozone, and the ozone is reinjected into the patient. It is used for pain and some degenerative diseases.

Physical therapy: Formerly used for rehabilitative therapy for both humans and animals, currently physical therapy refers to humans. Rehabilitative therapy, sometimes called Rehab, is the term now used for animals. (See Rehabilitative therapy.)

Prolotherapy: Injection of substances (usually including concentrated dextrose solution) to create scar tissue to help support joints. Commonly used in the back, hips, and stifles.

Pulsing magnetic field therapy (PEMF): Use of a machine that creates pulsed magnetic waves to alleviate pain, speed healing, heal non-unions and indolent ulcers, decrease edema, and decrease anxiety. Often the wave types are manipulated to have one main effect, such as anti-anxiety effect or speeding healing. That type of therapy is called targeted PEMF, or tPEMF.

Rehabilitative therapy (Rehab): Rehabilitative therapy is used to rehabilitate animals that have received injuries and to help strengthen animals that are disabled by age or disease. It consists of a number of different methods. Veterinary technicians and nurses can become certified in rehabilitative therapy and can perform some types of therapy themselves.

Reiki: Reiki is a Japanese technique to reduce stress and promote healing. It emphasizes application of "life force energy" through the hands placed on or above the animal.

Rife machine: A machine based on Royal Rife's work that emits various electromagnetic frequencies used to treat disease.

Traditional Chinese medicine (TCM): A system of Chinese medicine thousands of years old based on the concept of yin and yang, and organ functions that go beyond the Western understanding of how they work. It includes acupuncture and Chinese herbs as the main methods of treatment. TCM aims to bring the body back into balance and restore the flow of the body's energy (qi). The words and ideas of TCM may sound like superstition, but they are actually just a different way of looking at the body, which can lead to insights unavailable to veterinarians who only use conventional Western diagnostic methods. For example, the tongue is examined not only for paleness, but general color, shape, cracks, and coating. The pulse is taken on both sides of the body, not just the left (or right), and compared. One can sometimes make a diagnosis by using these methods alone (for kidney failure, for example). Sometimes potential problems can be seen here before they are seen by other signs (for example, pending heart problems from bloat surgery).

Trigger point therapy: Trigger point therapy locates trigger points (areas of tight and tender fibers) in muscles and releases them in a variety of ways. Some methods, such as chiropractic and acupuncture, must be performed by a veterinarian or licensed practitioner, but other methods, such as massage, can be performed by a veterinary nurse or technician.

TTouch: Tellington TTouch is based on circular motions made by the fingers and hands in a form of gentle massage applied all over the body. It also includes specific exercises. Its purpose is not to physically massage muscles but to reconnect an animal with its body. It is used to speed healing and to help with behavior problems.

Veterinary Orthopedic Manipulation (VOM): A type of manipulation using instruments similar to those used by some chiropractors (but not making adjustments by hand) that adjusts all joints, not just those with fixations.

Western herbal medicine: Based on a combination of European herbs and those found in the Americas, Western herbal medicine may use single herbs or combinations for various diseases. Common to other types of herbal medicine is the belief that the combination of dozens of factors in herbs has a more beneficial effect than a single drug (even if it is extracted from an herb) used for a single purpose. In addition, herbs as a group have fewer side effects than many drugs.

Appendix 3

Where to Go for More Help

Veterinary Technician/Nurse Organizations

National Association of Veterinary Technicians in America (NAVTA)
750 Route 202
Suite 200
Bridgewater, NJ 08807
Phone: (888) 996-2882
Email: info@navta.net
www.navta.net

British Veterinary Nursing Association (BVNA)
Suite 124
Arise Harlow
Harlow Science Park
Maypole Boulevard
Harlow, Essex
CM17 9TX
Phone: 01279 969281
Email: bvna@bvna.co.uk
https://bvna.org.uk

Veterinary Nurses Council of Australia
PO Box 7345
Beaumaris
Victoria 3193
Australia
Phone: 03 9586 6022
Email: admin@vnca.asn.au
https://www.vnca.asn.au/

Complementary Medicine for Veterinary Technicians and Nurses, Second Edition. Nancy Scanlan.
© 2024 John Wiley & Sons, Inc. Published 2024 by John Wiley & Sons, Inc.

Veterinary Organizations

Academy of Veterinary Homeopathy (AVH)
PO Box 9280
Wilmington, DE 19809
866-652-1590
www.theavh.org

American Association for Veterinary Acupuncture (AAVA)
PO Box 1048
Glastonbury, CT 06033
860-659-8772
www.aava.org

American Association for Veterinary Chiropractic (AVCA)
American Veterinary Chiropractic Association
442154 E. 140 Road
Bluejacket, OK 74333
918-784-2231
www.animalchiropractic.org

American Holistic Veterinary Medical Association (AHVMA)
PO Box 630
Abingdon, MD 21009
410-569-0795; e-mail: office@ahvma.org
www.ahvma.org

International Veterinary Acupuncture Society (IVAS)
1730 South College Ave.
Suite 301
Fort Collins, CO 80525
970-266-0666; e-mail: office@ivas.org
www.ivas.org

Veterinary Botanical Medical Association (VBMA)
6410 Highway 92
Acworth, GA 30102
e-mail: Office@vbma.org
www.vbma.org

Holistic Associations, Organizations, and Teaching Centers

Currently, there is no holistic association for veterinary technicians or nurses, but the AHVMA does have sessions for technicians at their annual meeting.

The organizations listed below support the ethical practice of holistic medicine. They educate veterinarians in the correct use of modalities and encourage investigation and research of their methods.

Occasionally, you may see something that has the appearance of a legitimate organization, but if you look more closely, you will find that they are often just a way to make money for the founders and to offer a fake degree or certification. Please support these following reputable organizations.

Academy of Veterinary Homeopathy (AVH)
www.theavh.org

American Association for Veterinary Acupuncture (AAVA)
www.aava.org

American Association for Holistic Veterinary Medicine, student chapter (SAHVMA)
www.Students.ahvma.org

American Holistic Veterinary Medical Association (AHVMA)
ahvma.org

American Veterinary Chiropractic Association (AVCA)
www.animalchiropractic.org

Chi University
www.chiu.edu

College of Integrative Veterinary Therapies (CIVT)
civtedu.org

Healing Oasis Wellness Center
www.healingoasis.edu

International Veterinary Acupuncture Society (IVAS)
www.ivas.org

Veterinary Botanical Medical Association (VBMA)
www.vbma.org

Books and Professional Journals

Journal of the American Holistic Veterinary Medical Association
   The Point (newsletter of the IVAS)
   The following books are a good foundation for the holistic veterinary library:

Gaeddart, Andrew. *Health Concerns Clinical Handbook*. Professional Health Concerns, Oakland, CA, 2010.
Goldstein, Robert, et al. *Integrating Complementary Medicine into Veterinary Practice*. Wiley-Blackwell, Ames, IA, 2007.
Hamilton, Don. *Homeopathic Care for Cats and Dogs*. North Atlantic Books, Berkeley, CA, 1999.
Karreman, Hugh. Treating Dairy Cows Naturally: Thoughts & Strategies. Acres U.S.A. 2007.
Pitcairn, Richard and Pitcairn, S.H. Dr. *Pitcairn's Complete Guide to Natural Health for Dogs and Cats*. Rodale Press Inc., Emmaus, PA, 2005.

Schoen, Allen. *Kindred Spirits: How the Remarkable Bond Between Humans and Animals Can Change the Way We Live*. Random House, New York, NY, 2002.

Schoen, Allen. *Veterinary Acupuncture: Ancient Art to Modern Medicine*, 2nd edition. Mosby, St. Louis, MO, 2001.

Schoen, Allen and Wynn, Susan. *Complementary and Alternative Veterinary Medicine*. Mosby, St. Louis, MO, 1998.

Schwartz, Cheryl. *Four Paws, Five Directions*. Celestial Arts, Berkley, CA, 1996.

Wynn, Susan and Fougere, B.J. *Veterinary Herbal Medicine*. Mosby, St. Louis, MO, 2007.

Wynn, Susan, and Marsden, Steve. *Manual of Natural Veterinary Medicine: Science and Tradition*. Mosby, St. Louis, MO, 2002.

Xie, Huisheng. *Chinese Veterinary Herbal Handbook*. Chi Institute, Reddick, FL, 2004.

Xie H. 2010. Xie's *Chinese Veterinary Herbology*. Wiley-Blackwell.

Appendix 4

Questions to Help Define the Scope of Your Practice

In order to help explain to the public the way your practice works, you need to understand the foundation of the practice: the types of medicine practiced and how all the pieces work together. There are a number of questions that can make this clear to you, and it can help pet owners who are "shopping" for a veterinarian. The answers to these questions are also useful when designing a brochure or website for the complementary veterinary practice.

1) How long has the veterinarian been using holistic medicine (or how long has he or she been using the modality of interest)?

   If the veterinarian has been using holistic medicine for a long time, he or she may be on the level of a teacher, which can help the technician and pet owners better understand the methods being used. Short-term users are still seeking and experimenting and may be more willing to try other new things. For pet owners who are looking for answers to unusual problems, sometimes an approach needs to be broadened to cover additional methods for the best results. Other times, it takes the experience of long-term use to produce the depth required for best results using a single modality.

2) What types of complementary medicine does the veterinarian use?

   The answer to this question can help prevent a lot of misunderstanding. Some veterinarians will use one single modality (such as acupuncture) but remain conventional for the rest of the practice. A person who comes looking for advice on raw diets or herbs may be disappointed here.

3) What diets does the veterinarian recommend?

   Advice on natural or raw diets can be a practice builder. If a veterinarian is somewhat interested, but not well-versed in all the pros and cons of natural versus commercial diets, a technician with additional knowledge can be very helpful here.

4) What does the practice recommend for vaccinations?

   A veterinarian's beliefs about vaccinations can be complicated by state law. Pet owners can also be confused and decide against *all* vaccines. A Tonkinese breeder lost all her breeding stock and kittens because she decided never to vaccinate, even the kittens. A good understanding of the practice's vaccination program, including the reasons for vaccination, how often, which are used, and why, is critical when communicating with the public.

Complementary Medicine for Veterinary Technicians and Nurses, Second Edition. Nancy Scanlan.
© 2024 John Wiley & Sons, Inc. Published 2024 by John Wiley & Sons, Inc.

5) How does the veterinarian diagnose a problem?

   This goes along with the types of complementary medicine used. With a general practice, most complementary medical veterinarians will start with some standard procedures (blood tests, radiographs, etc.) and add anything that they specialize in (TCM theory, homeopathic repertorizing, etc.). Some are so specialized that they only use complementary methods (such as repertorizing), but they may also expect the animal to already have had a regular diagnostic workup from an allopathic veterinarian.

6) Where did the veterinarian get his or her training?

   The best training is that which comes from an organization that makes the effort to offer as complete training as possible and that offers continuing education sessions in addition to the basic training. Nonveterinary practitioners who are licensed for human practice may also be good teachers, as long as they have had some additional training. (The anatomy of four-legged creatures differs in a number of ways from humans, as does their physiology—especially cats. Animals have been harmed by various types of physical therapy given by people who did not understand animal anatomy, and cats have been poisoned by nonveterinary practitioners who did not understand how different their metabolism is.) If there is a licensing or certification program available for practitioners, beware of anyone who claims to have had training but who has not been through one of these programs.

7) What continuing education sessions does the veterinarian attend?

   Just as for regular veterinary medicine, continuing education is important for complementary veterinary medicine. No one can learn everything about complicated systems in just a few months. Veterinarians, as well as technicians, need refresher courses to remind them about practices that they do not often use. Veterinarians also need the latest information about new developments and research in the field. In addition, there are some meetings that also welcome veterinary technicians and nurses. It is important for both technicians and veterinarians to keep up on developments in the field.

8) Is the veterinarian available to pet owners by telephone or fax for further information?

   Some veterinarians enjoy this part of their practice. If it is a substantial part of the practice, they will probably charge a fee for it (and if they do not, they should). If it is just a part of their normal patient follow-up, they may include it with their follow-up phone calls. If they find that it intrudes upon their ability to practice, the majority of these clients ask questions that can largely be answered by the informed technician or nurse. Often the questions have to do with clarification about herbs or other remedies that have been recommended, diet recommendations, whether or not exercise should be restricted, or the newest and latest recommendation from the neighbor or Internet. If technicians keep on top of these subjects, they can advise clients without intruding into the veterinarian's domain of prescribing and diagnosis.

9) Does the practice brochure explain what is covered by the practice? Is it in words the pet owner can understand?

   A well-written brochure is invaluable for introducing your practice to the public. It can be made available to health food stores and holistic pet stores (as well as regular pet shops) to give pet owners a choice when they are looking for a natural approach. If there is no brochure, the technician can be invaluable in designing one and making sure copies are distributed to the proper outlets.

10) Is the practice's website informative? Does it offer valuable information so that the public will return to it (and your practice) for their questions and needs?
A good technician will keep the website and its links updated properly. No matter how good a commercial service is, it is unlikely that anyone knows enough about complementary veterinary medicine to properly maintain the type of website your practice needs.

Appendix 5

Patient History Chart

Current symptoms: _____

_____

Five-element constitution type (fire, earth, metal, water, wood)

Circadian clock (when symptoms occur):

Hour _____ Season _____

Environmental influences (conditions when symptoms worsen or improve)

_____

Condition location:

  Exterior (acute): _____

  Interior (chronic): _____

Condition type: yin _____ yang _____

             hot _____ cold _____

Listening to sounds

  Breathing (loud, shallow, weak, dry, rapid): _____

  Coughing (deep, dry, moist): _____

  Voice (loud/strong, soft/weak): _____

Tongue

  color (pink, pale, red, spotted): _____

  coating (white, yellow, absent): _____

  shape/size (swollen, shrunken, teeth imprints): _____

Complementary Medicine for Veterinary Technicians and Nurses, Second Edition. Nancy Scanlan.
© 2024 John Wiley & Sons, Inc. Published 2024 by John Wiley & Sons, Inc.

Hair coat

(dry, oily, brittle, falling out): _____

Odors (scorched, rancid, rotten, sweet, metallic)

Breath: _____

Ears: _____

Nose: _____

Skin: _____

Genitals: _____

Discharges (clear, colored, thick, watery)

Eyes: _____

Ears: _____

Nose: _____

Genitals: _____

Pulse rate:	cats	small dogs	large dogs
Rapid	>180_____	>110_____	>80_____
Slow	<80_____	<60_____	<40_____

Shape (threadlike, large, knotted, normal, surface, deep):

_____

Force (strong, bounding, weak): _____

Gait: (strong, favoring) _____

Elimination habits:

Urination (frequency, color, odor, pain): _____

_____

Defecation (frequency, texture, color, odor, straining, blood, mucus):

_____

Mood/behavior changes (angry, fearful, restless, etc.):

_____

Qi assessment

Appetite: _____

Energy (am, pm): _____

Vomiting: _____

Yin assessment

    Thirst: _____

    Heat tolerance: _____

Yang assessment

    Cold tolerance: _____

Nutrition

    Current diet (raw, homemade, dry, canned, brands):

    _____

    Treats and snacks: _____

    Supplements: _____

Holistic treatments:

    Herbs: _____

    _____

    Homeopathy:

    _____

    Homotoxicology: _____

    _____

    Acupuncture: _____

    Chiropractic: _____

    Current medications: _____

Reprinted with permission (and slight modifications) from Cheryl Schwartz, DVM. *Four Paws, Five Directions*. 1996. Berkeley, CA: Celestial Arts.

Appendix 6

Consent Form

This consent form is based on several developed for AHVMA members (and available to AHVMA members on the AHVMA website). A consent form may be used to help protect practitioners and as an aid to discussing treatment risks and benefits before beginning treatment.

The original forms were developed in consultation with a lawyer (and so the language is rather stringent). Any practice using this form is advised to consult their state veterinary board and their own lawyer to be sure it meets their needs and the laws of their state.

CONSENT FOR VETERINARY TREATMENT OR THERAPY

I, _____ *[owner/owner's authorized agent]*, have engaged Dr. _____ (hereafter *"Veterinarian"*), a licensed veterinarian and the _____ *[veterinary facility]* to perform veterinary acupuncture treatment on my *[animal(s)]*, _____ *[name(s)* _____ *of* _____ *animal(s)]*, _____ *[breed(s) or other description(s)]*, *[license or tag number/i.d. chip number/ tattoo number]*, which treatment has been described and explained to me, to my satisfaction, by *Veterinarian*.

I hereby fully consent to and authorize the performance of such treatment by *Veterinarian*, including any preliminary, further, or additional treatments, therapies, tests, medications or injections that may be, in the judgment of *Veterinarian*, or any veterinarian associated with him/ her, considered advisable or necessary at any time while the treatment is being performed.

The intention of this *Consent* is to grant full authority to *Veterinarian*, and any veterinarian associated with him/her and their employees, assistants, or consultants, to perform and administer any and all treatments, drugs, medications, tests, or diagnostic procedures on my animal(s) that may be deemed advisable or necessary by *Veterinarian*, or any veterinarian associated with him/her.

I have been fully informed, to my satisfaction, by *Veterinarian* that this treatment is a complementary or alternative veterinary medical treatment, therapy, or procedure. Also, I have been advised that complementary and alternative veterinary medicine does or may be considered by some in the American veterinary profession as a philosophy or practice that does or may differ from current scientific knowledge, or whose theoretical basis and techniques do or may diverge, even considerably, from veterinary medicine routinely taught in accredited veterinary colleges in the United States.

Complementary Medicine for Veterinary Technicians and Nurses, Second Edition. Nancy Scanlan.
© 2024 John Wiley & Sons, Inc. Published 2024 by John Wiley & Sons, Inc.

I understand that this treatment: (a) is not like most conventional or drug therapies, in that it has or may have multiple effects on many systems in an animal at a time; (b) it may have no effect; (c) my animal(s) may experience some side effects such as diarrhea or discomfort from the treatment; (d) this therapy is usually, but not always, safe, and it may have side effects that may be the same or more severe than conventional drugs or other treatments; and (e) adverse effects may include, but not be limited to, illness, known or unknown interactions, nausea, vomiting, diarrhea, constipation, muscle spasms, or more serious, unforeseen effects.

I appreciate that my animal(s) may not respond nor benefit from this treatment. I also understand that it is important for me fully to follow *Veterinarian's* instructions on monitoring my animal(s) such as, but not limited to, blood, stool, and urine tests, over the course of its/their treatment and promptly and fully to report to *Veterinarian* or any veterinarian associated with him/her, any adverse effects or unusual behavior by my animal(s).

I further understand that if my animal(s) is seen by another veterinarian, not associated with *Veterinarian* while undergoing or having undergone this treatment, that I should fully inform the other veterinarian that my animal(s) is undergoing or has undergone complementary or alternative treatment, the nature of the treatment, and request the other veterinarian to contact *Veterinarian* or a veterinarian associated with him/her.

I HAVE FULLY READ THIS CONSENT FORM BEFORE SIGNING IT AND VETERINARIAN HAS ANSWERED, TO MY COMPLETE SATISFACTION, ANY QUESTIONS I HAVE ASKED HIM OR HER ABOUT COMPLEMENTARY VETERINARY MEDICINE, RISKS ASSOCIATED WITH COMPLEMENTARY VETERINARY MEDICINE, OTHER NON-COMPLEMENTARY TREATMENTS, THERAPIES, PROTOCOLS, OR PROCEDURES THAT ARE OR MAY BE AVAILABLE OR POSSIBLE FOR MY ANIMAL(S) AND I HAVE FREELY AND KNOWINGLY SIGNED THIS CONSENT FORM.

Dated: _____,
_____
[Owner / Owner's Authorized Agent]
Address: _____

Telephone: _____
E-mail: _____

Appendix 7

Vaccination Consent Form

Consent includes explanation of risks of vaccination and risks associated with failure to vaccinate.

(Clinic Name)

Date: _____

Immunizing your pet is an important procedure that in most cases will provide protection against an illness that may be life-threatening. In past years, veterinarians have followed the vaccine manufacturer's guidelines and recommended annual revaccination for diseases that were felt to be a threat to our patients. Recent studies have shown that annual revaccination may not be necessary for some diseases because many pets are protected for 3 years or longer when vaccinated. Although most pets do not react adversely to a vaccination, some have had allergic or other systemic reactions after receiving a vaccine. Occasionally, the allergic reaction can be so profound that it may be life threatening. Certain immune-mediated diseases such as hemolytic anemia (anemia caused by red blood cell destruction), thrombocytopenia (low blood platelet numbers), and polyarthritis (joint inflammation and pain) in dogs may be triggered by the body's immune response to a vaccine. In cats, a serious additional concern has been a "lump" forming at the site of the vaccination caused by a substance in the vaccine called an adjuvant. In some cats, if these lumps persist, a tumor may form called a fibrosarcoma that may have grave consequences if ignored. If your cat develops a lump under the skin following a vaccination that persists for longer than 4 weeks, you should have it examined as soon as possible.

Your decision to vaccinate your pet should not be taken lightly. A decision should only come after your pet's age and the risk of exposure to disease are considered by you and your veterinarian. Vaccinations given at the appropriate age and at the appropriate intervals will greatly benefit your pet and protect it against some life-threatening diseases.

The following vaccines listed are considered "core" and "non-core" by the AVMA, TVMA, AAHA, and Texas A&M College of Veterinary Medicine. The University of California at Davis and North Carolina State University Colleges of Veterinary Medicine also recommend vaccine protocols that consider core and non-core vaccinations. All pets should receive core vaccinations with boosters at appropriate intervals to be determined by exposure risk related to your pet's lifestyle. Non-core vaccinations should not be used routinely and are only administered if your pet's exposure risk warrants it.

Complementary Medicine for Veterinary Technicians and Nurses, Second Edition. Nancy Scanlan.
© 2024 John Wiley & Sons, Inc. Published 2024 by John Wiley & Sons, Inc.

For additional information regarding vaccinations and your pet, visit the website, www.dvmvac.com.

Core vaccinations for dogs:
__Distemper
__Hepatitis (Adenovirus-2)
__Parvovirus enteritis
__Rabies

Core vaccinations for cats:
__Panleukopenia (Feline parvovirus)
__Rhinotracheitis (Feline herpes)
__Rabies

Non-core vaccinations for dogs:
__Bordetella (Kennel cough)
__Leptospirosis
__Lyme disease
__Coronavirus (not recommended)
__Giardia (not recommended)

Non-core vaccinations for cats:
__FeLV–Feline leukemia virus
__FIV–Feline immunodeficiency virus (not recommended)
__FIP–Feline infectious peritonitis (not recommended)

Please check all of the statements that apply to your pet.
__ primarily indoors __ indoors-outdoors __ visits a boarding kennel frequently __ always outdoors
__ is groomed frequently __ (has) __ (has not) had a reaction to previous vaccinations
__ has exposure to wildlife (raccoons, opossums, skunks, snakes, etc.)

I certify that I have read the above information and I am now aware of the risks associated with failure to vaccinate my pet as well as the potential side effects associated with receiving the vaccination. By signing this consent form, I authorize the administration of the vaccinations checked on the form above to my pet. Because vaccination reactions are not predictable, I agree that the veterinarians at _____ shall not be held liable for any reactions related to the administration of vaccinations administered to my pet. I further agree to hold my veterinarian harmless when in the event the effort to reduce the frequency and minimize known complications of vaccination inadvertently increases my pet's risk when exposed to a disease and I shall be responsible for fees related to treating any of the diseases for which a vaccine was not administered.

Client/Owner _____
Witness _____

Appendix 8

Writing Case Reports

Practitioners of complementary veterinary medicine often get their best and latest information by discussing cases and methods with each other. It is difficult to find research on holistic methods and even harder to get conventional veterinary journals to publish it. Even if you do find research, it is more often a human study than an animal study. Thus, a practitioner must ask is this safe for a pet? Is a cat going to process this differently than a dog or human? What is the safe dose? Will it have the same effect? Even a failure can be instructive. For example, in humans, iodine can help with both hypothyroidism and hyperthyroidism as well as breast cancer. This also seems to hold true for dogs (for hypothyroidism and mammary tumors), but the effective dose in hyperthyroid cats is very close to the toxic dose and only seems to work for a short time. If we read this in a conventional veterinary medical journal, we might ignore it due to the bias of the journal, but when the advice comes from a holistic veterinarian, we are more likely to listen. This will help both our dog patients and our cat patients.

There are two groups of case reports: little snippets such as the information in the paragraph above and formal case studies, with references and scientific background included. The *Journal of the AHVMA* accepts both types, and the editor can help with formatting problems. A veterinary technician can help gather information for a single case that went especially well or can summarize treatments that their employer successfully uses. If the nurse or technician performs something especially well, they can help the profession by contributing their own items.

Richard Palmquist, DVM, has been dedicated to getting more of these case studies in print. He wrote the following article as a guide for anyone who wants to submit a formal case study to the *Journal of the AHVMA*.

Improving Evidence: A Brief Review of the Use of Clinical Case Reports in Complementary and Alternative Veterinary Medicine

Richard Palmquist, DVM. Centinela Animal Hospital, 721 Centinela Avenue, Inglewood, CA 90302. 310-673-1910.

> "... case reports are an important area of scientific enquiry and one that is entirely appropriate for the CAVM community. Robert Fletcher of Harvard Medical School states that 'case reports are not on the fringe of science and clinical practice, as they are sometimes believed to be. They deserve serious, scholarly consideration.'"
>
> *(Jenicek, 2001)*

Abstract

Evidence-based veterinary medicine (case studies) is being increasingly used to evaluate therapies. The research committee of the AHVMA has established the goal of increasing published case studies in CAVM. This will help practitioners of CAVM as well as be a guide to legislative bodies.

A publishable case report contains:

A brief *abstract* summarizing the case

A *title* that clearly describes the case, which is easily searchable by a database

Authors, with their contact information, in alphabetical order of their last names, except that a senior author may be listed first

An *introduction,* with references, summarizing present knowledge and treatment of the condition, with expected results

The *case report,* containing

    Patient description

    Chief complaint

    Patient history, including environment and diet

    Client views and goals

    Results of diagnostic procedures

    Differential diagnosis, prognosis, and treatment plan

    Follow-up exams and progress

    Final outcome

Discussion, including opinion and assessments of the treatment

References, in the form required by the journal

Introduction

Veterinary medicine is moving rapidly toward an evidence-based medicine system for use in evaluating the appropriateness and usefulness of therapies available to practitioners and researchers. Increasing discussions of evidence-based veterinary medicine (EBVM) appear regularly in professional medical and legal journals (Hardin and Robertson, 2006; Kochevar and Fajt, 2006; Working Party of the Royal College of Physicians, 2005). As the veterinary research literature expands, EBVM will play a significant role in assisting veterinarians in evaluating data presented as useful in the treatment of animals. The purpose of this article is to introduce basic information about EBVM and the use of case reporting to the complementary and alternative veterinary medicine (CAVM) community and to encourage increased use of this material in publication and lectures created by our membership.

The AHVMA Journal can be used by veterinarians and other interested parties to demonstrate effective clinical uses of CAVM, as well as to assist legislative and regulatory bodies such as state boards in properly evaluating consumer complaints and legislative requirements regarding CAVM practitioners and practices (AHVMA Journal, 2024). The journal has worked to increase the number of high-quality, useful pieces of literature that can be used to establish the validity and applicability of CAVM and sees this as an important action at this time. It is hoped that competent CAVM clinicians and researchers will use EBVM to document their successes. Establishing proper scientific literature and making it more readily available allows for more interested parties to learn about many of the miraculous results seen in CAVM practice (AHVMA, 2006). Doing such actions allows for the expansion of knowledge, the expansion of CAVM acceptability, and the improvement of our profession, and EBVM depends utterly upon having access to correct, current, and complete information for its best functioning.

CAVM is by definition, "a heterogeneous group of preventive, diagnostic, and therapeutic philosophies and practices. The theoretical bases and techniques of CAVM may diverge from veterinary medicine routinely taught in North American veterinary medical schools or may differ from current scientific knowledge, or both." (AVMA, 2006) An excellent review of the history of CAVM and EBVM is contained in Allen Schoen and Susan Wynn's textbook on CAVM, which is the foundational text introducing CAVM to broader publics (Schoen and Wynn, 1998). The CAVM community often consists of professionals who continue to seek out additional methods of assisting patients. Conventional veterinary medicine does not have answers to all cases that are presented for assistance. Professionals and consumers of CAVM are often dissatisfied with certain aspects of conventional medicine. Such dissatisfaction can arise from many sources, including

1) poor or no results in a particular area or case;
2) failure of conventional methods to address the cause of a condition, thus concentrating on merely suppressing symptoms without more permanent relief of disease condition;
3) reliance on medications or surgeries that may have toxic, damaging, or unpleasant side effects;
4) paradigmatic conflicts between conventional medicine and psychological or spiritual views of the patient or consumer;
5) positive experience by consumers with CAVM; and
6) disagreements with a conventional practitioner.

Studies of human medicine have shown that complementary and alternative medicine users have higher personal income, higher levels of education, and desire more personal approaches to their health-care needs (Gray et al., 2002; Tindle et al., 2005). Few such studies exist in the veterinary profession, but clinical experience suggests similar reasons exist in our profession.

Case reports consist of simply presenting data from the clinic. They can be used for many reasons:

1) presenting a new disease
2) presenting new treatment options
3) summarizing case responses for clinic medical rounds
4) summarizing case results and treatments for legal reasons such as in lawsuits or in reviewing and planning legislative or regulatory actions.

Each form of case report contains slightly differing material, and a good summary of these is contained in Jenicek's text, which forms the foundations of this article (Jenicek, 2001).

Clinical case reports have been incorrectly perceived to be less important, or even not important, in the present environment of scientific literature, as they form a lower level of scientific evidence. However, case reports are an important area of scientific enquiry and one that is entirely appropriate for the CAVM community. Robert Fletcher of Harvard Medical School states that "case reports are not on the fringe of science and clinical practice, as they are sometimes believed to be. They deserve serious, scholarly consideration" (Jenicek, 2001).

Case reports are especially appropriate in CAVM as they serve importance in reporting first occurrences of particular diseases or therapeutic responses to novel therapies, as well as in reviewing the application of various modalities in integrative practice. Well-done case reports are highly desired by epidemiologists and researchers in identifying areas for further research. Once a case report appears, researchers can examine case series studies and then design appropriate procedures for better testing materials useful in diagnosis and treatment. This is a totally appropriate course of evaluation by scientific methods and leads to strong evidence and eventual support of such procedures. Such steps were seen in the recent recommendation by boarded internists regarding the use of the milk thistle extract (silymarin) and SAMe by conventional medicine in treatment of hepatitis patients, a practice used by CAVM doctors for quite some time.

Jenicek defines evidence as "any data or information, whether solid or weak, obtained through experience, observational research or experimental work (trials). This data or information must be relevant either to the understanding of the problem (case) or to the clinical decisions (diagnostic, therapeutic or care-oriented) made about the case" (Jenicek, 2001). EBVM is heavily interested in well-done case reports that provide evidence as defined above and case reports are incredibly important in the advance of CAVM. Competent, bright clinicians are perfect sources of such information. With the advent of clinical professorships in integrative veterinary medicine, such as that of Narda Robinson at Colorado State University, it is hoped that greater cooperation may be achieved in the future as clinicians provide areas for more productive research by academic medicine. Interest in such material is at an all-time high.

A good clinical case report will contain the following information:

1) A *title* that clearly describes the case and modality used. An author wants his or her materials to be readily accessible to those interested. This is important to those accessing databases and doing literature searches (Cockcroft and Holmes, 2003). Descriptive titles read as a sentence (e.g., The use of photo-acupuncture in treatment of feline nasal squamous cell carcinoma: a case report). A person interested in finding references about photo-acupuncture could readily search under "photo-acupuncture" and return useful references. Another person interested in finding treatment options for squamous cell carcinoma could also find references, although the results of such a broad search would likely be massive (PubMed yields a daunting 81,104 references). Narrowing the search by including species in the title reduces the number of references to 196, which would be more helpful to a busy clinician interested in treatment options for a client's cat. Addition of photo-acupuncture yields only seven articles, and none has to do with squamous cell carcinoma in cats. Spelling is a critical issue as searching under "photoacupuncture" results in no articles, while searching "photo acupuncture" provides 1400 articles for examination. Treatments should be named generically, not as a brand name. This enables a search for all instances of that treatment. In addition, those who are not familiar with a brand name will not inadvertently omit a specific product in their search.

2) An *introduction* that summarizes quickly the present knowledge about the medical condition described and its conventional therapy, as well as expected results of that treatment. Statements of fact that are not obvious must be referenced. This section establishes why the information might be useful to veterinary medicine. There is an obvious need for reports about improved conditions in cases where conventional therapy and diagnosis fail to completely, safely resolve a medical condition and where CAVM procedures have succeeded. While such cases cannot establish the effectiveness of the modality used, they provide primary evidence suggesting a need for further research. They also give other clinicians secondary options to choose in cases where established therapy is undesirable, has failed, or has been declined by the animal's steward. In the case of herbs, nutraceuticals, homeopathy, homotoxicology, etc., descriptions of a product should include ingredients and their form (powder, tincture, etc.), with a footnote for the brand name and manufacturer. Some journals request a summary or abstract that encapsulates the entire paper in a few paragraphs. This allows readers to quickly preview the article to see if it meets their needs before investing larger amounts of time and effort involved in reading the complete work. Such summaries usually precede the introduction section.

3) *Case report presentation* includes the following:

Patient identification and demographic data (species, breed, age, sex, vaccine status, neutering status, and special uses or environmental issues).

Chief complaint or reason for the medical presentation.

Patient history (travel, residence, environment, prior illnesses, and treatments).

Client views about the issue, prior therapy, personal treatment goals, or other personal issues as applicable to the case. Physical examination results.

Paraclinical evaluation (results of diagnostic procedures such as laboratory, imaging, and other objective evaluations).

Clinician's impression and working or provisional diagnosis.

Treatment plan and orders with general reasoning behind that course of action, including entire treatment used (e.g., including diet as well as specific modalities).

Differential diagnosis and diagnostic and therapeutic planning.

Prognosis and priority assessment of present problems.

Follow-up examinations, tests, and progress.

Final outcome and evidence of the treatment plan's causation in the final outcome.

4) *Discussion of the case.* This is where the authors can review further literature and correlate their opinions and assessments with the case presented. All literature must be referenced and footnoted. Such discussions usually originate new questions for further investigation and evaluate the data presented, suggesting possible uses for the data.

5) *References.* References serve several purposes. They provide the reader with useful reading and direct their attention to information that may not be widely known, but that is important to the subject. They also allow the reader to evaluate the data presented for its usefulness and reliability.

Discussion

CAVM contains many useful theories, techniques, and treatment options that CAVM practitioners use daily to assist patients in their search for health and longevity. Critics frequently invalidate CAVM for its lack of scientific literature and for ideas that disagree with mainstream medicine. Dialogue with hardcore skeptics can amount to a waste of time as some of these individuals have no real desire to approach CAVM with an open mind or actual scientific evaluation, but there are valid criticisms of the CAVM community regarding our lack of published and researched materials. These discussions have been well reviewed elsewhere and are not the center of this paper (Wynn and Wolpe, 2005).

Case reporting is one way that CAVM practitioners can record their results publicly so that others can benefit from their labors. We know that investigator bias can affect research results, and quantum physics has clearly demonstrated that the observer can affect the results of phenomena in the physical universe. This effect can lead to positive results that are not repeatable by others, as well as negation of procedures due to improper environment. Science consists of an orderly progression and categorization of data about the physical universe. Once material is known and verified, it can be organized into useful applications, which are known as technology. All veterinarians, whether CAVM, conventional, or integrative practitioners, have an interest in seeing proper scientific method applied to our field, but improper science can rapidly lead us to erroneous and even harmful conclusions.

Critics of CAVM are quick to point out the lack of double-blind randomized studies in our field, often without recognizing the situation present in conventional veterinary practice. In many situations, this type of study is not readily applicable to CAVM processes as therapy is individualized to each specific patient's particular situation. As an example, homeopathic cases are not easily studied in this manner, while acupuncture and herbal medicine can be. CAVM literature frequently consists of case reporting, and these reports are often correctly criticized as being incomplete or improper for use by EBVM. Since case reports are often disregarded by those searching the literature for evidence, CAVM doctors have become discouraged and ceased to make concerted efforts to publish in the conventional literature, and this is unfortunate indeed.

As an example of the problems faced by those attempting to provide evidence, Epstein recently attempted to publish a very well-done case report in a conventional journal. The case report documented complete clinical remission of chronic nasal Aspergillosis in a canine treated with classical homeopathy. The response to therapy was remarkable and noteworthy, but the conventional literature refused to publish the article because the author and client had not done repeated anesthetized imaging and biopsy procedures to document the regression of fungal lesions in the case. The board-certified reviewer stated that this was the level of proof required for a new therapy, even though the case was deemed incurable and hopeless, and the literature contains not one case of spontaneous resolution. The author and client felt that such "diagnostic" invasion had strong probabilities of depressing immune response and lowering chances of healing. They ethically refused to subject the patient to such invasive and unnecessary practice (Epstein, 2006). Massive medical ethics discussions ensue following such situations, and they frequently frustrate CAVM doctors for understandable reasons. Critics respond that they must have adequate evidence before allowing such articles to access respected literature.

Clinical research is not done to satisfy critics but rather to satisfy our quest for effective knowledge, which has applicability in assisting our patients stay healthier, recover faster, or in providing further options for use by veterinarians in difficult situations. Case reporting is done to establish where something appears to have worked and how it happened. The CAVM community needs to spend less time battling with professional skeptics and more time documenting and enquiring into our methods and results. In pursuing such activity, we forward truthful information for use by others to expand our practices and our profession.

A recent Gallup Poll (2006) placed veterinarians as number 3 on the list of respected professions by the public (after nurses and pharmacists and before physicians). If our profession continues to offer well-thought out, results-oriented treatments to our patients and clients, we will continue to bask in this popularity. Research, when properly done, expands truth, and truth properly applied leads to improved survival. At a recent AHVMA meeting, Sagiv Ben-Yakir urged people to stop fighting skeptics and associate with Nobel prize winners. That is good advice, and publishing well-done clinical case reports is a beginning. If we simply obtained two well-done case reports from each modality this year, we could rapidly advance the literature available to CAVM. The research committee of AHVMA believes this is possible and hopes this article will move things forward.

CAVM procedures do work. We all see this daily. Because of the increasingly cooperative efforts by board-certified referral practices and CAVM practitioners, it is hoped that such barriers to publication will be minimized in the future as more and more cases are occurring that have excellent conventional and alternative documentation. Case reports have been perceived to be less important in the present environment of scientific literature, as they form a lower level of scientific evidence. However, case reports are an important area of scientific enquiry and one that is entirely appropriate for the CAVM community.

References

AHVMA Journal, AHVMA Journal Submissions. Accessed online at 1/19/2024 https://www.ahvma.org/journal-submissions.

AHVMA, 2024. American Holistic Veterinary Medical Association website. Accessed online at 1/19/2024 https://www.ahvma.org/association.

American Veterinary Medical Association (AVMA). 2006. Guidelines: AVMA Guidelines for Complementary and Alternative Veterinary Medicine. Accessed online at 1/19/2024 https://www.avma.org/resources-tools/avma-policies/complementary-alternative-and-integrative-veterinary-medicine.

Cockcroft, P. and Holmes, M. 2003. *Handbook of Evidence-based Veterinary Medicine*. Maltden, MI: Blackwell Publishing.

Epstein S. 2006. Nasal Aspergillosis treated homeopathically in the dog. *JAHVMA* 25(3):9.

Gallup poll. 2006. Most Trusted Professionals. Accessed online at 9/6/2010 https://www.galluppoll.com/content/?ci=25888.

Gray C. M. et al. 2002. Complementary and alternative medicine use among health plan members. A cross-sectional survey. *Eff Clin Pract* 5(1):17–22.

Hardin L.E. and Robertson S. 2006. Learning evidence-based veterinary medicine through development of a critically appraised topic. *J Vet Med Educ* 33(3):474–478.

Jenicek M. 2001. *Clinical Case Reporting in Evidence-Based Medicine*. New York: Oxford University Press.

Kochevar D.T. and Fajt V. 2006. Evidence-based decision making in small animal therapeutics. *Vet Clin North Am Small Anim Pract* 36(5):943–959.

Schoen A. and Wynn S. 1998. *Complementary and Alternative Veterinary Medicine*. St. Louis, MO: Mosby.

Tindle H.A., et al. 2005. Trends in use of complementary and alternative medicine by US adults: 1997–2002. *Altern Ther Health Med* (1):42–49.

Working Party of the Royal College of Physicians. 2005. Doctors in society. Medical professionalism in a changing world. *Clin Med* 5(6 Suppl 1):S5–S40.

Wynn S.G. and Wolpe P.R. 2005. The majority view of ethics and professionalism in alternative medicine. *J Am Vet Med Assoc* 226(4):516–520.

Appendix 9

Special Diets for Disease Problems

Recovery From Disease Causing Weight Loss

(High-protein, high-fat diet, sometimes increased vitamin levels, especially B vitamins)

Hills A/D
Purina Critical Care and Critical Nutrition CN
Royal Canin Recovery

Allergic Conditions that Cause Itchy Skin

There are two approaches to diets for food allergies:

Novel proteins (such as kangaroo or rabbit or other proteins they have not been exposed to before)
Hydrolyzed proteins, where the proteins are partially digested down to short pieces or amino acids

There are four problems with novel protein diets:

1) It is increasingly hard to find a novel protein that a pet never has been exposed to because regular dog foods have included more and more of what used to be exotic unusual proteins
2) If they are a dry diet, the "digest" that is sprayed on the surface of kibble might have a different protein in it, since a company does not have to declare what is in the spray.
3) A food that sounds like it has one single novel protein might have a second one hidden way down in the ingredient list.
4) Grain-free food made with pulses (usually peas) has been associated with Dilated Cardiomyopathy, including in breeds that do not normally have this problem.

Novel Protein Foods

Hills Prescription D/D diets—there are lots of combinations (note that their Derm Complete has one whole protein AND a different hydrolyzed protein, so I am not putting it in this list)
Natural Balance Limited Ingredients formulas
Purina DRM (trout-based)
Royal Canin Selected Protein—a lot of flavors

Hydrolyzed Diets

Hills Z/D
Purina HA (hydrolyzed proteins) and EL (amino acids)
Royal Canin HP and Ultamino

ARTHRITIS

(Usually based on increased glycosaminoglycans and/or increased omega-3 fatty acids. May have antioxidants also.)

Hills J/D
Purina JM, OM Plus Joint Mobility
Royal Canin Advanced Mobility Support

Cognitive Dysfunction

(High antioxidants)

Hills B/D
Purina NC neurocare

Diabetes

(High-fiber or low carbohydrates)

Hills W/D or M/D
Purina DM (for cats)
Royal Canin Glycobalance cat food

Heart Disease

(Low protein, low salt)

Hills H/D, G/D (heart plus kidney)
Purina CC
Royal Canin Early Cardiac

Irritable or Inflammatory Bowel Disease

(Low fiber or high fiber or novel proteins)

Hills I/D (low fiber) or W/D (high fiber) or Z/D (modified protein) or GI Biome
Purina EN (balanced soluble and insoluble fiber), and HA (modified protein)
Royal Canin HP and Ultamino (modified protein); Selected protein PR; Gastrointestinal High
  Fiber, Gastrointestinal Low Fat

Kidney Disease

(Low protein)

Hills K/D, G/D (heart plus kidney)
Purina NF
Royal Canin Renal Support

Kidney and Bladder Stones and Urinary Crystals

(For dogs, may have increased salt, but not for cats because they do not have a good thirst mechanism. Should contain nutrients to acidify the urine or turn it more neutral, depending on the type of stone.)

Hills S/O (struvite) and U/D (non-struvite)
Purina NF (for dogs with oxalate stones)
Purina UR St/Ox(for cats with struvite stones), UR Ox/St (for dogs with struvites)—both also help
  prevent calcium oxalate formation
Royal Canin Urinary SO 14 (for oxalates), Control (for struvites), Urinary UC 18 (for cystine and
  urate stones), and Vegetarian (for urate stones)

Liver Disease

(Moderate levels of easily digested proteins)

Hills L/D (dogs), A/D (cats)
Royal Canin Hepatic and Recovery

Obesity

(Low-calorie, high-fiber, both soluble and insoluble)

Hills R/D and W/D
Purina OM
Royal Canin Satiety Support for weight loss for obesity, and slightly lower calorie Calorie Control
  to maintain a lower weight

Tartar

(Harder kibble, which may be modified so it does not shatter as easily)

Hills T/D
Royal Canin Canine Dental

Appendix 10

Analysis of Some Homemade Diets

You may see diets similar to those below recommended as ideal for feeding your pet. They are based upon people's concept of wild diets but do not include some items of true wild diets. (See Chapter 8, Holistic Diet and Nutrition.) In addition, they ignore the fact that dogs have been domesticated for thousands of years and may actually have evolved to use diets with more carbohydrates and less meat (since meat has been much more important to people and was less likely to have been given to dogs in primitive societies).

Diets 2 and 3 do contain carbohydrates, but they have other problems. Diet 3 is closer to a balanced diet, but it is deficient in some minerals. (It is also low in calories, but this can be remedied by feeding a little more.) Diet 4 shows a problem with diets that try to address specific disease problems without a thorough analysis of whether they actually do so. Low-protein diets have been shown to prolong survival time for patients with kidney disease. However, they do not prevent the onset of kidney disease and do not prolong the life span of elderly animals without major disease problems. In addition, although egg whites are considered the ideal protein (with an ideal balance of amino acids), you still need about the same amount of egg whites as you do meat protein.

These diets were analyzed by Sally C. Perea, DVM, MS, DACVN, a member of Davis Veterinary Medical Consulting, Inc., 606 Pena Dr., Suite 700, Davis, CA 95618. This is the company that owns Balance IT, an online service that will formulate a balanced diet for you, including substitutions you can make for various items (to vary the diet). Their formulations include the addition of their supplements, available as powders to be added to the diets. (Without the powders, the diets are not balanced.)

Dr. Perea warns that her analysis is based on USDA tables with some additional recommendations. The USDA tables do not commonly include choline, chlorine, vitamin D, or iodine for many foods, so the estimations for these nutrients may be a little low. (The comments on these diets ignore these items if they are too low.) USDA tables usually consider chopped vegetables, not ground, and do not include bone in their ground meat. Dr. Perea use BARF World's estimates of mineral content for chicken necks in her analysis of recipes that include chicken bones, but she admits this might not be exactly the same as the mineral contents of other parts of the chicken (when feeding a whole chicken, for example, or chicken backs as a calcium source). This makes obvious some of the problems involved in trying to analyze a new dog food, which is why actual feeding trials tell us the most about a food.

Analysis was based upon USDA recommendations for adult animals and was done on both a dry matter basis and per 1000 megacalories (Mcal) of energy.

The Association of American Feed Control Officials (AAFCO) recommendations for percentages of nutrients are reported on nutrients per megacalories. A high-fat diet has many more calories per mouthful than a low-fat diet. If the diet is analyzed as nutrients per quantity (such as a teaspoonful), then a nutrient (such as vitamin E) may very well measure as normal in each teaspoon. But if the diet is analyzed as nutrients per calorie and one compares the two diets, then the actual quantity of food measured will be less if it is high fat. If the high-fat diet has four times as many calories as a low-fat diet, then when the nutrients per calorie are measured, the comparison will be the nutrients in 1/4 teaspoon of a high-fat diet to nutrients in 1 teaspoon of a low-fat diet. Vitamin E content, when measured this way, will also be reported as 1/4 as much, rather than as the same per teaspoonful. One of the diets below is so high in fat that it looks like it has a lot of deficiencies (especially when analyzed in terms of nutrients per megacalories), but in part that is just because it is such a high-fat diet. When there were deficiencies, Dr. Perea included a breakdown of the contribution of each item for that nutrient and indicated where she had no information, allowing the author to judge whether the analysis may have been too low. (A laboratory analysis of a food made from the complete recipe costs about $3000 per analysis; thus, it is outside the resources for this book. Dr. Perea went to great lengths to make her analysis as accurate as possible.)

Diet 1 (Both Cats and Dogs)

1 cup ground vegetables (1/10 cup of each of the following: broccoli, squash, romaine lettuce, cauliflower, cabbage, celery, kale, chard, parsley, and pumpkin)

4/5 cup ground organ meats (equal parts of beef heart, liver, kidney)
4/5 cup ground fat
2/5 cup ground lean beef
(all of the above are raw)
1 1/2 tsp cod liver oil
Calcium/magnesium supplement (3 : 1 Ca/Mg) containing 1000 milligram calcium

Analysis for Cats

This diet has eight times the recommended amount of fat for cats. When analyzed on a dry matter basis, there is only 64% of the recommended amount of calcium (and half that when analyzed per megacalorie). Because of the high-fat content, the analysis for this diet is somewhat misleading, so results have been recalculated by omitting enough fat to correct the calcium supplied to 100% of the recommended amount. This would revise the amount for other trace minerals upward by about 30% of their calculated value. Even so, there is not enough taurine in this diet, and only 90% of required methionine. Other amino acids are present in more than sufficient quantities. The diet is also lacking in thiamin and vitamin E, but it has 10 times the recommended amount of vitamin A and 6 times recommended amounts of vitamin D. In addition, 4 times the recommended amount of copper is present.

Fish oils greatly increase the need for vitamin E. Until about 1970, one could see vitamin E deficiency in cats fed diets consisting of pure tuna, especially red meat tuna (available as cat food with vitamins and minerals added). Because of this, AAFCO increased the recommended amount of vitamin E in cat foods and we no longer see this problem with commercial diets. Liver and cod liver oil are also especially high in vitamins A and D, and cats on pure liver diets develop vitamin A toxicity. Cat diets do need a source of eicosatetraenoic acid (EPA) and docosahexaenoic acid (DHA), but it is safe to provide this with fish body oil (such as salmon oil) rather than fish liver oil.

Analysis for Dogs

For dogs, the amino acids are all available in sufficient quantities. However, this diet has 20 times the recommended amount of fat. There is only 10% of the recommended amount of vitamin E for dogs. Just as for cats, this diet is too high in vitamin A, 13 times: vitamin D, 8 times; and copper, 3 times the recommended amount.

Diet 2 (Dogs)

71% ground whole chicken, including bones and giblets
29% ground vegetables/fruit (mix of equal parts of: celery, parsley, zucchini, yellow squash, carrots, sweet potato, bell pepper, cabbage, broccoli, mango, apples)

This diet contains 6 times the fat and 2.5 times the amount of protein recommended for dogs. However, the amount of energy per cupful is a little low (because of the vegetables), and thus an owner would want to feed a little more of this diet than if they were feeding canned food. The recommended amount of protein varies depending on which nation is doing the recommending, so for a young, healthy dog, this is probably not a problem.

The problem lies in the mineral and vitamin content. This diet is low in copper, iron, and manganese. (It is probably also low in iodine, but there is not enough information available to confirm this.) It is also low in vitamins D, E, and B_{12}. It also has 10 times the recommended amount of zinc. An increase in zinc leads to an increased requirement for copper, so it increases the imbalance.

A good diet recommendation usually includes some type of concentrated source of vitamins and minerals in a form that allows the calculation of exact amounts more precisely.

Diet 3 (Dogs)

Amount recommended: 2 cups daily for a 30-pound 2-year-old cocker spaniel

2 C millet
6 C water
Cook 30 minutes
Remove from heat, add:
1 pound raw ground turkey
1 C finely minced combination of: zucchini, sprouts, carrots
1.4 heaping tablespoonfuls nutritional yeast
0.75 tablespoonful lecithin
0.5 rounded teaspoonful bone meal powder
0.12 tablespoonful kelp
2 tablespoonful flax seed oil
200 IU vitamin E
10,000 IU vitamin A

This diet contains a good source of carbohydrates and a number of concentrated sources of vitamins and minerals. The energy content is good. This diet contains adequate iodine.

However, the calcium is low: only 22% of the recommended amount, and the calcium/phosphorus ratio is low (0.28). This is similar to the zinc/copper ratio problem because high phosphorus will increase the bad effects of low calcium. The iron, potassium, and zinc levels are also low, as are vitamins A and D.

Diet 4 (Senior Cats)

Recommended amount: 3/4 cup daily for 16-year-old 9-pounds cat

1 C millet
3 C water
Cook 30 minutes
Remove from heat and add:
1 egg
1 tablespoon butter
1.1 heaping tablespoonfuls nutritional yeast
.6 tablespoonful lecithin
.4 rounded teaspoonful bone meal powder
.09 tablespoonful kelp
1 teaspoon flax seed oil
200 IU vitamin E
10,000 IU vitamin A

There are two main problems with this diet. First, the diet has only 13% protein on a dry matter basis. The recommended protein level for cats with kidney failure is about 26% on a dry matter basis. (For dogs, it is about 13%.) Cats need a much higher protein level than dogs, even if they have kidney problems. Most of the amino acids are far too low for a cat on this diet, fed at the recommended level. Most sources now recommend additional taurine for all cat diets, even if the protein level is sufficient.

The second problem for cats is that they need an animal source of omega-3 fatty acids; flax oil is a plant source. Cats can't convert this into the final EPA and DHA form, so they would suffer from a deficiency.

The diet is low in vitamins A, D, and K. It also needs more calcium, zinc, potassium, selenium, and iron. Even though some supplements were added, cats need more.

Appendix 11

Doses for Herbs

There are many different, often conflicting, herbal doses for animals published in books, magazines, and on the Internet. The problem with recommending doses is that herbs come in powders, tinctures, fluid extracts (infusions and decoctions), capsules, and tablets of varying strengths and sizes. Extracts are made using different proportions of herbs to water or alcohol. Doses of "one drop" differ depending on the size of the dropper and the viscosity of the substance. Some herbs work best dried, some fresh, some as a type of extract, and so on. The methods and their pros and cons are well summarized in Wynn and Fougere's *Veterinary Herbal Medicine*, on pages 232–236 (Tables A11.1 to A11.3), but a more thorough discussion is beyond the scope of this book.

Another complicating factor is that although many herbs are best dosed three to four times a day, owners may only be able or willing to administer doses once or twice a day. Sometimes the daily dose recommended has the additional instruction "in divided doses." This means if giving the herb twice a day, divide the initial dose by two to determine each dose. If giving three times a day, divide by three for each dose, and so on.

Some animals are sensitive to herbs. Most often, this is seen as diarrhea, or sometimes inappetence or vomiting. Often herbs will still work at lower doses, but it will take longer for results. With the permission of your veterinarian, explain this to the owner, recommend they stop the herb until the problem has stopped, and then start with a decreased dose and try again. Occasionally, you will see hives or other signs of allergies. In this case, it is best to stop giving the herbs.

This book will ignore the question of which is the best form of herb. It assumes that the prescriber or the manufacturer has enough knowledge that the correct form and strength are already present in whatever the practice uses. Instead, recommendations are based primarily on a proportional method, and liquids are recommended in terms of cubic centimeters (cc). (Doses for dogs and cats are in proportion to doses recommended for humans.) Cats and small dogs may need proportionally a little more, and very large breeds may need proportionally a little less. One must be very careful in cats with herbs processed through the liver because feline livers are deficient in some detoxifying enzymes, and they process these items more slowly than dogs or humans do. (This is why one tablet of acetaminophen can easily kill a 5-kilogram [11-pounds] cat, whereas a 5-kilogram dog may be very sick but much less likely to die from the same dose.) Consult a good text on veterinary herbalism to see which herbs these might be.

Complementary Medicine for Veterinary Technicians and Nurses, Second Edition. Nancy Scanlan.
© 2024 John Wiley & Sons, Inc. Published 2024 by John Wiley & Sons, Inc.

Table A11.1   Liquid herb doses.

Human dose	Dose in Milligrams (mL) Per Day for Dogs or Cats, Per Kilogram (kg) of Bodyweight					
	5 kg	10 kg	15 kg	20 kg	30 kg	40 kg
1	0.05	0.15	0.2	0.3	0.45	0.6
2	0.2	0.25	0.45	0.5	0.9	1.0
3	0.25	0.3	0.5	0.6	0.9	1.2
4	0.3	0.55	0.85	1.1	1.7	2.2
5	0.35	0.7	1.05	1.4	2.1	2.8
6	0.4	0.8	1.2	1.6	2.4	3.2
7	0.5	1.0	1.5	2.0	3.0	4.0

Source: Adapted from the proportionate dose table from Wynn, S. and Fougere, B., 2007. *Veterinary Herbal Medicine.* Mosby, St. Louis, MO.

Table A11.2   Herb doses for tablets and capsules.

Human dose	Tablet Amounts for Small Animals Per kg Bodyweight					
	5 kg	10 kg	15 kg	30 kg	40 kg	50 kg
2 Tablets	1/4–1/2	1	1.5	2	2.5	2.5–3

Table A11.3   Herb doses for Chinese tea pills.*

Weight of pet	Tablet Amounts for Small Animals Per kg Bodyweight					
	5 kg	10 kg	15 kg	30 kg	40 kg	50 kg
No. of tea pills given twice a day	1–2	2	3–4	4	5	6

* Small pills that look like black BBs.

Bibliography

Wynn, S.G. and Fougere, B.J. 2007. *Veterinary Herbal Medicine.* St. Louis, MO: Mosby.

Appendix 12

Dosing Schedule for Homotoxicology Formulas

Species and Dose	Tablets	Tinctures	Ampoules 5 mL	Oral Vials/ Ampoules	Ear Drops	Ointment/Gel
Horse/cow	4–5 tabs 2–3×	10–20 drops 2–3×	1 vial 2–3×	1–3 vials 2–3×	1 vial 2–3×	Apply topically
Large dogs	1–2 tabs 2–3×	10–15 drops 2–3×	1/4–1/2 vial 2×	1/2–1 vial 2–3×	1 vial 2–3×	Liberally, as needed
Medium dogs	1 tab 2–3×	8–10 drops 2–3×	1/4 vial 2–3×	1/2–1 vial 2–3×	1/2–1 vial 2–3×	
Small dogs/ cats	1/2–1 tab 2–3×	5–8 drops 2–3×		1/4–1/2 vial 2–3×	1/2 vial 2–3×	
Puppies/ kittens	1/2–1 tab 2–3×	5 drops 2–3×		1/4–1/2 vial 2–3×	1/2 vial 2–3×	
Pocket pets	1/2 tab 2–3×	2–5 drops 2–3×		1/4 vial 2–3×	1/4 vial 2–3×	

Source: From Goldstein R., ed. 2008. *Integrating Complementary Medicine into Veterinary Practice.* Wiley-Blackwell, Ames, IA.

Complementary Medicine for Veterinary Technicians and Nurses, Second Edition. Nancy Scanlan.
© 2024 John Wiley & Sons, Inc. Published 2024 by John Wiley & Sons, Inc.

Appendix 13

Alphabetical List of Bach Flower Remedies

Agrimony (*Agrimonia eupatoria*)—oversensitive, act jolly, and hide their feelings

Aspen (*Populus tremula*)—vague fear that something is going to happen

Beech (*Fagus sylvatica*)—see beauty in all things

Centaury (*Erythraea centaurium*)—want to serve others so much they neglect themselves

Cerato (*Ceratostigma willmottianum*)—no confidence in themselves to make the right decision

Cherry plum (*Prunus cerasifera*)—fear of being too stressed

Chestnut bud (*Aesculus hippocastanum*)—keep repeating past mistakes

Chicory (*Cichorium intybus*)—over-care for the welfare of others

Clematis (*Clematis vitalba*)—no great interest in life

Crab apple (*Pyrus malus*)—feels like something is dirty in their body that they have to get rid of

Elm (*Umus campestris*)—think whatever they are trying is too hard to achieve

Gentian (*Gentiana amarelle*)—easily discouraged

Gorse (*Ulex europaeus*)—unable to believe that anything can be done

Heather (*Calluna vulgaris*)—always need to be with others

Holly (*Ilex aquifolium*)—jealousy and suspicion when there is no need for it

Honeysuckle (*Lonicera caprifolium*)—living in the past

Hornbeam (*Carpinus betulus*)—fear they are not strong enough to go on

Impatiens (*Impatiens roylei*)—want everything done faster; excruciating pain

Larch (*Larix europaea*)—think they are never as good as others

Mimulus (*Mimulus luteus*)—ordinary everyday fears

Mustard (*Sinapis arvensis*)—clinical depression

Oak (*Quercus pedunculata*)—fight strongly to get well, even though their case is hopeless

Olive (*Olea europaea*)—have given up on life

Pine (*Pinus sylvestris*)—always blaming themselves

Red chestnut (*Aesculus carnea*)—fear for others

Rescue Remedy contains: Impatiens, star of Bethlehem, cherry plum, rock rose, clematis

Rock rose (*Helianthemum vulgare*)—terror and the feeling there is no hope

Rock water (*Aqua petra*)—carry self-denial to an extreme

Scleranthus (*Scleranthus annuus*)—inability to decide between two things

Star of Bethlehem (*Ornitholagum umbellatum*)—sudden misfortune brings great unhappiness

Sweet chestnut (*Castanea vulgaris*)—life is unbearable, can't endure anymore

Vervain (*Verbena officinalis*)—fixed ideals that they think others should share

Vine (*Vitis vinifera*)—very self-confident, think others would do well to adopt their way of doing things

Complementary Medicine for Veterinary Technicians and Nurses, Second Edition. Nancy Scanlan.
© 2024 John Wiley & Sons, Inc. Published 2024 by John Wiley & Sons, Inc.

Walnut (*Juglans regia*)—too easily influenced by others

Water violet (*Hottonia palustris*)—aloof and independent

White chestnut (*Aesculus hippocastanum*)—obsessed with unpleasant thoughts

Wild oat (*Bromus asper*)—want to do something great, but no great calling toward anything

Wild rose (*Rosa canina*)—gliding through life

Willow (*Salix vitellina*)—can't accept misfortune without resentment

Appendix 14

How to Find a Holistic Veterinarian

Pet owners may be confused when trying to find a practitioner of complementary veterinary medicine who matches their concept of what a holistic veterinarian is. The points below can be adapted to create a handout for clients, for prospective clients, or for a lecture you might give on the subject.

You can't find a holistic veterinarian until you know what you are really looking for. Some people think of this as "either/or"—the veterinarian in question is either holistic or not. However, to be a good holistic veterinarian you also have to be a good veterinarian. For this reason, you will also see the terms *complementary* or *integrative* used in the same way as *holistic*.

Holistic medicine encompasses a wide variety of subjects. Just as in regular medicine, no holistic veterinarian is expert in all of them. Some are general practitioners, using many modalities, and some are expert in one single area. This means that their general outlook about subjects such as vaccination and diet may be very conventional, or it may encompass a totally different way of looking at things.

You can't practice good holistic medicine without some kind of training. There is no single course on holistic medicine that is taught in veterinary schools. Many schools offer elective courses, but students are not required to take them. However, for graduate veterinarians, there are several options. There are a number of useful, in-depth texts with extensive references written by veterinarians for veterinarians.

For other subjects, there are specific courses that have been created by experts in the field. To gain a certificate from these courses, a veterinarian must spend many hours in classes, pass a written exam and often an oral or practical exam, spend time as an intern with another veterinarian who is certified in that subject, and submit case reports using the modality being studied. Often, the courses have been recognized by the Registry of Approved Continuing Education (a committee of the American Association of State Veterinary Boards). In addition, some have state accreditation by the appropriate board of education, or they may be recognized by the state veterinary board.

After receiving their initial training, veterinarians are expected to continue their education not only by attending sessions held by the certifying institutions but also by being present at meetings that are organized by state and national veterinary associations. Most have agendas limited to one specific modality, but the annual meeting of the AHVMA tries to cover all the main types of holistic medicine, as well as at least one that is less well-known.

How do you decide what you want for your dog? Read about the different types of treatments available, see what you are comfortable with, and then find a holistic veterinarian who will help you explore it further. After all, if you faint at the thought of needles in your pet, no matter how tiny they are, it does not make a lot of sense to start with acupuncture.

Complementary Medicine for Veterinary Technicians and Nurses, Second Edition. Nancy Scanlan.
© 2024 John Wiley & Sons, Inc. Published 2024 by John Wiley & Sons, Inc.

The following are some of the more common holistic treatments used by veterinarians.

Acupuncture—insertion of *very* thin needles into specific spots to help pain and other problems.

Chinese medicine—encompasses both acupuncture and Chinese herbal medicine. Also known as TCM or TCVM. Adds Chinese methods of diagnosis to conventional medicine, which can sound strange if you are not used to concepts such as yin and yang.

Chiropractic—manipulation of joints to help with pain (and behavior associated with pain).

Herbal medicine—uses herbs in a way similar to drugs. A good herbalist knows about drug interactions and toxicity as well as the proper use of herbs and is aware of species differences, such as the high sensitivity of certain breeds to some herbs. There are a number of types, such as Ayurvedic, American Indian, Chinese, Western (which includes a number of European as well as American herbs), and South American. A good herbalist will be acquainted with the theory behind the herbal system, rather than just use them like drugs.

Homeopathy—The use of dilute amounts of substances that in larger amounts cause the signs you are trying to treat. For example, arsenic in large amounts can cause diarrhea, but in minute amounts can help it. In Western medicine, digitalis is similar: an overdose causes heart problems, but dilute amounts can help. A good homeopath will take a *very* complete history of your animal's problems and base treatment on that. Classical homeopaths often dispense just one remedy at a time.

Homotoxicology—Emphasizes detoxification as well as treatment of disease. Multiple homeopathic remedies are used.

Nutraceuticals—Nutritional supplements used to help various problems.

Rehabilitation therapy—In the holistic spirit, it incorporates a number of different modalities, and a therapy team to help rehabilitate injured animals and those who have had surgery. Uses treatments such as acupuncture, massage therapy, swim therapy, underwater treadmill, stretching, etc., to achieve these goals.

Appendix 15

Inventory Management

Proper management of inventory can make the difference between holistic products acting as black holes that absorb money and a major part of productive income for the practice. The properly trained registered veterinary technician (RVT) or veterinary nurse is ideally suited for this role in a number of ways. You are less easily swayed by the claims of the newest and best supplement for diseases that are difficult to treat.

As the person filling prescriptions, you can see what is really being used and what is just sitting there. As the person responsible for keeping the veterinary pharmacy organized, you can literally see what is gathering dust and what is active. In addition, you can save your employer money by carefully examining "bargain" sales that require buying more than is really needed. And finally, you are indispensable in helping explain the proper storage and use of holistic herbs and supplements as well as what each actually does. This frees up your employer's time to do more of the things he or she has been trained to do: diagnose, prescribe, and perform specific treatments that require veterinary training.

Ordering

Some veterinarians prefer to order items themselves, whereas others are happy to leave this chore to the RVT or veterinary nurse. Even if you do not order items, you can help your employer be aware of items that are needed, excess inventory, and items on sale.

Some products are ordered through veterinary distributors, whereas others must be ordered from the company themselves. Distributors and large companies usually have salespeople who will visit the practice with information on the latest new items and any items that are on sale. You may have to order from other companies by telephone or on the Internet. You should have a file of all companies, distributors, and salespeople that you deal with, including name, address, telephone number, and website (if appropriate). Keep this file in the area of the dispensing pharmacy.

Items that need to be ordered should be placed on a "want" list that should also be kept in the area of the dispensing pharmacy. There should be lists corresponding to major distributors or large companies and one or two smaller lists corresponding to items ordered less often from small companies. The smaller lists may contain items that are from several separate companies.

There must be some way to note items that need to be ordered, items that have been ordered but not received, and items that have been received. One way to do this is to write down items that need to be ordered, check them off when ordered, then cross them out when they have been received. Another way is to use sticky notes on an appropriate surface such as a nonstick marker board. Items to be ordered are placed on the left. Once ordered, the note is moved to the right. When received, the note is removed.

When a box is received, items in the box should be checked against the packing list that comes with the box. If the wrong item has been sent, if an item or its packaging is damaged, or if the number received does not match the number on the packing list, the company should be notified immediately. If you do so, they will be happy to rectify the situation, replacing wrong orders or sending additional bottles as needed. If you wait for weeks, they will be justifiably suspicious of your request. An item that should have been cold but is hot when it is received may no longer be active. Consult your employer to see whether the company should be contacted and the item returned.

An item may be placed on back order, which means that it is not in stock at the moment but will be shipped as soon as possible. Most companies will give you a time when the shipment is expected. Some may not ship after an item has been on back order for a certain amount of time. Make a note of back-ordered items, incorrect orders, when you called the company, and when the items are expected, and post it in the area where your ordered items are posted. All packing slips should be saved to check against invoices. When an invoice is received, it should be checked against the corresponding packing slip. If it is correct, the packing slips can be discarded. Invoices should never be discarded.

Any box that has warnings about requirements for refrigeration should be opened first, and items should be immediately placed in the refrigerator. Boxes with herbal items should be opened next. Although they can be stored at room temperature, they are especially vulnerable to excessive heat. During hot summer months, if overheated, they may need to be placed in the refrigerator for a time to cool down quickly. Otherwise, volatile elements can evaporate, some herbal tablets can become sticky, colors (which usually are from phytoactive chemicals in the herbs) can fade. This makes these supplements less active and effective. If this becomes a problem, be sure you are ordering at a time of the week when products will be received in the shortest time possible. You may also need to request that an ice pack be included in the shipment (or an extra pack, if they are already doing this).

Inventory Arrangement

There are a number of ways to arrange a veterinary pharmacy. Obviously, some items must be refrigerated, while other items can stay on a shelf. Some items are for use only in the veterinary hospital and others are primarily to be dispensed. Some items require mixing at the time they are dispensed, some must be poured out or counted, and some can be sold intact in the bottle in which they came. The arrangement should match the way your employer practices and the way that is easiest for dispensing and ordering. These two requirements are not always compatible, and compromise may be needed.

The following is a system that has worked well for, and can be adapted to most practices. No matter what item you stock, everything should be arranged so that items with the closest expiration date are be placed in front of items with a date that is farther away. Check dates of everything that comes in. Sometimes, especially if you have taken advantage of a special offer for short-dated items, the expiration for incoming items is sooner than the expiration of items you already have. Check the dates of items on the shelf. If an item has expired, it should no longer be used. For some things, this can be highly critical. If you are still using herbs that are outdated and notice that the colors or smells have faded, then the active principles are fading also, and the herbs will not work as well, if at all. The same can be said for pharmaceutical items.

Pharmaceutical items and nutraceutical or herbal items that have become mainstream (such as glucosamine products, Denamarin, lysine, etc.) are kept together, usually in alphabetical order. They can be ordered from a few distributors of veterinary products and so are easiest to use and order when kept together. Tablets and capsules are kept alphabetically in one area, ointments and creams for ears and skin are kept alphabetically in another, and drops and ointments for eyes are kept in a third area.

Chinese herbs should have a separate area. These are often subdivided by the company they come from (because they are usually ordered directly from the company) and are filed alphabetically in each section. Acupuncture needles, moxa, and small electroacupuncture and laser equipment may be kept in the same area, or the equipment may be housed elsewhere. Homeopathic items also have a separate area and may or may not be separated by company, depending on preference and ease of finding these items. Nutraceutical items may also be in a separate area if your employer uses a lot of them and may be separated by company if your employer uses many items from separate companies. Otherwise, they may be interspersed with pharmaceuticals or with herbs.

"Just-In-Time" Rotation

The just-in-time inventory rotation system, invented by Japanese automakers, can be used to a certain degree in a veterinary practice. To successfully employ it, you need to know how quickly you will receive items from a company or distributor and how many items you use in a week or a month. As less money is tied up in inventory, more money is available to spend on fixed expenses, equipment purchase and repair, building upkeep, and staff salaries and benefits. In addition, there will be more available to spend for new items and items available on sale. However, you must make sure you have enough critical items on hand at all times. Without the appropriate needles, animals can't be treated properly with acupuncture. If herbs are often unavailable, clients will go elsewhere or find them on the Internet. Just-in-time works best for items that are used the most. The "80–20" rule applies here: 80% of items dispensed will be from about 20% of the items in stock. As long as you primarily keep track of this 20%, you will do well with inventory control.

The idea of just-in-time inventory is to keep just enough stock on hand to fill all prescriptions and to order so that another bottle will arrive just as you are using the last bottle of an item. To do this properly, you must have an idea of how fast items are used up. If you have just begun to work for a holistic veterinarian, you may know which common drugs work this way, but you may not know which holistic items may have a fast turnover. There are four things that determine turnover: what conditions are most commonly treated by your employer, what items are most commonly recommended to treat them, which companies supply these items, and how often the clients buy these items on their own.

Check with the veterinarian to see what is treated the most and dispensed the most frequently. You can confirm this with invoices. When you are first deciding what to order this way, keep track of individual items with the date ordered and the number ordered. You should be able to determine an average amount to order by using 6 months of invoices.

Talking to Salespeople

Just because something is for sale doesn't mean it is a bargain. If you have to buy 12 to get a discount, and you only use 12 in 1 year, this is not a bargain. If you use 12 in 1 month, it can pay to buy more than one dozen.

When you are working with individual small companies, if you are ordering large amounts of their products each month, try to negotiate a larger discount. Companies give a bigger discount to distributors than to individual practitioners. If the practice you work for uses large quantities of a company's products, they may be willing to give you a distributor's price. Usually, they require that you buy a minimum amount each month and then will give an additional discount. It is *not* worth ordering more than you need just to get the discount.

Salespeople can alert you to upcoming sales, so you can hold off on a big order until a sale is in effect. They can also let you know about new products and give you information for your veterinarian. Many will give you a free sample for your employer to try. Never use one without your employer's permission and input about safety and efficacy.

Prices and Markup

Veterinarians use items that really work. If they don't work well, we will not use them. Veterinarians judge what works by published research, case studies, and by attending lectures and conferences that are given by experts in the field, as well as by how these items perform for them. Companies that want to sell to veterinarians must have products with the correct amount and form of ingredients, without contamination. In the United States, companies that are especially concerned with product safety and efficacy are members of NASC (National Animal Supplement Council). Because of the quality and care taken in the manufacturing process, these items are often more expensive than many items available over the counter. When a client buys from your hospital, they are buying quality.

In addition, veterinarians want items that are not readily available to the general public. Big box stores such as Walmart and Petco have much greater buying power than a veterinarian and can buy items for lower prices than the veterinarian can negotiate. It does not make sense to do all the work of diagnosis, educating a client in a product's use, and then recommending a specific product that the client will go buy at the nearest discount store. This is another reason why veterinarians are particular about which brands they recommend.

Everything that is used or sold in a veterinary hospital must contribute to the cost of running the hospital. A veterinary hospital has a higher overhead than a herb store, so the prices charged for herbs and supplements may be higher than prices charged in the herb store or on the Internet. In addition, the items that are used by a holistic veterinarian contain the proper type and amount of herbs, and this is not necessarily true for the cheaper herbs and nutraceuticals found on the Internet. Whenever an item is dispensed, the price should cover the cost of the label, the container, part of the cost of computer, software, and label printer involved, and the salary of the person during the time it takes to fill the prescription. All of this contributes to the quality of holistic medicine that the patients receive.

For these reasons, prices charged may be higher than those seen in shops because there is a built-in "packaging fee" (although this is not noted on a client's receipt). In addition, for small dogs and cats, because only part of a bottle may be dispensed, the price per pill is higher than if you just sell the bottle. This price includes all the items mentioned above, So the price of 1 pill may be the same as the price of 5 or 10 because most of the cost of dispensing this amount is related to your activities instead of the activity of a cashier in a shop.

When clients complain about prices, they are not interested in these reasons. However, they are more willing to spend money if they believe they are paying for quality. Quality service includes taking a little extra time to explain how to use an item and making sure they understand the proper time and way to give them and how to store them. (See the appropriate chapters for each item.) Do this, and you will not have to defend your hospital—clients will be praising it instead!

Client Education

If the people who visit your veterinary hospital come to your employer for advice but believe that all vitamins, treats, diets, and supplements are equal, then someone is not doing a good job of education, and clients will use cost as their guide when shopping. We know that some companies are more ethical than others. With both melamine and *Salmonella* found as contaminants in pet food and pet treats (Burns, 2007; Dobson et al., 2008; Osborne et al., 2009) and FDA concerns about contaminants found in some Chinese herbal formulas, pet owners have become aware that source of origin can be important. In addition, many supplements on the market have a large number of ingredients that sound good for a disease condition, but often only one to three of them are present in amounts large enough to help the problem.

If a client has stopped buying herbs or nutraceuticals from your veterinary hospital, ask why. If they have found the same item (same brand, same company) for sale cheaper elsewhere, there is no good answer. If this happens to a great extent with a single item, you may want to consider not stocking it anymore or decreasing the markup (with your employer's permission).

On the other hand, if your client has bought something that they consider to be the same thing, ask them to bring in the bottle or jar. Compare it to the product that you stock. The actual ingredients or amounts may be different, or they may have to take more tablets (in one "serving size") to get the same amount. In that case, point this out and let them know that your employer has found that the product that your hospital dispenses is one that she has found to be superior. If the amounts of the ingredients in their bottle are much lower than yours, point this out also. A client brought me a glucosamine product, which cost 25% less than the one we sold. It recommended 1 tablet per 50 pounds of body weight. There was only 250 milligram of glucosamine per tablet, whereas ours had 500 milligram. I showed her the difference, and we figured it would actually cost 50% *more* to use her product instead of ours. If you are good at math, you can show clients the actual figures. If you are not so good, you can still point out the difference in quantity. This again shows your establishment to be one of high quality.

References

Burns, K. 2007 Researchers examine contaminants in food, deaths of pets. *J Am Vet Med Assoc* 231(11):1636–1638.

Dobson, R.L., et al. 2008. Identification and characterization of toxicity of contaminants in pet food leading to an outbreak of renal toxicity in cats and dogs. *Toxicol Sci* 106(1):251–262.

Osborne, C.A., et al. 2009. Melamine and cyanuric acid-induced crystalluria, uroliths, and nephrotoxicity in dogs and cats. *Vet Clin North Am Small Anim Pract* 39(1):1–14.

Appendix 16

Medicating and Grooming

One thing a veterinary technician can do to help out clients is show them how to give medication to their pets. Dogs are easier than cats, but many dogs figure out that pills may be hidden in treats and eat the treat while spitting out the pill. Cats are infamous for their methods of refusing medication, and owners may face serious damage when trying to pill a cat. Their ability to generate foam when they do not like the taste of something is alarming to owners who are unfamiliar with this reaction.

Pills can be hidden in something tasty if the animal loves food, if the pill is small enough, and if it doesn't taste too bad. Greenies Pill Pockets® are designed to do this, but they have an artificial preservative and some ingredients that are frowned upon by holistic nutritionists (such as corn syrup and wheat gluten). If an animal is an eager eater, pills can be hidden in pieces of nitrite-free hot dogs, cheese, or other special treats.

The best things overall to hide a pill in are tasty and sticky, so cream cheese, butter, and nut butters often work well. Nut butters are often not sticky enough, but if you use the natural type and let the oil separate out, the top of the solid layer is stickier and works better. Another thing you may want to try is feeding foods that let the pill slip down. Vanilla ice cream can work well: the coldness dulls the sense of taste, so they don't taste the medication as easily, and it melts as it goes down, helping the pill to slide down more easily.

When using this method, owners should always follow it with a pill-free treat. This ensures that the pill will reach the stomach and not be stuck in the esophagus. They may also want to "prime the pump" by starting with a pill-free treat, to start the flow of saliva (especially true for cats). The three treats should be given in rapid succession.

When the pet is wise to hidden pills, or does not eagerly accept treats, the only recourse is to push the pill down the throat. There is skill involved, but it can be taught. The method for dogs and cats is different, but both start with a pill that is coated with something slippery. The two best coatings are butter and vanilla ice cream. Oil can be used, but you can't apply a thick coat of it.

Dogs

To pill a dog, you must be able to open his mouth. For some dogs, this is easy, but others have jaws that they have learned to clench shut with the force of a steel trap. To easily open a dog's mouth, first locate the space behind the canine tooth (Figure A16.1).

Complementary Medicine for Veterinary Technicians and Nurses, Second Edition. Nancy Scanlan.
© 2024 John Wiley & Sons, Inc. Published 2024 by John Wiley & Sons, Inc.

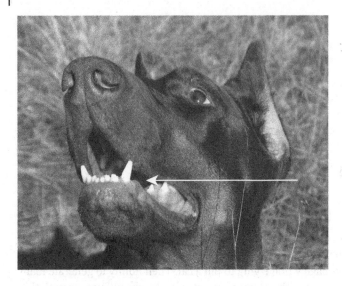

Figure A16.1 There is a space just behind the canine teeth where the teeth are small and farther apart.

Insert your thumb in this space and press on the roof of the dog's mouth. He will open his mouth. If he fights you and bites down, the space is large enough that you will get a slight pinch rather than a puncture wound, as long as he has a normal mouth where the canine teeth mesh together. In the case of an underbite (seen in dogs such as pugs and Pekingese), there may be no such space.

When the dog opens his mouth, quickly poke the coated pill down the middle of the mouth. At the end of the tongue, there is a slight hump. The pill must be pushed just past and over that hump to ensure that it will be swallowed. If it does not go that far, the dog may still be able to spit it out (although many dogs are so cooperative that they will swallow it anyway). When the dog swallows the treat, he will lick his nose. If you hold his mouth shut, tip his head up, and rub his throat, it may be harder for him to swallow. (Try swallowing when your face is pointed to the ceiling, and you will see what I mean.)

Follow this with a treat, poked down the same way. The treat should be soft, moist, and small. For example, you can use a piece of a dog vitamin coated with butter, or you can use a small piece of cheese. This gets the dog used to having something small and tasty poked down, and makes future pills easier to give. It also increases the flow of saliva, ensuring that the pill slides all the way down to the stomach.

If the owner has difficulty doing this, or if the dog is uncooperative, owners can practice with small pieces of canned food, cheese, or other treats that will slide down easily. Once the dog figures out that this is a new, strange way to get something tasty, he will be more cooperative. This is something you can have the owners do for new puppies as part of puppy training.

Cats

Cats must be handled differently, and the proper procedure requires a little more dexterity. They are more likely to bite and scratch when you try to open their mouth in the way you would for a dog. In addition, a pill is much more likely to stick in the esophagus of a cat than in the dog. For that reason, it is essential to lubricate the pill before giving it, preferably with a little butter. It is also helpful to give the cat a very small bit of something tasty, to make their saliva flow. Follow up with additional water to help the pill slide down all the way.

Figure A16.2 Grasp a cat's head just below the cheekbones.

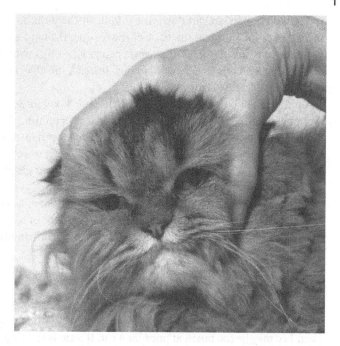

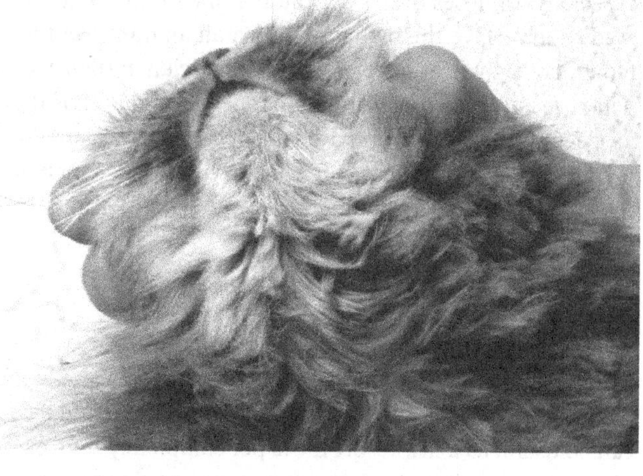

Figure A16.3 Tilt the head so the nose points toward the ceiling and the neck is straight.

Instead of trying to pry open a cat's mouth, grasp the head just below the cheekbones (Figure A16.2). Tilt the head so that the chin points toward the ceiling and the neck is stretched out (Figure A16.3).

Some cats just keep the neck and head in their normal positions and elevate their body. This does not work, and if owners say the cat's mouth does not open, this is probably why. If done properly, the lower jaw relaxes. With one finger, gently open the jaw, then push the lubricated pill straight down the middle of the tongue, over the hump at the back of the tongue. Release the head immediately—it is difficult for a cat to swallow when its head is stretched out. Then squirt in 0.5–1 cc of water with a syringe or eyedropper.

If you do not go straight down the middle of the mouth, you can get bitten. If you do not push the pill over the hump at the back of the tongue, the cat will push it right back out. The trick for pilling a cat is speed. Again, the owner can practice this with small amounts of tasty food. Unlike dogs, the cat will not look forward to this. Instead, the object of the lesson is to increase their cooperation and decrease struggling.

A pill gun can be used instead of your fingers. Look for one that will grasp a pill easily without dropping it and that is small enough to fit in a cat's mouth. To make a cat open its mouth, you still use the same strategy, but put the pill gun in the mouth instead of your fingers.

If a cat protests with claws, wrap the cat's body in a towel first. Place the cat on the towel, then bring the sides up over the cat's back to wrap it. (If you place the towel on top and wrap it under the cat, it is easier for them to escape.)

Another option is to put the cat in a restraint bag such as the Cat Sack™. Owners can buy this from large pet stores and via the Internet. The best type of bag will allow you to unzip various areas to be able to pull a single leg through. This is handy for trimming nails if a cat will not cooperate.

Liquid Medication

The biggest mistake that people make when giving liquid medication is to give too much, too fast. Even 1 cc may be too much at once for a cat. If a cat is fighting a typical dose of 1 cc at a time, have the owner try giving 0.5 cc, waiting for the cat to swallow, and then giving the second 0.5 cc.

There are two spots to place the medication: in the space between the cheek and the teeth and in the space behind the canines (see Figure A16.1). A syringe is easier to use than an eyedropper, especially for doses over 1 cc, and the practitioner may want to dispense a syringe along with the medication. Have the owner give a small amount, wait for swallowing, then give a little more. If too much is given at once, pets will often clench their teeth, set their tongue, and the medication will ooze out of their jaw and onto the owner's hand. If the amount of liquid is large (for example, an electrolyte solution) and does not need to be measured exactly, then a curved-tip syringe is often handier to use. The owner will need to snip 1/8–1/4 inch off the end with a pair of scissors because the hole at the end is too small to let much liquid through.

How to Force-Feed

There are several ways to force-feed dogs and cats: poking food down as if it were a pill, sticking it on the roof of the mouth, smearing it on the paws, and feeding with a syringe. The syringe method can be useful as a last resort if the pet completely refuses to eat. However, because of the amount that it must be diluted, much more must be fed to supply the proper amount of calories.

For dogs, you can roll their regular food into a meatball and poke it down as if it were a pill. Dogs will often take food this way with a minimum of fuss. If they fight you, use something that has a paste consistency, such as strained chicken baby food. Put some on your finger, insert your finger into the space behind the canine tooth, and stick it onto the roof of the mouth. They will usually swallow this. Keep in mind this is not a balanced food; thus, it is a temporary method.

Dogs are not as obsessed with cleanliness as cats are, so smearing a substance on their paws does not work nearly as well as for a cat. Feeding with a syringe (without a needle) can work, however. Dilute a pasty food with just enough broth to let it go easily through the end of a syringe. Insert the tip of the syringe into the space just behind the canine teeth and inject a *small* amount onto the

Table A16.1 Calories needed to maintain weight.

Body Weight (lb)	Kilocalories (Calories) Needed
11	400
22	700
44	1300
66	1500
88	2100
132	2900

Note: This is an average. More is needed with increased activity or for animals left in the cold. Less is needed for sedentary animals and older animals as well as breeds that gain weight easily.

Table A16.2 Calories in baby food.

Strained beef	16 calories per tablespoonful
Strained chicken	14 calories per tablespoonful
Strained lamb	15 calories per tablespoonful
Strained turkey	17 calories per tablespoonful

tongue. Owners often underfeed using this method. Instead of tracking the number of syringes fed, they should note the number of ounces or cans of food fed. To keep an animal's weight up, they must be fed the amount of calories needed for maintenance. (See Table A16.1.) To find out how much must be fed, divide the number of calories needed by the number of calories per can or jar. For example, if a 22-lb (10 kg) dog needs xxx calories, and the amount of calories in a jar of baby food is yyy, the formula is xxx/yyy or zzz cans. (See Table A16.2 for a list of calories in some baby foods and cat and dog foods.)

When cats are sick, they often stop eating, and if this goes on long enough, they may develop liver damage (hepatic lipidosis). Often, if they are not vomiting, you just need to "prime the pump" with a little food and they will start eating again.

Chicken hearts, whole or in pieces (depending on the size of the cat) slip down easily. Liver also is easily swallowed. You can give these the same way as you would give a pill. (See above.) Some cat foods can be formed into a ball and used in this way also. Anything that has the consistency of paste can be stuck onto the roof of the mouth in the same way as you would for a dog. They can also be fed with a syringe in the same way as for a dog.

Use of a Feeding Tube

Cats who have hepatic lipidosis can stop eating for as long as a month. It may take this long with force-feeding to heal their liver and bring back their appetite. If regular force-feeding is impossible, your veterinarian may place a stomach tube, either through the nose (nasogastric, or NG tube) or through the pharynx or esophagus. Cats tolerate the esophageal tube much better than the NG tube. In addition, the NG tube is smaller in diameter; thus, it is more difficult to push food through it.

To feed through a feeding tube, food must be liquid enough to easily inject. After the last syringe, some water should be syringed through it to rinse the tube and prevent clogging. The biggest mistake when using these tubes is to inject too fast and to inject too much. Both of these will result in vomiting. A cat's stomach holds only 20 cc per pound of bodyweight (45 cc per kg) at the most, and less if not allowed to expand slowly. An esophagus needs enough time to continue the whole swallowing reflex and push food down to the stomach. Multiple, small meals, given slowly, is the best way to go, and will prevent the vomiting problem.

Furminator

People sometimes believe that a heavy-coated animal should not be shaved. This can result in a pet with thick, matted fur with dandruff, fleas, and inflammation or even infection under the matted areas. Even if they are properly groomed, they may be too hot in the summer. The coat gives some protection from the sun, which otherwise would beat down on the naked skin, but it also seals heat in, making it harder for a pet to cool off in the summer. Encourage owners of uncomfortable dogs to have them shaved.

Proper grooming of a dog or cat with a thick coat requires specific tools. If their coat is not matted, two tools are especially useful: a comb and a Furminator® deshedding tool. The comb quickly removes hair but can pull and cause pain if there is an excess of coat. The comb part of the Furminator is shaped like a clipper blade and takes the top layer off a little at a time, causing less discomfort while removing mats, and ultimately removes more hair closer to the skin.

If a pet is hopelessly matted, so that the fur is like a large piece of felt, it is best for their health to have all the matted area shaved off. Owners should be encouraged to have this done to prevent severe skin infections and to help with flea control.

Complementary Medicine for Veterinary Technicians and Nurses

Webliography

Academy of Veterinary Homeopathy
www.TheAVH.org
Information and approval of certification courses in classical homeopathy.

American Academy of Veterinary Acupuncture
AAVA.org
Association for education about traditional Chinese veterinary medicine.

American Holistic Veterinary Medical Association
AHVMA.org
Devoted to information about all modalities, annual meeting with tracks on all major modalities, annual homotoxicology meeting.

American Veterinary Chiropractic Association
AVCA.org
Training in veterinary chiropractic.

Angels Gate
https://www.angelsgate.org/animalhospiceguide.htm
Guidelines for hospice care.

Animal Rehab Institute
https://animalrehabinstitute.com/
Training for Certified Equine Rehabilitation Assistant (CERA) for Registered Veterinary Technicians

Animal Reiki Source
https://www.animalreikisource.com/
Education in animal Reiki.

Aromaweb
www.aromaweb.com
Website with lots of information about aromatherapy.

Complementary Medicine for Veterinary Technicians and Nurses, Second Edition. Nancy Scanlan.
© 2024 John Wiley & Sons, Inc. Published 2024 by John Wiley & Sons, Inc.

Ashi Aromatics Inc.
School for Animal Aromatherapy & Flower Essence Studies
https://www.animalaromatherapy.com/
individual courses and certification

Assisi Animal Health
https://assisianimalhealth.com/
Manufacturers of the Assisi loop

Association for Pet Loss and Bereavement
https://www.aplb.org/
Provides support, support groups and referrals for those with elderly animals and for those seeking
   help with memorials, memorial ceremonies, etc.

Ayush Herbs
https://ruved.com/blogs/rooted-in-health
Source for Ayurvedic herbs for pets. Their blog (above) has information about Ayurvedic medicine
   for humans and animals

Bach Flower Remedies
https://www.bachflower.com/
Source of Bach flower remedies, made according to the original methods of Dr. Bach.

Boiron
https://www.boironusa.com/education/online-training/
Boiron is a manufacturer of homeopathic remedies. Their website has webinars about various
   aspects of homeopathy.

Canine Rehabilitation Institute
https://www.caninerehabinstitute.com
(For veterinary technician graduates of a 2-year veterinary technology program, they award a
   Canine Rehabilitation Veterinary Nurses certificate (CCRVN); for non-credentialed veterinary
   technicians, it awards a Canine Rehabilitation Assistant certificate (CCRA); for veterinarians
   and physical therapists, the institute awards a CCRT certificate)

Chi University
www.chiu.edu
Association for education about traditional Chinese veterinary medicine; certifies veterinarians in
   acupuncture and Chinese herbal medicine and also offers a tour of China, with sites of interest
   to veterinarians.

College of Integrative Veterinary Therapies (CIVT)
https://civtedu.org
Offers online courses in integrative veterinary therapies for veterinarians, veterinary technicians
   and nurses, and animal lovers.

Color Matters
https://colormatters.thinkific.com/courses/color-psychology-for-logos-and-branding
Psychological properties of colors and how they affect us.

Consumer Lab
consumerlab.com
Independent organization that tests and reviews health products.

Directly From Nature
https://www.directlyfromnature.com/
Bach Flower Remedy products, information, and short courses.

EBSCO Publishing
https://www.ebsco.com/products
Their health •library is a subscription-based library accessible online, including alternative medicine sources.

Equissage
https://www.equissage.com/
Equissage is the oldest trainer of animal massage therapists in the world.

Grayfield Optical, Inc.
https://www.grayfieldoptical.com/
Company which has created microscopes with characteristics of Rife's microscopes, but which use white light, not UV light.

Handicapped Pets.com
https://www.handicappedpets.com
A site for products, services, and support for handicapped pets. Their About section has links to videos, articles, and forums.

Healing Oasis Wellness Center
www.HealingOasis.edu
Training in veterinary chiropractic and animal massage.

Heel, Inc. for animals
www.heel-vet.com
Information about homotoxicology for animals.

Herbalist and Alchemist
https://www.herbalist-alchemist.com
Herbal products, links to associations, courses, other Western herbal medicine resources.

Homeopathic Pharmacopoeia of the United States
https://www.hpus.com/
legal standards of strength, quality, purity, and packaging as well as identification and quality standards of homeopathic starting materials and tinctures.

I Love Veterinary blog
https://iloveveterinary.com/blog/vet-nurses-in-the-uk/
Source of information for and about veterinary medicine in the UK

Institute for Functional Medicine
https://www.ifm.org/
Information and resources for human functional medicine; useful for animals also.

International Association of Animal Massage & Bodywork
https://iaamb.org/directory/iaambacwt-preferred-educational-provider/#!directory/map
Provides a list of member schools.

International College on Applied Kinesiology
https://www.icak.com/
Information about applied kinesiology and practitioners of it, and certification in Applied Kinesiology.

International Veterinary Acupuncture Society
www.IVAS.org
Association for education about traditional Chinese veterinary medicine; certifies veterinarians in
acupuncture and Chinese herbal medicine.

JennScents Aromatherapy
https://jennscents.com/aromatherapy/aromatherapy-for-animals/guidelines
Guidelines on aromatherapy for animals.

Mayo Clinic Herb and Drug Guide
https://www.mayoclinic.org/drugs-supplements
One of the best online references for herbs including interactions with drugs, from a physician's
point of view. Information for humans, but applicable to animals.

Nambrudipad's Allergy Elimination Technique (NAET)
https://www.naet.com
Website with explanation about NAET and links to training.

National Animal Supplement Council
www.nasc.cc
Supplement manufacturers who work with the FDA to ensure safety of supplements for pets and
to ensure the contents match the labels.

National Association of Myofascial Trigger Point Therapists
https://www.myofascialtherapy.org/
Website specifically about myofascial release.

National Association of Veterinary Technicians in America
navta.net
Veterinary Technicians dedicated to advancing the profession of veterinary nursing.

National Center for Homeopathy
https://homeopathycenter.org/training-practice/
Information about homeopathy, homeopathic schools, and training programs.

Natural Pet Rx
http://www.naturalpetrx.com
Source of Western herbs, and links to videos, slide shows, webinars, and articles about Western
herbal medicine.

Northwest School of Animal Massage
https://www.nwsam.com/programs/
Provides distance learning classes and training. Has a certification course for Animal Massage.

Online Pet Health
https://onlinepethealth.com/resources-for-the-veterinary-rehabilitation-therapist/
This page has a long list of links to various resources for veterinary rehab.

Options for Animals
www.animalchiro.com
Training in animal chiropractic for veterinarians and chiropractors.

Prolotherapy.com
www.prolotherapy.com
Information on prolotherapy for humans.

Quantum Immunotherapy
https://quantumimmunotherapy.net/
The site of IAT therapy today.

ReikiOne.com
https://www.reikione.com/
Information and resources for Reiki practitioners.

Respond Systems
https://respondsystems.com/pemf/how-it-works/
The company makes PEMFT beds for dogs and blankets and wraps for horses.

Sechrist Veterinary Health
https://sivethealth.com/product-details/
Hyperbaric chambers for animals and information about hyperbaric oxygen therapy for pets.

Senior pet products.com
https://seniorpetproducts.com
Web site for items for senior dogs and cats: braces, stairs, raised bowls, etc.

Standard Process
https://www.standardprocess.com
Whole food supplements including glandulars and powdered plant parts. Has products for animals.

Tellington TTouch Training
https://ttouch.com/
https://learn.ttouch.ca/
Training on how to learn Tellington TTouch.

The Bach Centre
https://www.bachcentre.com/en/
Home of Dr. Edward Bach and the Bach flower remedy system.

The Biological Medicine Institute
https://www.biologicalmedicineinstitute.com/
source of information about homotoxicology and related practices.

The Bodyworker.com
https://www.thebodyworker.com/
Information on general bodywork methods, including trigger point therapy.

The Medical Acupuncture web page
https://med-vetacupuncture.org/english/
Primarily a site about scientific support about veterinary acupuncture, web page also has information about prolotherapy. Author is Phil Rogers, MRCVS, not Narda Robinson.

The National Association for Holistic Aromatherapy
https://www.naha.org/safety.htm
Good article on safety for use of aromatherapy at this website for practitioners of aromatherapy.

Thorne Research
https://thornevet.com/
Nutritional supplements for animals, some information (tends to be hard to find on this website).

UK government website Veterinary Nurse authorization page
https://www.gov.uk/find-licences/listed-veterinary-nurse-authorisation-all-uk
Includes information about what is required for a veterinary nurse to perform surgery.

Undersea and Hyperbaric Medical Society
https://www.uhms.org/
Interesting information about hyperbaric chambers.

University of Tennessee College of Veterinary Medicine rehab certification
https://www.u-tenn.org/ccrp/
(Awards a CCRP certificate for canine rehabilitation, and a CERP certificate for equine rehabilitation. The labs are available worldwide, and classes are available online).

Veterinary Botanical Medical Association
www.VBMA.org
Information and training in herbal medicine; welcomes all types, certification in Western and Chinese herbal medicine.

Veterinary Information Network
vin.com
veterinarypartner.vin.com/
Sources of information on veterinary practice. Vin.com is for veterinarians. Veterinarypartner. vin.com is in-depth, accurate information about pet health for owners.

Vetriscience
http://www.vetriscience.com
Makes a number of nutritional supplements for animals.

Vluggen Institute for Equine Osteopathy and Education
https://www.vluggeninstitute.com
Information and courses for Equine Osteopathy.

VOM Technology
https://vomtech.com/
Information and classes on VOM.

Index

a

AAFCO. *See* Association of American Feed Control Officials, Inc.

Academy of Veterinary Homeopathy (AVH)   179, 250, 251, 301

N-Acetylcarnosine   145

N-Acetyl-cysteine   145

Acupressure   32, 62, 65, 68
  for clearing allergens   35
  courses for   73
  definition of   66, 69, 182
  description of   70, 183–184
  history of   63, 70, 182
  points for   70–71
  purpose of   69, 182
  technician experience with   72
  veterinarian experience with   72

Acupuncture   5, 6, 8, 25, 35, 241, 245, 261, 288
  American Academy of Veterinary   186, 301
  as anesthetic   182
  in cats   268
  courses for   186
  definition of   10–11, 182, 241, 245
  description of   183–184
  electro-   37, 182, 237, 241, 246, 291
  history of   182
  IVAS   182, 186, 188, 191, 250, 251, 304

legal implications of   25
medical   184
needles for   xxx, 78, 183, 291
for pain   xxix, xxx, 106, 182–184
photo-268
points of   8, 10–11, 32, 36, 37, 41, 45, 63, 65, 66, 69–72, 74, 77, 163, 164, 182–184, 212, 213, 237, 241, 242, 246, 247
purpose of   182
technician role in   184–185
use of   3, 53, 78
veterinarian's role in   184

Aflatoxin   92, 241

Agrimony   209, 285

AHVMA. *See* American Holistic Veterinary Medical Association

Albumin   91, 241

Allergens, acupressure clearing   206

Allergic dermatitis   113, 114, 116, 207

Allergies   35, 76, 205
  to food   114, 116, 273
  itchy skin from, diets for   273
  Natural Balance   114
  qi energy in   205
  test for   114, 205, 206

Allopathic   67, 175, 180, 219, 241

Alpha lipoic acid
  for dogs   148–160
  use of   148